YOU'RE DOING IT WRONG!

YOU'RE DOING IT WRONG!

Mothering, Media, and
Medical Expertise

BETHANY L. JOHNSON
MARGARET M. QUINLAN

RUTGERS UNIVERSITY PRESS
NEW BRUNSWICK, CAMDEN, AND NEWARK,
NEW JERSEY, AND LONDON

Library of Congress Cataloging-in-Publication Data

Names: Johnson, Bethany L., 1974– author. | Quinlan, Margaret M., author.
Title: You're doing it wrong! : mothering, media, and medical expertise / Bethany L. Johnson
    and Margaret M. Quinlan.
Description: New Brunswick, New Jersey : Rutgers University Press, [2019] | Includes
    bibliographical references and index.
Identifiers: LCCN 2018031138 | ISBN 9780813593791 (cloth) | ISBN 9780813593784 (pbk.)
Subjects: LCSH: Motherhood. | Child rearing. | Medical care. | Social media.
Classification: LCC HQ759 .J6226 2019 | DDC 306.874/3—dc23
LC record available at https://lccn.loc.gov/2018031138

A British Cataloging-in-Publication record for this book is available from the British
Library.

♾ The paper used in this publication meets the requirements of the American National
Standard for Information Sciences—Permanence of Paper for Printed Library Materials,
ANSI Z39.48-1992.

www.rutgersuniversitypress.org

Manufactured in the United States of America

For Hazel, Otto and Erik; Sweeney, Teddy and James

There's a crescendo of voices saying,
"If you don't do X or Y, you're doing it wrong,"
. . . and it's amplified by the Internet and social media.

—Dr. Catherine Monk, psychologist and associate professor
  at Columbia University Medical Center

CONTENTS

PART IV

Infant Loss and Early Childhood

YOU'RE DOING IT WRONG!

INTRODUCTION

The woman who is a good wife, a good mother, is entitled to our respect as is no one else; but she is entitled to it only because, and so long as, she is worthy of it.
—*President Theodore Roosevelt, 1905*

The authors of this text (in no particular order) are scholars, mothers, and givers and receivers of unsolicited and solicited expertise. One of us ingested Robitussin to get pregnant; the other had four years of infertility treatment. One had gestational diabetes, while the other had a nausea-free pregnancy. One used Pitocin while in labor; both of us had an epidural. One labored with a doula and midwives, while the other's baby was resuscitated in the first hour because of an "incorrect" breastfeeding position. One had an episiotomy that made intercourse painful (thus infrequent) for over a year, while the other was back to her workout routine six weeks postpartum. One took encapsulated placenta (supplements made from one's placenta, thought by some to increase milk supply); the other covered her legs to avoid seeing the afterbirth. Both have a family history of postpartum depression. While both of us had unhealthy thoughts and high anxiety, one took anxiety medication during the postpartum period. One had at least one glass of wine a night since their child was born, without "pump and dump"; the other drank Diet Coke while breastfeeding. One pumped for more than a year after returning to work; the other never used a bottle or a pacifier. One uses liquid arnica, while the other uses Tylenol; both of us gave our babies antibiotics. One always used disposable diapers, while the other tried cloth for five months. One practiced near constant baby wearing, while the other loved the Bumbo. One family coslept for ten months; one did sleep training. One had in-home childcare at four months, the other after ten months; one put her child in part-time daycare at 16 months, the other at almost three years. One feeds her child fried chicken, while the other avoids white sugar. One has a toddler who eats a wide variety of foods; one does not. One's husband buys all of the baby's clothing and does a majority of childcare, while the other has a partner who works long hours and travels. One doesn't allow screens and automated toys in the house; the other takes her child to a kid-friendly movie night. We both read about respectful parenting; one does short timeouts in a crib, and one of us only uses the crib for sleeping. One spent the night away from her child after 27 months, while the other took a work trip when the baby was 10 months old. Both of us had to create our own support networks as we have no family close by. One has job security but went without health insurance for months when on unpaid family medical leave; the other has no paid leave or job security. One of us has a toddler who likes to cuddle, while the other does not. One of us has a PTSD diagnosis due to a series of childhood traumas, while the other has multiple (mostly invisible) disabilities.

Are We "Good" Mothers?

Who is the "good" mother? Do you think you can break this list into two categories? Are you certain the person that had Pitocin is also the person who drinks Diet Coke? Are you scandalized that while one birthed with a midwife both had an epidural? Are you horrified that one coslept for ten months? Or does the Tylenol bother you more? In short, do you need more specific details or an "answer key" to the list above before you can judge our narratives? Like most parents, we too questioned every decision, ended up in situations we never dreamed of, and understood that our choices would be judged with scrutiny exercised in few other arenas today. We both felt guilty, had regrets, sought expertise from all manner of practitioners, Googled for information, joined public and private "moms' groups" on Facebook (FB) for support, and questioned when and how to "trust our guts."

To begin to contextualize and analyze our experiences, we must begin by acknowledging our enormous privilege. Our children arrived in relative economic stability (middle- to upper-class homes), with parents in their mid-30s to early 40s; we have advanced degrees and are white. We are cis, heterosexual females (meaning sex and gender correlate), and we "pass" as able-bodied. Our privileges allow us significant freedom, access, and agency within American culture; we do not face the particular (intersectional) forms of oppression rooted in race, class, gender, and sexual orientation (Crenshaw, 1991). On the other hand, we contend with gender-based oppression and inequality, as well as the challenges of invisible illness. Meanwhile, all American mothers/parents face structural and policy challenges like adequate, affordable childcare, family leave, and cultural expectations about "good" motherhood. Perfection in motherhood is an old dictate, but in the social media landscape it becomes particularly barbed, as anonymity may breed harsher criticism and the ability to be constantly "plugged in" heightens expert surveillance and self-surveillance. As mothers, we do not claim technical, lay, or any other expert status; we are writing this book to navigate motherhood-specific health information, disseminated through various forms of expertise, to illuminate the discourses of acceptable motherhood in selected moments in the American past and on social media today. We also write to contend with our own experiences.

This is not a parenting book. We do not offer parenting advice, provide expertise, or suggest the use of products, methods, medicines, or treatments. What interests us is the exploration of the ways in which public and private discourse have and continue to influence how individuals communicate about motherhood and childcare. Throughout, we engage historical texts (e.g., doctor's notes, family papers) and present-day, social media texts (e.g., comments, hashtags) to discover how such discourses have and continue to interrupt the technical/lay expertise binary. For instance, in our experiences as new mothers, we sought expertise from a variety of sources; on social media platforms we had difficulty fully uncovering the context of information exchanged and, as a result, remained unsure what information to trust.

Alongside individual and collective experience and anecdotal evidence, we know from decades of scholarly research on mothers and motherhood that both the cis female body and motherhood are continually critiqued and disciplined through legal sanction as well as through more diffuse forms of control, such as peer pressure or public shaming (Apple, 2006; Duncan, 1994; Kukla, 2005; Lupton, 2003; Smith-Rosenberg, 1985). Whether sought or imposed, medical expertise results from cultural discourses that create, entrench, and deflect beliefs and expectations around women's health, reproduction, and motherhood (Jensen, 2016; Koerber, 2018; Robbins, 2009). The "expert" gaze continues to maintain a long-term focus on the cis female body and the assumed ability—and necessity—of that body to conceive and carry children (Ehrenreich & English, 1978; Jensen, 2016; Lupton, 2003). Moreover, a disproportionate share of medical expertise, perhaps because of the fragility of new life for much of history, has been directed toward mothers. Even as definitions and constructions of motherhood shift, "social and legal rules have historically governed who can be a legitimate mother" (Solinger, 2005, p. 12). Though cis male bodies play a central role in the biological process of conception and now in child rearing, cis male individuals are also considered part-time caretakers or "babysitters" instead of full parents (Toalson, 2016; Wood, 1994). Thus, many cis and trans males who parent are not subject to the same scrutiny and medical expertise from expert communities as cis female individuals are (Doucet, 2017; Koerber, 2018; Medved, 2016). We most often use the term "mother" in this book, to reflect historical terminology, self-identification, and the direction of the medical gaze, yet we acknowledge that gender is a continuum and motherhood is a state of flux. This word is both sufficient and wholly insufficient to describe the experiences of many today. Given our intersectional approach, we attempt to examine how power and oppression impact individuals who wish to identify as a mother or identify themselves as mothers or parents across diverse social strati (see also Griffin & Chávez, 2012).

The investigation of both technical and lay expertise, across time, offers a unique insight into the history of womanhood, motherhood, and the development of expertise, before and after the advent of the Internet. Technological developments play a central role in constructing and reconstructing societal expectations and behavioral patterns. In an age of "big data," "old" advice can reappear, supported by different, new, or "better" data. For example, in 1933, Dr. Martin Couney suggested that "delicatessen lunches" were one of the root causes of an uptick of premature births (Baker, 2000; "Scolds," 1933); today, women are instructed not to eat lunch meat to avoid possible listeria infections. Must we all agree then that lunch meat is a great evil of our time? The pregnant women in the postwar 1950s seemed to eat a good deal of it, and the vast majority carried their children to term. So how might individuals find the best expertise (see Oster, 2013)? And does the interactive experience of giving and receiving medical expertise to mothers with young children reinforce or challenge social hierarchies based on gender, race, class, ability, and sexuality?

Historically, white cis men have had vastly disproportionate claims to credentialed "expertise," creating and disseminating so much of what counted as authoritative maternal advice (Ehrenrich & English, 2008; Koerber, 2018). Given that context, throughout the book we look for instances where expertise empowered and/or disempowered cis female individuals. We also explore points of failure or resistance, such as the inadequacy and inaccuracy of pregnancy behavioral dictates, particularly for those with disabled bodies (chapter 3) or the sharing of images of deceased infants on FB to draw attention to infant loss and publicly celebrate a life lived (chapter 7). This is not a traditional historical study or historiography, but a comparative work in which we depend on archival materials to contextualize contemporary discussions about motherhood and public understandings of health and reproduction within the historical record. Within each topographical chapter, we find vestiges of nineteenth- and early twentieth-century medical expertise (lay, technical, and other), emerging or reemerging in current social media discourses.

The Life Cycle of Early Motherhood

Conceptually and methodologically, we focus on the life cycle of early motherhood as a way to offer a fresh perspective for scholars interested in the study of motherhood and mothering rhetorics in historical and present-day variations. This life cycle begins with preconception and moves through conception, pregnancy, childbirth, the postpartum period, and the toddler years (e.g., when most toddlers begin to practice rudimentary forms of self-care such as dressing and feeding). During these stages, the mother-child dyad confronts particular health difficulties and potential crises and is the subject of much cultural anxiety. Historically, this period in the lives of mothers and children was recognized as uniquely vulnerable and weighted with cultural, political, and even religious meaning. The seemingly capricious nature of female fertility, the dangers of childbirth, and the high U.S. infant mortality rate (well into the twentieth century) underscored this vulnerability (Marsh & Ronner, 1996; Morbidity, 1999; Stern & Markel, 2002; Vandenberg-Daves, 2014; Zelizer, 1994). Today, many mothers and children move through this period without a major, life-threatening incident. However, some individuals experience miscarriage, do not conceive, and adopt or foster, or opt to be child-free; some do not carry and use a surrogate. At the other end of this "life cycle," when (most) children grow out of the need for constant caregiving, there are individuals who have lost children, and/ or there are children who have needs requiring long-term, intensive care. Varying experiences and outcomes within the life cycle of early motherhood ensure that expert knowledge is particularly loaded, given the enduring idea that a "good" mother always knows what to do or when to seek and submit to the (correct) expertise.

(RE)DEFINING LAY AND TECHNICAL EXPERTISE: TECHNOLOGICAL INTERRUPTIONS

In this book, we tackle very sensitive, complicated issues; each chapter focuses on potential health crises in which parents might seek medical expertise, due to conception difficulties, premature birth, or infant loss, among others. Throughout the book we reveal the porous nature of the boundaries between lay and technical expertise with respect to the specific experiences of the life cycle of early motherhood, drawing attention to the shifting definitions of both "lay" and "technical" across time and how they intersect with notions of ideal motherhood, race, class, and gender and, in the present day, hetero- and cis normativity. There are limitations to all language, some of which we complicate throughout the book, in an effort to reveal the ever-shifting contours of expertise. We hope to move beyond a binary-based understanding of expertise and lay knowledge by investigating both the overt and covert ways forms of expertise intersect, impact one another, or circumvent one another. Our investigation of dissemination through various forms of media (historically and in the present) allows us to illustrate the nonbinary nature of expertise during the life cycle of motherhood.

Scholarly definitions of technical or lay knowledge (or advice, expertise, spheres) differ; we define both technical and lay expertise as discursive tools wielded by individuals in public and private spaces. Previous scholarship often studied technical and lay expertise (and experts) as partners or adversaries; the historical progression seems to bend toward further entrenchment and bifurcation into the categories of "technical" or "lay." We recognize that, historically, conflicts around expertise often ensured the ascendancy of technical-professional language (Abbott, 1988; Johnson & Quinlan, 2015; Jordan, 1997; Koerber, 2005), particularly in the policing of cis female bodies from first menses until menopause. As Jordan (1997) posited, in the modern period, lay experts and their knowledge are labeled "alternative," and thus "backward, ignorant and naïve" (p. 56). Yet, technical and lay medical expertise cannot be simplistically bifurcated, though they are often depicted as jockeying images of "mainstream" versus "alternative" medicine, or "legitimate" versus "quack" science (see also Derkatch, 2016). This division reflects neither the history of medical concepts and directives toward female bodies nor the distribution of such knowledge on and through social media platforms. Moreover, women utilizing social media today must navigate exponentially numerous, complicated, and competing claims of expertise.

Many mothers over the last century and a half turned to advice books on fertility, prenatal health, and infant and toddler care (Ehrenreich & English, 2005; Grant; 2012; Guttmacher, 1962; Hoffert, 1989; Kellogg, 1891; McMillen, 1990; Melendy, 1904). Much of the public embraced advice manuals, and some, marked with the legitimacy of credentialed medical researchers and practitioners and twentieth-century versions such as *What to Expect When You're Expecting* (now available on eReaders and in a smartphone app), sold millions of copies. Historians and health communication scholars have analyzed "baby books" and parenting books (Apple, 1995; Dobris & White-Mills, 2006; Dobris, White-Mills, Davidson, & Wellbrook, 2017; Ehrenreich & English, 2005; Grant, 2012; Vandenburg-Daves, 2014).

While books were popular in the nineteenth century and throughout the twentieth, newspapers were more accessible through both price and availability, though neither reached illiterate populations. In late nineteenth-century magazines, "protoscience journalism" (e.g., journalists educating the public on childbirth practices such as Twilight Sleep) (Tomes, 2002, p. 630; see also Johnson & Quinlan, 2015, 2017) emphasized hygiene, child rearing, and domestic health; this style of journalism expanded in the early twentieth century to explore infectious disease, new and emerging health threats, and scientific research, translated for the widest possible readership (Tomes, 2002). Book-length texts have less in common with social media posts today, which are much shorter (e.g., 280-character limit on Twitter tweets). Newspaper and magazine articles are not social media posts, but also have length limitations. Today, social media play a role in popularizing historical figures, but as length limitations prohibit proper context, posts can create new mythologies and perpetuate ongoing misinformation. For example, Martin Couney appears on Twitter, Instagram (IG), and FB each year when Coney Island celebrates its history. Most posts identify him as a medical doctor—in chapter 5, we question the label and analyze the potential impacts of his mythology. The media sources we investigated are analytically valuable because, unlike advice books, newspapers and magazines and social media applications and platforms represent the dissemination of expertise and folklore without clear distinction.

Therefore, we do not investigate advice books as media sources of expertise dissemination in their own right. In chapter 3, we engage historical advice books in an effort to trace the sources of information disseminated on social media today. Instead, we concentrated on the "golden age of newspapers," roughly 1830 to 1930 (Douglas, 1999), though we focused closely on the late nineteenth century and early twentieth and the rise of social media applications and platforms, which emerged in the early 2000s. About a century apart, these two critical "ages" in media (print and digital) reshaped the ways we understand expertise and even knowledge itself (Cho, Hunt, Beckjord, Moser, & Hesse, 2009; Douglas, 1999; Hardey, 1999; Hawn, 2009; Tomes, 2002). The rise of mass-produced newspapers and popular magazines in America in the nineteenth century (Johnson & Quinlan, 2017; Schroth, 1974; Tomes, 2002) and the advent of the Internet and social media have each significantly altered the transmission of technical and lay expertise and the nature of expert-led health discourse in the public sphere (Eastin, 200; Ostherr, 2013).

Importantly, these media can convey information to mothers directly (Tomes, 2002; see also Hawn, 2009), and both blurred the lines between technical and lay expertise. If the first stage of "blurring" came with the rise of the newspaper and protoscience journalism, then the rise of the Internet with the growth of digitized and publicly available data, access to scholarly works, and the prevalence of social media blurred the lines between technical and lay even further (Hardey, 1999; Hawn, 2009). Our focus highlights the important role these specific textual media play in disseminating authority, lay expertise, and protoscience journalism. For example, in chapter 8, which explores baby contests, we note the role of newspapers in advertising the events and health rankings. In chapter 4, we cite books addressing Twilight Sleep, but it was newspapers like the *Brooklyn Eagle* that fielded reader queries regarding local hospital access, while organizations like the Twilight Sleep Association sent (lay) magazine articles to women asking for information (Dennett Papers, 1874–1945). Similarly, most parenting or baby advice books didn't include sections on premature birth, the subject of chapter 5, but newspapers like the *New York Times* provided ample coverage of Martin Couney's work saving premature babies in an exhibit on Coney Island.

Inasmuch as this is not a parenting book, it is also not a book about advice. Advice is generally offered freely (e.g., from family members and friends), with ranging expectations for the success or applicability of said advice and a varying burden to follow it. It seems everyone has advice to offer (e.g., opinions, recommendations, and/or guidance as a way to elicit behavior or thought), particularly for individuals seeking to become pregnant, expecting, or caring for young children. Conversely, medical expertise is often sought out in times of crisis, regularly comes with a monetary fee, is provided and received in a relationship of unequal power, and includes some expectation that said expertise, whether implicitly or explicitly stated, will be followed and/or adhered to as a way to address a problem, make a decision, or manage a situation. As such, the transmission of expertise through media outlets to the public may directly impact individual health behaviors, ranging from the choice of health providers based on their ability to provide a "family-centered cesarean" (Family Centered Cesarean, 2017) to the use of fertility apps (e.g., Kindara and Ovia) to maximize conception efforts (Kindara, 2017; Ovia, 2017).

We found that social media platforms both continue and interrupt the dissemination of expertise. Smartphones, which provide access to apps and social media platforms, are not available to everyone, but they remain accessible to many without other resources such as cars and laptops/home computers. The entry point is more accessible for smartphones than it is for computers, so more of the American public is likely to use these forms of technology. Now more individuals, with a broad range of backgrounds, levels of trainings, and schools of thought, are citing themselves as experts and providing their expertise for free (e.g., through their IG accounts) as well as for payment (e.g., eCourses on natural fertility treatment). Alternatively, health professionals (e.g., labor and delivery nurses) provide their expertise for free through their personal social media accounts (e.g., their private FB accounts) while providing their employment details (e.g., which position at which hospital). We use the term "expert advice" throughout the book to delineate this categorically fuzzy combination of lay and technical expertise, and the ways this new delivery of expertise is transforming and/or maintaining knowledge structures entrenched over the last century and a half.

Furthermore, expert advice directed at cis female individuals in the life cycle of early motherhood is confusing, contradictory, vast, and swiftly changing. The amount and availability of medical information exploded with the introduction of social media. Recent examples include the "Science of Mom" blog and the author's translation of medical research on skin-to-skin touch (Callahan, 2013, 2015), "Moms in Charge" FB groups offering advice on fevers and selling homeopathic teething tablets currently under investigation by the FDA (Malinda, 2016; Ray & Haller, 2016), and health-related IG postings that include photographs of personal cervical mucus during fertility treatments.[1]

Yesterday's "musts" (do *not* pick your child up if she is crying) are today's "nevers" (you must *never* leave a child to cry). Over the course of U.S. history, some practices disappeared from both the technical and lay compendium—for example, experts from all backgrounds now frown upon giving diluted whiskey to infants, toddlers, and young children. Still, one can never say when "old" methods will return: for example, the ancient custom of baby wearing is popular again today.

We are not the first scholars to wade into the complicated, and sometimes messy, literatures about women's health, childbirth, and motherhood, nor will we be the last. Below, we outline available historical and health communication scholarship and discuss how we build on previous findings to examine motherhood in the digital age.

Review of Literature

From the nineteenth century through the twenty-first, "expert" advice surrounding women's health and reproduction altered not only how scientists, medical professionals, and policy makers (technical experts) viewed cis females, but also how (lay) individuals conceptualized womanhood, motherhood, and "the female" in public and private spaces. Given that the public engages health and reproduction through socially constructed linguistic and symbolic systems that translate into corporeal and material consequences for individual bodies, it is imperative that we address both historical and contemporary discourses of expertise on women's health (Weedon, 1996). Accordingly, our inquiry is linked to the study of reproductive medicine and the historical, social construction of motherhood as the pinnacle of womanhood. To explore medical expertise dissemination on social media outside of the context of medical history would be to obfuscate how expertise on social media is both an extension of and a turn from previous trends.

The Historiography of Medical Expertise and Gendered Health Advice

Vast monographs address American women's history, women's medical history, and the history of motherhood. Margarete Sandelowski (1984, 1993, 2000) studied the history of medical care, childbirth, and infertility and conducted qualitative research on couples' experience with infertility treatment. Other scholars used archival resources to navigate the history and impact of the technical medical gaze on female bodies, the history of women's medical care, women in medicine, Victorian constructions of female health, the social history of American medicine and medical care, and the history of motherhood (Breslaw, 2012; Curry, 1999; Grant, 2012; Herzig, 2005; Hoffert, 1989; Janik, 2014; Kline, 2001; Leavitt, 1984, 1986; Morantz-Sanchez, 2000; Smith-Rosenberg, 1985; Starr, 1982; Ulrich, 1990; Weiner & Hough, 2012). Several scholars offer a useful context for understanding constructions of race, class, sex, and gender in America during the periods of our focus (Adickes, 1997; Bederman, 1995; Kerber, Kessler-Harris, & Sklar, 1995; Kline, 2001; Rosen, 2007; Smith-Rosenberg, 1985; Washington, 2006; Weiner & Hough, 2012). These texts have informed and framed our historiographical perspective, allowing us to contextualize present-day health, reproduction, and motherhood dialogues on social media platforms. However, none of these groundbreaking manuscripts wrestled with the complexity of medical expertise and lay knowledge as transactional; this critical distinction is one way our work extends available scholarship on the dissemination of medical expertise.

Broadly, significant trends and developments that directly impact our research include the "modernization" of American health care, beginning in the nineteenth century and extending into the early twentieth century; the golden age of public health and bacteriology (1880–1920); and the rise and integration of psychology into medicine in the first half of the twentieth century (see also Breslaw, 2012; Starr, 1982). Historian Paul Starr (1982) intimated that these periods might be categorized as the rise of "professional sovereignty," followed by the development of medicine as a sprawling industry (p. IX; see also Bonner, 1990, 1995; Burnham, 2015; Janik, 2014; Vandenberg-Daves, 2014; Washington, 2006; Weiner & Hough, 2012). During the nineteenth century, medical practice became more sectarian, professional organizations formed, and a changing understanding of disease shifted from systemic pathology to local pathology (e.g., instead of a poor constitution one has heart disease). Eventually, these changes radically altered medical practice. Exciting new discoveries and increasing methodological rigor transformed medicine from art to science in the late nineteenth century. The rise of germ theory and bacteriology alongside the emergence of antiseptic and then aseptic surgery, and the invention of new serums, vaccines, medicines, and other treatments transformed medical practice. Paralleling and intersecting with these periods are major populist, patient-driven (lay), and/or alternative movements that embraced, rejected, or circumvented traditional (technical) medicine or created new medical systems and theories altogether (e.g., hydropathy). We examine moments in which these technical and lay systems intersected and transacted, specifically where developments created treatment systems for the mother-child dyad in the life cycle of early motherhood (e.g., conception, birth, recovery).

Monographs addressing lay and technical expertise, including lay expertise as a form of agency for women and mothers, have provided an overview of medical expertise and the impact of various practitioners in and across communities, where individuals and groups partnered with, embraced, or rejected traditional practitioners (Curry, 1999; Leavitt, 1999; Leavitt & Numbers, 1997). Scholars explored southern and rural lay understandings of health, medicine, the body, and expertise, some with an eye to the experiences of women in the antebellum period (McMillen, 1990; Weiner & Hough, 2012); others studied women as lay practitioners within and outside enslavement (Abel, 2002; Fett, 2002). Historians have identified the ways women adopted and/or rejected advice from various experts as arbiters of health care within the mother-child dyad (Grant, 2012; Hoffert, 1989; Marsh & Ronner, 1996). We reviewed historiography focused on "stages" within the life cycle of early motherhood, which offered various perspectives on the history of childbirth and fertility treatment, providing research foundational to our understanding of historical and contemporary expertise (Caton, 1999; Leavitt, 1986; Marsh & Ronner, 1996, 2010; Wertz & Wertz, 1977; Wolf, 2009).

Our work contributes to a rich tradition of interdisciplinary analysis of women's health with a historical perspective. Given the numerous sources available that address various threads in our analysis, there are monographs that directly overlap with some of the topics we examine in our text. Sandelowski's *With Child in Mind* (1993) paired a historiographical study of infertility with qualitative research to significant acclaim. Ehrenreich and English's (1978, 2005) groundbreaking work *For Her Own Good* probed (technical) expertise on women's health, from childhood through maturation and menopause. Vandenberg-Daves's (2014) *Modern Motherhood* addressed motherhood in the nineteenth and twentieth centuries, expertise directed at mothers, as well as the ways that technical medical expertise allowed for increased control of and access to cis female bodies. Hoffert (1989) provided a useful model for interrogating the life cycle of early motherhood from 1800 to 1860.

Like Ehrenreich and English's (1978) original volume, now 40 years old, we study medical expertise from the nineteenth century to the present. However, our purpose is not to debunk technical expertise. Instead, we explore and shed light on the processes by which expert advice is defined today as "technical" or "traditional" versus "lay" or "alternative," and how these categories prove inadequate to express the fluidity and interactive nature of expert knowledge, past and present. Our research draws on Ehrenreich and English's (2005) historiographical research and Sandelowski's (1993) use of qualitative data in that we include archival resources, but also personal narratives culled from popular social media platforms and social media analysis through Radian6 (R6). Additionally, an analysis of contemporary social media discourse is not available in these monographs (Ehrenreich & English, 1978, 2005; Sandelowski, 1993). Building on the work of Ehrenreich and English (1978, 2005), Hoffert (1989), and Vandenberg-Daves (2014), we interrogate the categories of "lay" and "technical" across time, demonstrating the interactional nature of expertise even when experts are competitive or combative. We extend Hoffert's (1989) study of lay and technical expertise as partners or foes and examine how health crises particular to the life cycle of early motherhood challenge binary notions of expertise and practitioner-patient relationships.

In contrast with both Vandenberg-Daves (2014) and Hoffert (1989), we interrogate the very categories of "lay" and "technical" across time, demonstrating the interactional nature of expertise, even when experts are competitive or combative. Unlike some researchers of the history of motherhood, we do not explore motherhood in the political realm, within a particular group or within a specific region. We focus on the mother-child dyad, often realized and performed in the private and less structured spaces governed by lay expertise (e.g., the bedroom, the bathroom, the private FB group). Yet the policies, procedures, grassroots movements, and social media conversations we address throughout the book uphold the adage that the personal is political. We acknowledge that long-term historical trends, which privatized and geographically isolated many nuclear families—and held up this isolation as a cultural ideal—have shaped modern mothers' experience of maternal expertise (Vandenberg-Daves, 2014). But with the advent of social media, the potential health crises mothers and children face in the life cycle of early motherhood are both intensely isolated (e.g., unlikely to live near family) and intensely public (e.g., birth announcements and hospital pictures posted to FB). Again, extending these works, our research augments more traditional historiography, which is not meant to analyze the present; we use historical research to extend the study of medical expertise directed toward mothers into the Internet age.

Finally, we draw from texts that explore topics beyond the history of motherhood but offer great insight into alternative expertise dissemination (see also Derkatch, 2016). Historical monographs such as Kathy Peiss's (1998) *Hope in a Jar* and Herzig's (2015) *Plucked* illuminate aspects of gender history in the United States not specific to mothering, yet they offer striking examples of the interplay between technical and lay expertise, as well as how these types of expertise reach and impact public health knowledge and individual decisions. Peiss (1998) traced the medical roots of cosmetics and the nature of (eighteenth- and early nineteenth-century) lay expertise passed between friends and relatives, who "traded" time-worn recipes, methodologies of personal hygiene, body care, and plant lore. Our book maps the internecine conflict between technical and lay experts, as well as the multiple influences (e.g., public, private, technical, lay) that inform individual health choices as well as the shifting categorization of medical expertise as neither technical nor lay on social media today.

Our focus on potential crises and challenges that may emerge during the life cycle of early motherhood foregrounds the advance of technical expertise, achievements in medicine, and the emergence of social-media-based lay expertise as a counternarrative to what some perceive as an overreach by technical experts and American allopathic medicine. We address some familiar territory (e.g., the use of pain-relieving medication during labor), but we reframe these topics as contestations and resulting redefinitions or reorganizations of expertise. For example, in our chapter on early twentieth-century Twilight Sleep (TS), we assess the role of lay experts in altering technical expertise, and ultimately hospital birth, across the nation. We then follow this impact into the mid-twentieth-century "natural childbirth" movement and onto social media today. Pregnancy, breastfeeding, childbirth, and the nutrition of young children are well represented in histories of medicine, childhood, and motherhood. The history of neonatal units, "better baby" contests, infant-loss photography, preconception, and postpartum care are less studied. In part, these "new" crises speak to the successes of turn-of-the-twentieth-century medicine in the United States. The crises and challenges we explore result from medical advancements and the potential of lay expertise to educate, inform, and empower parents, changing outcomes and expectations. Premature birth is not the same sort of crisis it was in the nineteenth century because, in the case of prematurity, death was the expectation, not the exception. Today, the expectation of carrying a pregnancy to term and having that child live through early childhood makes premature birth a different type of crisis.

Yet the technological and practitioner apparatuses that accompany premature birth were as jarring in the early twentieth century as they are now (e.g., a baby living in a mechanical box). Similarly, given extraordinary advances in medicine and sanitary living conditions, infant loss is unusual today. Parents grieved then and now, but today infant death is an aberration, rather than a constant possibility (Zelizer, 1994). As with other topics, we juxtapose the power of textual media in the nineteenth and early twentieth centuries with the influence of digital media (especially social media) today, in exploring the ways parents grappled and continue to grapple with these crises as they encounter expertise through social media.

Historians of American medicine and gender (Curry, 1999; Grant, 2012; Morantz-Sanchez, 2000; Weiner & Hough, 2012) continue to call for further inquiry into the history of health and health care in America. We answer this call by examining the shifting conceptualization of and interplay between technical and lay expertise during the ascendancy of both textual and digital media in America, with a focus on mothers as consumers of medical expertise, negotiators, and creators. With this monograph, we seek to extend available scholarship both temporally, by considering the role of contemporary social media, as well as substantively, by focusing mainly on the continuity and disruption of various forms of expertise focused on the crises possible during the life cycle of early motherhood.

Rhetorics of Motherhood

Alongside our historiographical research, we turned to health communication scholars to help us understand technical and lay rhetorics around health, reproduction, womanhood, and motherhood. Lynn O'Brien Hallstein's *Women's Studies in Communication* (2017) special issue on "Mothering Rhetorics" overviews rhetorical facets of motherhood and mothering from intersectional perspectives (e.g., Adams, 2017; Dickenson, Foss, & Kroløkke, 2017; Mack, 2013; Morrissey & Kimball, 2017; see also Mack, 2013). Communication studies scholarship has focused on the political and cultural performativity of motherhood, discourses of care, institutional mothering, and the challenges of motherhood and mothering in light of intersectional oppression (e.g., queer, impoverished, ability, terminal illness) (Buchanan, 2013; Demo, Borda, & Kroløkke, 2015; Enoch, 2012; Hayden, 2003; Hundley & Hayden, 2016; O'Brien Hallstein, 2010; Schely-Newman, 1999; Seigel, 2014; Tonn, 2001). Other scholars interrogate the navigation of health issues during stages of the life cycle of early motherhood (Dubriwny, 2012;

Dubriwny & Ramaduri, 2013; Jensen, 2016; Seigel, 2014) and the ways mothers are represented in the media (Hundley & Hayden, 2016; Mack, 2016; O'Brien Hallstein, 2011, 2015).

Projects by Douglas and Michaels (2004), Lay (2000), Meyer, Oberman, and White (2001), and Taylor (1996) discussed elements of mothering and motherhood in a heavily news-mediated and/or wireless social context. Available research addresses trust and credibility of health information online; however, much of that research focused on the Internet more broadly and is more than a decade old—hardly fresh given the pace of technology change (Briggs, Burford, De Angeli, & Lynch, 2002; Eastin, 2001; Kata, 2010; Sillence, Briggs, Harris, & Fishwick, 2006). More recent Internet research fails to account for the ubiquity of platforms such as IG, which has hundreds of millions of users and involves the exchange of health advice and even medicine.[2] Douglas and Michaels's (2004) *The Mommy Myth* referred to the "maternal panopticon," a space that houses the self-surveillance technology required for today's intensive, selfless mothering (p. 171). Throughout our book, we examine this increasingly intensified self-surveillance, resulting from social media platforms and smartphone apps.

The challenge we pose here to the binary nature of expertise/lay wisdom today enhances research on the rhetorics of motherhood. None of the communication studies mentioned above probe the interplay between technical and lay expertise and how these forms of expertise influence each other and rhetorics of motherhood across time (see also Mack, 2013). Further, we contribute new understanding to this literature through our examination of how social media can both entrench and upend historical expertise hierarchies. Hence, our focus offers a unique perspective on the role of social media as a space in which technical expertise moves through lay channels and lay experts access power in new ways.

Expertise in the Age of Social Media: Opportunities and Challenges

As we discuss throughout this monograph, the enormous impact of social media on the dissemination and reception of medical expertise during the life cycle of early motherhood remains misunderstood, underestimated, or simply not considered. For example, when labor and delivery nurses use their expertise to direct patients through their own personal FB accounts, how is medical expertise functioning here and what are the implications for health care delivery? Currently, 46% of patients use social media for health information and 40% find information online that influences their choice of doctor (Khouri, McCheyne, & Morrison, 2018, p. 975). It is established that social media platforms such as FB, IG, Twitter, and others are a pervasive influence on daily life, for good or ill (Khouri, McCheyne, & Morrison, 2018; Landry, 2014; Ridgeway & Clayton, 2016; Sillence, Briggs, Harris, & Fishwick, 2006). Research on the impact of the Internet on public health information began shortly after the advent of the World Wide

Web; scholars interrogated the practices of individual users seeking health advice online, navigating accurate and inaccurate information collected by search engines, and more (Briggs, Burford, de Angeli, & Lynch, 2002; Eastin, 2001; Kata, 2010; Sillence, Briggs, Harris, & Fishwick, 2006). Earlier public spaces on the Internet included search engines such as Yahoo with attached email accounts and chatrooms, online forums, and instant messaging (e.g., on AOL), which composed the bulk of personal interaction. The advent of social media and smartphone applications ("apps") drastically increased mobile, instant, interactive communication (Johnson, 2014; Khouri, McCheyne, & Morrison, 2018).

Recent research has begun to uncover the importance of social media platforms and apps (sometimes self-contained and sometimes integrated with social media platforms such as FB) to new mothers and caretakers of infants. For example, Bartholomew, Schoppe-Sullivan, Glassman, Kamp Dush, and Sullivan (2012) reported that childbirth prompted a significant increase in the use of FB. More strikingly, Edison Research (2013) found in a sample set of over 300 self-identified mothers that 90% can access the Internet, although the study failed to distinguish wider Internet use from social media platform use. Further, 95% of those surveyed used smartphones to access the Internet, including sites like FB (Edison Research, 2013). A Pew Research Center (2016) study revealed that FB use among adults increases, with 79% of online adults regularly accessing the site. Conversations about pediatricians, payment plans for giving birth, postpartum care, infertility treatment, and more are readily available on social media platforms, and users engage in these dialogues seeking expertise, particularly in moments of crisis. Scholars cite the need to create and maintain social support as a primary reason for increased use (Madge & O'Connor, 2006).

There is available scholarship on the pervasiveness and socioemotional impact of social media platforms specifically, though the research largely addressed use by young adults and/or focused on health issues we do not address here, including disordered eating, body image, diabetes management, and more (Fergie, Hilton, & Hunt, 2015; Khouri, McCheyne, & Morrison, 2018). In our work, we explore how social media platforms utilized through tablets, smartphones, and other wireless technologies collapse the boundaries between public and private, as well as between technical and lay (Johnson, Quinlan, & Marsh, 2018). For example, in chapter 3, on pregnancy behavior, we recount the claim of an FB poster that caffeine consumption caused chromosomal abnormalities. This claim, delivered as incontrovertible fact without supporting evidence and presented as if all of medical science agreed, illustrated a lay expert who referenced medical research (technical expertise) without citing a single source. Perhaps the most unfortunate impact of social media is the false confidence these platforms provide—a unique combination of some level of anonymity and limitations on post length allows individuals to make confident claims devoid of context and lacking sufficient explanation. These increasingly common posts can add to the stress and anxiety of parenting, as claims are hard to assess and expertise is increasingly challenging to define and ultimately to trust.

Documenting Our Sources

Investigating the role of social media platforms in disseminating expertise and creating new forms of medical expertise afforded us rich material for historical comparison in the book. Using these sources also provided some challenges, including with citation. We are familiar with both Chicago and American Psychological Association (APA) styles of citation. While Chicago style is better suited to the archival materials we cite throughout the text, it is a system less flexible for social media sources, including Twitter tweets, IG posts, FB comment chains, and posts on websites like Amazon, below online articles, and on blogs. The APA style model allows us (with some tweaking) to engage with this material as text, as a contemporary form of medical expertise, and as technical and lay expertise expressed through protoscience journalism in early twentieth-century magazines and newspapers (Tomes, 2012). Hence, we chose APA style to cite both historical and contemporary sources.

Unfortunately, the amount of data we collected through R6 and in our preliminary research left us with an unwieldy number of sources, given that each text and each comment can be cited independently—one R6 search produced 9,000 possible data points, each requiring a citation if we chose to use them. To elucidate the particular interdisciplinary methods we use throughout the book, we included a Methodological Appendix. We also integrated some Chicago-style elements in the bibliographic section, supplementing APA formatting and citation and allowing us to adequately explain our materials. We include both a "master" reference list (APA style), which includes full citations of sources used in more than one chapter, as well as a selected bibliography, which reduces other source material, including social media posts to be included in truncated form, and organized by historical and contemporary categories (e.g., early twentieth-century newspapers, Twitter accounts). As we cite hundreds of sources, a master reference list and a selected bibliography allow us to address our citations. The full citations for each chapter are available digitally, to ensure full access to readers. Below, we provide an overview of our interdisciplinary methodology; specifics and examples are available in the Methodological Appendix.

An Interdisciplinary Methodology

In tracing the history of both technical and lay expertise as it pertains to the life cycle of early motherhood in America, we approach each chapter "topologically," viewing time as flexible and interconnected, acknowledging that constructions of the past are not divorced from constructions of the present or the recent past (Jensen, 2016; see also Serres & Latour, 1995). We recognize that comparative discussions easily become anachronistic, and throughout the text we diligently address the contextual (e.g., social, economic, political) differences across time, even while we identify ideas that continue to reappear in new forms with varying impact. Our archival research helps illuminate the ways that social-media-based technical expertise and lay expertise are both an extension of—and distinct from—historical medical information dissemination in public and private spheres. This book project began with two overarching research questions that guided our data collection and analysis:

RQ1: How does social media help, hinder, or complicate the propagation of medical expertise/knowledge popularized since the nineteenth century?

RQ2: In what ways does the expression of expertise on social media today continue or depart from historical patterns and power structures?

In conversation with primary and secondary sources, our work examines present-day constructions that reproduce apprehension and uncertainty around early motherhood. By examining seemingly "modern" worries in parallel with their historical roots, readers gain a sense that while the format of expertise dissemination has changed, the crisis framing of the stages within the life cycle of early motherhood (e.g., conception, the postpartum period) represents an important continuity. For all the expertise received (and ignored) by mothers over time, most individuals biologically mature, babies continue to be born, and children still grow into adulthood. Still, some admonitions (e.g., sanitation practices) revolutionized parenting and saved lives.

Given our particular focus on technical and lay expertise in historical and present-day contexts, we include data and findings from three qualitative/rhetorical studies, and the use of the program R6, which assisted us in gathering social-media-based data on technical and lay expertise dissemination. Our qualitative work includes 25 interviews on doctor-patient communication and a survey study and resulting patient support materials for people experiencing infertility treatment based on lay (patient) expertise. It also includes rhetorical analyses of over 200 IG images, as well as a study of historical newspaper articles discussing TS. In all our research, we privilege the voices of those we study and draw on our narratives, reflecting Ellis's (2004) contention that systematic self-reflection is vital to investigating cultural experience. Throughout our research, we conducted interviews with individuals whose perspectives were missing or underrepresented (e.g., a trans man who gave birth) to interrogate the ways in which less powerful groups, such as mothers who are poor, mothers of color, mothers who are immigrants, and mothers who are queer, are policed and engage in self-surveillance. Finally, we studied technical and lay expertise in individual papers and doctors' notebooks and records to understand how different practitioners (traditional and eclectic) viewed disease and recorded patient interactions.[3]

In each chapter, we outline our definition of lay and technical (medical) experts and (medical) expertise, emphasizing the ways these definitions change across time and contexts. We deconstruct the binary of technical and lay, exposing the ways in which this binary impedes access and agency for those already disadvantaged by traditional hierarchies. Throughout the text, we warn against the embrace of technical expertise as "gospel," or lay expertise as value-neutral, necessarily "radical," or true a priori in opposition to technical expertise.

OVERVIEW

This book consists of four sections, topically representing each stage in the life cycle of early motherhood through analysis of both historical and contemporary discourse: (1) conception and (in)fertility, (2) pregnancy and birth, (3) the post-partum period or the "fourth trimester," and (4) infant loss and early childhood.

The first chapter, titled "On Preconception, the Beginning of the Life Cycle of Early Motherhood," is a brief discussion that homes in on sex selection as one aspect of preconception advice and illuminates the complexities of technical and lay expert knowledge, including the ways they can overlap and/or mimic one another. In chapter 2, "A State of Mind? Fertility Treatment(s) and Expertise," we trace the historical progression of (in)fertility treatments while focusing on the long history of mental or "psychosomatic" infertility. Central to our analysis is the question of infertility patients continually being asked to mentally discipline themselves to achieve pregnancy. We trace language and ideologies popular in the late nineteenth and early twentieth centuries, then resurfacing in the twenty-first century through online eCourses and disseminated on social media platforms.

Part II explores pregnancy- and childbirth-related crises. Chapter 3, "Red Underwear, Genes, and Monstrosity: Pregnancy and Social Media Surveillance," addresses the social surveillance of gestating bodies in public and on social media. We show how, as construed within the traditional gender binary, pregnancy is performative; it is also imbued with class, race, ability, and gender expression privilege. We interrogate how experts of all types demand performative pregnancy and explore what this means for pregnant individuals using smartphone apps and engaging with social media platforms today. Social media may be increasing self-surveillance practices during pregnancy, but the advice is often more than a century old. Chapter 4, "'You Women Will Have to Fight for It': Twilight Sleep and Transactional Childbirth Expertise in Twentieth-Century America," centers on the popularity of the TS birth method in the early twentieth century. Comparing the campaign for TS in hospitals to mid-century efforts to move births away from a hospital-centric model, we investigate how lay experts transact with and circumvent technical experts' expertise in the birthing room. We end by exploring interactions on social media between lay experts and technical experts about circumventing Baby-Friendly Hospital Initiatives, which lay experts fought for just a few decades ago.

Part III addresses the postpartum period, or the "fourth trimester." Chapter 5, "'One of the Most Curious Charities in the World': Infant Incubation as Sideshow and/or Medical Specialty," focuses on "Dr." Martin Couney, a turn-of-the-twentieth-century practitioner who cared for premature babies in incubators at Coney Island and various World's Fairs (1900s–1940s). His pronouncements on mothering illuminate the power of technical expertise in defining the life cycle of early motherhood in early twentieth-century print media. We analyze Couney's recent resurgence as a social media sensation and debunk him as a "maverick" among technical experts. Finally, we explore the ways the Couney myth complicates or obfuscates the experiences of NICU (Neonatal Intensive Care Unit) parents today. In chapter 6, "Not Just Baby Blues: Historical Realities and Social Media Accounts of Postpartum Care Today," we interrogate how late nineteenth- and early twentieth-century (no-cost) postpartum care through in- and outpatient programs compares with present-day postpartum care. Materials collected via Radian6 allow us to analyze social media accounts of support desired (by mothers) and support received in the first six weeks after birth (e.g., news stories, tweets, blogs) for comparison to historical patient records. We discover that the comparison is not just between systems of postpartum care in particular contexts but also between health care and the absence of health care.

Part IV focuses on infant care and early child rearing. Chapter 7, "Memento Mori in the Victorian Era and on Social Media: The 'Right' (Way) to Grieve," delves into the tragedy of child loss. In the mid-nineteenth century, the emergence of photography allowed for emphasis on imaging the deceased as a powerful tool for remembering. We assess the practice of memento mori specifically for infant and early childhood (toddler) loss. We consider the role of technical and lay observers in these cultural practices, and then we interrogate how viewing is misconstrued as expertise to police grief on social media today. The final chapter, "'Better Babies': Early Twentieth-Century Scientific Babyhood and Constructions of Twenty-First-Century Infancy on Instagram," questions the role of social media in perpetuating baby contest ideals. Here we examine nineteenth-century beauty contests for babies, twentieth-century "better babies" contests, and social media platforms such as IG, which create modern-day "better babies" contests online. We study the role of both lay and technical experts in designing these events and in creating the judging materials. We use these materials to frame the "tyranny" of pediatric perfection and the long-term impact of milestones on perceptions of "normal" child development, now realized in social media spaces.

To close, we summarize the practical and theoretical implications emerging from our work. The conclusion includes a call for a reexamination of categorizations of (medical) expertise in the social media age, as well as a template for engaging on these platforms without increasing self-surveillance or replicating social hierarchies; we include ruminations from those mothering at the margins as well. Finally, we interrogate the potential for net neutrality to limit this developing conversation and silence social media expertise in ways we cannot yet foresee.

We begin the book with a discussion of sex-selective conception myths to consider the ways in which gametes are gendered in medical research and in the wider society, impacting our ideas of conception. What we aim to highlight is that medical myths transcend forms of expertise—gaining currency in lay and technical medical communities, and impacting public perceptions, folk medicine, and even formal research (Keil, 2010). More broadly, the sex selection debate provides a pathway into more obvious questions and examples, which we explore in subsequent chapters. So how is this niche sex selection debate (via conception methods or genetic testing) a crisis? How is sex selection implicated in "preconception"? The potential crisis for mothers is another layer added to the already significant pressure to create the "perfect baby" (e.g., free of chromosomal abnormalities, able-bodied) or families "balanced" around a traditional gender binary (one girl, one boy), a pressure that begins during preconception and frames cis female bodies as "good" or "bad" sites for conception, pregnancy, birth, and child rearing.

As we explore throughout the book, expertise dissemination on social media platforms and in smartphone apps can increase the pressure to "achieve" a socially accepted, performative motherhood, shifting the focus from systemic injustice and oppression to individual responsibility, while increasing self-surveillance. Simultaneously, these technological tools offer wider access to medical information and democratize expertise, which allows for alternative mothering discourses with parallel collective action.

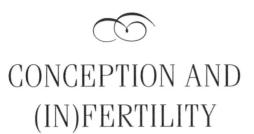

PART I

CONCEPTION AND (IN)FERTILITY

CHAPTER 1

ON PRECONCEPTION, THE BEGINNING OF THE LIFE CYCLE OF EARLY MOTHERHOOD

Do you care enough about your (potential) future children to perfect your health today? As new mothers, pressure around proper preparation for conception continues to grow (Stephenson et al., 2014), even for "pre-mothers." Have you taken the proper steps to ensure conception including taking prenatal vitamins? Do you "eat clean" to maintain and protect your fertility? Are you exercising regularly and getting sufficient sleep? Have you even considered sex selection techniques to ensure you create the family of your design? Are you controlling your stress level to create the optimum gestational environment? Have you been screened for potential genetic issues? Are you informed about your fertility health/status? Discussions of preparedness for pregnancy and the emergence of "preconception" as a life stage that is either achieved or failed frames this "stage" as a time imbued with potential crisis, and prescriptive behaviors for preconception now begin during the teen years (Ayala & Freeman, 2016). Problematically, this extends the life cycle of early motherhood drastically, with the preconception stage alone lasting potentially a decade or more (Ayala & Freeman, 2016). Failure to prepare for possible conception denotes numerous negative potentialities, few of which are proven or even demonstrable in available research. For example, failure to "achieve" healthy preconception behaviors could prompt fertility issues, high-risk pregnancies, or a nonoptimal environment for fetal development, with worrisome yet inchoate outcomes (see Ayala & Freeman, 2016). Thus, preconception is a crisis in which either you prepare for the conception of healthy children or your preparation is inadequate and you become a "bad" mother prior to conception.

The notion of preconception as a stage in which women need to prepare their minds and bodies, through products and practices most accessible to educated, middle- and upper-class, white, cis, able-bodied women, reflects long-held notions of the proper work and roles of females as potential mothers in our society as well as the particular assumptions of "good" motherhood bounded by race, class, education level, and gender (Ayala & Freeman, 2016; Breslaw, 2012; Smith-Rosenberg, 1985; Vandenberg-Daves, 2014). This framing extends, in its focus on middle-class whiteness within a heterosexual nuclear family, back to the mid-nineteenth century (and before). Curiously, the "failure" of so many women to meet these emerging preconception standards underscores the blurred lines between technical and lay expertise, as experts of all kinds continue to offer more specialized preconception products and services, angling for market share in the wellness economy. Products and services offered by lay experts online to best prepare the body for conception (e.g., eCourses, preconception nutrition plans, meditation practices, yoga courses, and workouts) are available, albeit different from those available in a traditional doctor's office (e.g., prenatal vitamins, blood tests for egg "age," genetic testing). There is also an emerging market for smartphone apps tracking menstruation, ovulation, and optimal fertility (e.g., Kindara, Ovia). The burgeoning number of expert practitioners addressing preconception also increases awareness about this new life stage, and the advent of social media advertising and outreach ensures that potential parents are bombarded with preparation messaging (see Anderson, 2017; BabyCenter, 2017; Mama, 2017; Rhythms, 2016; Weeks, 2013).

BabyCenter (with the website tagline "expert advice") is a popular parenting website with a similarly popular pregnancy smartphone app. An article on this website offers a list of 17 actions women can take before trying to conceive, including visiting the doctor for a "preconception visit," monitoring one's caffeine intake, stocking one's fridge with healthy foods which include "clean" foods such as kale and spirulina and other "superfoods" like maca, which were previously known mostly in indigenous communities and are now repackaged largely for middle- and upper-class (predominately white) consumers shopping at high-end grocery stores. Other actions include maintaining a workout regimen, and even considering "genetic carrier testing" (BabyCenter, 2017).

This BabyCenter list prompted us to research preconception further, and we were surprised to find the topic of sex selection, sometimes related to genetic carrier issues, occupying a lot of "space" on social media sites when preconception presented in the discourse. Maggie encountered a large number of such discussions during her preconception journey and received contradictory information from the technical and lay experts she consulted before the conception of her first (and second) child. On the topic of sex selection, there are inconsistent findings on how prevalent social-media-based information is or what kind of impact it has on personal decisions for conceptive practices. Similarly, there are no available data on how social media discourse impacts other individual decisions regarding preconception, including dietary or exercise choices. Anecdotally, Instagram and Facebook (FB) offer a wealth of options for supporting preconception health, including food products, exercise classes, mindfulness courses, and sex selection techniques.

In this chapter, within the discussion of sex selection and preconception, we define "lay experts" as those individuals who offer preconception advice, products, or sex selection techniques outside of a traditional doctor's office (e.g., individuals posting folklore or formal research findings on social media platforms, in chatrooms, etc.). Technical experts include researchers conducting studies and publishing on sex selection as well as practitioners who can assist couples in choosing the sex of their baby through embryo transfer (e.g., reproductive endocrinology and infertility [REI] specialists). Historically, technical experts on sex selection included traditionally trained doctors and lay experts included eclectic medical practitioners (e.g., homeopathic physicians), faith leaders, and observers of atmospheric conditions (e.g., lunar calendars for sex selection in China) (see also Derkatch, 2016). Below we examine the fluidity of technical and lay expertise and the nature of preconception knowledge particularly for sex selection techniques and document how this fluidity confounded Maggie when she sought information during her preconception periods.

Maggie turned to both technical experts and lay experts to address her preconception concerns, such as her baseline health and ability to conceive, including posting questions on social media platforms such as FB. As the BabyCenter post suggested, Maggie (and her partner) also pursued genetic carrier testing, which resulted in a deep dive into the niche dialogue regarding sex selection as a part of preconception. Born into a family with carriers for the gene (CFTR) for cystic fibrosis (CF), Maggie chose testing, having witnessed the struggle and eventual death of some of her classmates with the disease in her all-girls high school. CF is a disease that impacts organ function through the overproduction of mucus (Cystic Fibrosis Foundation, n.d.). Individuals with CF struggle with persistent lung infections, breathing difficulty, and complications in other organs, including severe stress on the pancreas (Cystic Fibrosis Foundation, n.d.). Maggie learned that cis females with CF have a decreased life expectancy and are likely to have "worse outcomes with common CF pathogens" and become "colonized with respiratory pathogens" slightly earlier (Harness-Brumley, Elliot, Rosenbluth, Raghavan, & Jain, 2014, pp. 1012, 1017). She and her partner also worried about their ability to care for a child with CF monetarily; therefore, they decided if they were both carriers, they would either not have children, adopt, or seek fertility treatment with sex selection (see U.S. Department of Health and Human Services, 1995). It was not a decision they had to make. Maggie is a CF carrier; however, her husband James is not. Maggie carried two children to term, and they did not find out the sex before delivery during either pregnancy.

As Maggie and James awaited their CFTR testing results, a colleague provided her with a copy of Weschler's (2006) *Take Charge of Your Fertility*, which she read on the beach with a magazine disguising the front cover. Weschler wrote her book after Googling "how to increase your chances of conceiving a boy" and coming across several links and chatrooms dispensing advice on sex-specific conception. Her book details the Shettles Method, which originated in the 1960s and in the 1970s became the book *How to Choose the Sex of Your Baby* (Shettles & Rorvik, 2006; see also Shettles, 1960, 1961). By following Shettles's advice and tactics (e.g., to conceive a boy, time intercourse close to ovulation and use a vaginal rear-entry sexual position), a couple could reportedly increase their chances of the desired outcome (from about 75% to 90%). However, during her second preconception stage, Maggie remained curious about the efficacy of sex selection and the preoccupation with it on social media, so she contacted her practitioner directly for more information. In April 2017, she sent a password-protected email to her obstetrician/gynecologist (OBGYN). As part of their conversation, her doctor stated, "Because male sperm is the faster of the two, some suggest having intercourse as close to ovulation as possible. If you have sex several days before ovulation, the male sperm may die off." Two other doctors in this same OBGYN practice classified these claims as myth; reproductive endocrinology and infertility specialist Dr. Lauren Johnson (2017) recalled these claims in texts but concluded, "Recent data refutes Shettles' and Billings' original hypothesis."[1]

Questions about Shettles's (and other scholars') sex selection research have resurfaced in medical literature for nearly 40 years. In 1978, the *New England Journal of Medicine* concluded that insemination on different days of the menstrual cycle does lead to variations in the sex ratio (e.g., boys conceived closer to ovulation) (Corson, 1979). It was hypothesized that Y sperm are slightly more likely to fertilize (due to their speed), causing a distorted primary sex ratio. However, later research concluded that natural sex selection methods are not successful (Grant, 2006; Gray et al., 1998). In 1991, Gray published a meta-analysis of sex-selective intercourse practices, including Shettles's methods, and concluded that "the selection of male offspring by intercourse around the time of ovulation . . . is contradicted by scientific data" (p. 1984). A 1995 article in the *New England Journal of Medicine* reported that timed intercourse and ovulation had no impact on the sex of the baby (Wilcox, Weinberg, & Baird, 1995). In 1998, *Human Reproduction* published an article in which researchers recorded acts of intercourse and signs of ovulation, then assigned the most probable time of conception based on the provided data (Gray et al., 1998). The research team concluded that "manipulation of the timing of insemination during the cycle cannot be used to affect the sex of offspring" (Gray et al., 1998, p. 1397). In a 2006 editorial in the *British Medical Journal*, Grant dismissed the Shettles Method: "It was not until the development of computer-assisted sperm analysis (CASA) that reliable observations could be made. So far, researchers have found no morphological differences between human X sperm and Y sperm. . . . Y bull sperm do not swim faster than X sperm" (p. 919; see also Hossain, Barik, & Kulkarni, 2001; Moruzzi, Wyrobek, Mayall, & Gledhill, 1988; Penfold et al., 1998). Yet the expertise Maggie received from various doctors contradicted the last 20-plus years of research. With little consensus, it is difficult to know what to believe (see also Ovia, 2017).

Importantly, Shettles's study attributed traditional, gender-specific traits to X (female) and Y (male) chromosome sperm, informing readers that Y or "male" sperm are said to be faster and smaller but die faster; X or "female" sperm are slower and better able to withstand the acidic cervical environment (for a summary of Shettles, see FertilityFriend, n.d.; Gary, 1991). Without gendered gametes, sex selection would be more difficult to predict in the Shettles Method. The notion that sperm are inherently "male" and ova are "female" and that these cells act with gendered behavior undergirds all sex-selective recommendations on social media, at family reunions, and, as we've seen, in the doctor's office. The idea that timed intercourse can work for sex selection stems from assumptions about Y ("male") sperm being more robust and swimming more quickly than X ("female") sperm. The implication is that male offspring might have these same characteristics, an assumption that circles back into problematic sex preferences. As Emily Martin (1991) noted, the vast majority of medical textbooks depict sperm as masculine and exhibiting strength, virility, and aggressive behavior, while the egg is portrayed as a "damsel in distress" passively awaiting "her" rescue via penetration. The egg "is swept" or "drifts" (pp. 491, 489); women "shed" or lose eggs while men "produce" sperm (Martin, 1991, p. 486). And the impact of these medical teachings doesn't end with doctors—Barnes's (2014) work recounted men revealing the pressure they feel to "gush sperm" to prove their virility (p. 5).

Unfortunately, even after extensive studies at leading research institutions showed that egg and sperm both played an active role in conception and other studies found that protein structures placed the egg in the role of aggressor, descriptive language sustained the notion of gametes as operating within the gender binary (Martin, 1991). Citing the new discovery that the sperm is drawn to the ova and then sticks to it, powerless to extract itself from the surface, researchers focused on the harpoon-like head of the sperm (see Schatten & Schatten, 1983). Even when researchers frame the egg and sperm as partners, gendered language remains, parsing the egg into weak, disconnected parts and the sperm into a cohesive, logical whole (Martin, 1991). Again, these same characteristics and constructs are used to define the behavior of X and Y spermatozoa, despite research illustrating no differences exist.

Rooted in these gendered constructions, Shettles's original hypothesis is popular in obstetrics textbooks in use at many medical schools today (see Cunningham, Leveno, Bloom, Spong, & Dashe, 2014) but also prevalent on social media platforms and in smartphone apps. At the beginning of her search, Maggie could find only arguments in support of Shettles's work, from both lay and technical experts, or online "experts" whose expertise background was not apparent. We found one chat board that attempted to debunk Shettles's conclusions. Baby42015 (2014) said, "Male sperm do not swim faster than female sperm"; the poster used scientist Valerie Grant's (2006) letter to the editor in the *British Medical Journal* to support her point: "The number of gender based medical falsehoods I keep hearing in and around my pregnancy is just staggering. This one seems to be prevalent too, that male sperm swim faster and female sperm slower." While technical experts acknowledge the lack of consensus, lay experts also acknowledge varying research conclusions. Positioning herself as a lay expert, Baby42015 (2014) utilized Grant's arguments (which seem to fall in line with the most up-to-date medical findings) and then chided other lay experts posting on social media for spreading misinformation. However, this supposed misinformation still holds sway with some technical experts. It is clear from Maggie's experience that some misinformation or outdated information is received at the doctor's office and then potentially broadcast to personal networks on social media.

Currently, the impact of this gendered framing is apparent among lay experts on social media, in discussion threads trading "techniques" and medical expertise to achieve sex selection during conception. Despite the prevalence of gendered gamete language, individuals are also criticized for engaging in sex selection. For example, a social media uproar (mostly among lay experts) occurred when John Legend and Chrissy Teigen announced the sex of their baby conceived via in vitro fertilization (IVF). Because of IVF, couples can learn the sex of their embryos and can decide which to implant (PeDahl et al., 2006). Teigen's feed prompted a lot of personal critiques; she defended her preconception choices on Twitter, attempting to educate the public on her views about IVF and sex selection during that process. As Teigen responded to critics: "we didn't create a little girl. we had multiple embryos. girls and boys. we simply chose to put in a female first (and second)," and "we didn't 'throw away' anything and still would love to have more of both in the future. hard to explain such a complicated process here" (also cited in Lee, 2016).

As with other medical technologies, embryo sex selection is available only to individuals with financial means to undergo IVF with the added cost of testing embryos for sex selection. Infertility is not easy for any couple to face. For parents with class privilege (e.g., access to funds or capital to take loans for treatment) encountering this challenge, to be able to select a gender may be a small "perk" of an emotionally and physically demanding and socially isolating experience. Not all individuals have fertility privilege (the ability to conceive without difficulty) (Johnson, 2016), and very few have the luxury of engaging in preconception preparations that include sex selection. Some medical professionals continue to promote this embryo testing for sex selection, although in 1999 the American Society for Reproductive Medicine (ASRM) stated that using IVF treatment for sex selection should "not be encouraged" and in 2015 urged clinics to develop clear policies for sex selection services (ASRM, 2004, p. S247; see also Storrs, 2016, n.p.). In Canada and the United Kingdom, there are bans on sex selection used for social reasons, such as to promote family balancing (one of each sex) (see Genetics and IVF Institute, 2017). Sex selection is allowed for medical situations, such as for parents seeking to avoid chromosome-linked diseases or genetic mutations like CFTR, provided individuals can afford and/or access these technologies.

For centuries, personal and social forces, including a sexist preference for boys, encouraged individuals in many societies to attempt sex selection for non-medical reasons. By the late 1980s, ethicists such as Dorothy Wertz and John Fletcher (1989) disputed prenatal testing for purposes of sex selection because of systemic, structural gender discrimination. They argued forcefully that sex selection and selective abortion identify gender as a liability. These practices, Wertz and Fletcher said, "[undermine] the major moral reason that justifies prenatal diagnosis and selective abortion—the prevention of serious and untreatable genetic disease. Gender is not a disease. Prenatal testing for nonmedical reasoning makes a mockery of medical ethics" (p. 24). Despite the ethical issues with sex selection and gender-binary-based descriptions and depictions of human gametes (Martin, 1991), some individuals still attempt sex selection as part of preconception. Furthermore, since traditionally trained doctors and researchers (technical experts) continue to disagree about the effectiveness of the Shettles and other methods to choose or predict the sex of a child, genetic testing is the only certain method for gaining this information. There are multiple issues here. First, as stated, it is difficult to ascertain the actual success of timed intercourse for sex selection. Second, using these techniques and/or genetic testing and, potentially, selective abortion contributes to current preference for male children in much of the world, creating misery and suffering for millions of girl children and provoking demographic crises (and thus economic and social ones) only now coming to the fore (Eftekhaari et al., 2015). Third, the very knowledge underpinning the Shettles, Billings, and other methods reflects the sexist, binary biology with deep roots in traditional Western medical theory, acknowledging only two genders. Additionally, these methods assume that individuals who time intercourse will give birth to a child with the sex of their choice, but that does not ensure gender (e.g., children who identify as transgender, nonbinary, agender, and other nonconforming identities). And yet this binary is deeply interwoven into our understanding of conception, even down to the language used to identify or describe gametes.

Individuals will consider sex selection based on their own needs, deeply held beliefs, and ethical systems. Some may attempt sex selection, which others would never consider. But beyond this singular issue, the wider social pressure to engage in preconception rituals for perfect, healthy babies remains and continues to increase, and along with that has come an explosion in the market for products and services for individuals seeking to conceive. Expectations of personal responsibility as the main predictor of reproductive outcomes continue throughout conception, pregnancy, childbirth, and childhood. We are not advocating for or against expanded access to sex selection; instead, we are questioning the growing emphasis on sex selection as yet another addition to the laundry list of responsibilities potentially pregnant bodies must shoulder in the preconception life stage.

Similar to every other topic we explore in this book, gendered descriptions of gametes and advice on sex selection techniques are not specific to the twentieth and twenty-first centuries. If any improvement is discernible, it is that medicine has begun to complicate the gendered framing of gametes instead of mapping binary gender stereotypes onto all reproductive organs. However, research produced in the last decade still contains outdated medical concepts from more than a century ago. For example, in 1891, Dr. Kellogg surmised that the ovum could "lose its way," though the sperm "retain their vitality and efficacy for a number of days after copulation" (pp. 78–79). A gendered, sexist understanding of the gametes apparent in descriptions of sex-selective intercourse practices is also nothing new. In the early twentieth century, Dr. Mary Melendy (1904) noted one "belief" on "sex in generation": "If the wife is in a higher state of sexual vigor and excitement at the time of coition, boys will be conceived" (p. 373). So even heightened arousal in a female, suggestive of sexual aggression and virility, was sure to produce males. Nearly 60 years later, Dr. Louise H. Branscomb wrote,

Sex determination, Female
1—coitus up to 2–3 days before ovulation, not during ovulation time
2—coitus without female orgasm
3—shallow penetration at omission
4—before coitus drink 1/4 cup whole omega to get to uterus (p. 99)[2]

While we know Branscomb recorded this information in her private notebook, it is unclear whether or not she advised her patients to use these methods. Still, the inherent sexism in these recommendations is striking. Using "shallow penetration" and "coitus without female orgasm" to conceive a female seems rooted in the pervasive myth of the "cold" or "prudish" (white) woman—called "frigid" in the 1950s and blamed for marital dissatisfaction and even infertility. How is it that a "less aggressive" penetration leads to a female child? How can this be a sound medical theory? Despite CASA-based observations showing no differences in gametes, the notion of gendered gametes has been and continues to be pervasive, imbuing all conception research with this gender binary and impacting public perception as well (Martin, 1991).

As we will explore in the ensuing chapters, historical understandings of medical expertise, including conception, pregnancy, premature birth, infant loss, and early childhood milestones, continue to impact parents in person and online, particularly on social media platforms where historical myths are often perpetuated out of context. The question remains whether or not experts of all kinds understand or acknowledge this reality. Moreover, these historical constructions can impact individual health choices in ways that are difficult to quantify and/or counteract. Throughout our book, we contest the notion that lay and technical knowledges are separate, siloed, or merely combative. In 2005, medical researchers published an article that sought a linkage between moon cycles and vaginal pH (Sarkar & Biswas, 2005). The authors concluded that the full moon favored the conception of male babies (Sakar & Biswas, 2005). Regardless of the findings or the methods of this study, one must acknowledge the fluidity between lay and technical knowledges and the construction of expertise based on them. Misunderstanding this fluidity leads to narrow definitions of expertise and the impact of medical expertise on individual health choices, particularly among individuals who frequent social media sites and use smartphone applications. Thus, we remain unaware of the complexity of expertise in an age of social media, particularly for those traversing the life cycle of early motherhood. To begin to disabuse us of a binary understanding of expertise, we turn next to the crisis of infertility on the road to parenthood.

CHAPTER 2

A STATE OF MIND?

FERTILITY TREATMENT(S) AND EXPERTISE

I was at the point where I was like, if you want me to wear clown shoes to get pregnant, that's what I will do.

—Arlene, interviewee, 2014

Tasha Blasi (2017), a former biology teacher and now a vlogger with a YouTube channel, provides a website and eCourse on how to make "IVF [in vitro fertilization] easier, smarter, and cheaper." In one video, Blasi recounted getting pregnant after an IVF cycle in which she followed the advice of a woman who urged, "You're too scientific about it. You need to think outside the box" (n.p.). This exchange culminated in Blasi spending a week applying molasses to her abdomen, removing it with a piece of watermelon, and throwing that watermelon into the ocean tied in a yellow cloth. Blasi concluded, "Now there were many other variables during that round too, but I can't discount the watermelon technique" (n.p.). In a crisis, Blasi "kept on trying anything" to support her goal of becoming pregnant. She is not alone.

In the United States, tens of thousands of cis females seek traditional fertility testing, diagnosis, and treatment annually (Christensen, 2014; Johnson, Quinlan, & Marsh, 2018), many while also attempting to get pregnant using methods, information, and advice that are not necessarily based on scientific evidence. The World Health Organization (WHO) and the American Society for Reproductive Medicine (ASRM) recognize male and/or female factor infertility as a disease. The CDC (2016) reported that the percentage of infertile women (ages 15–44) in America is 6.1%, while 12.3% have some form of "impaired fecundity" and 11.3% (ages 15–44) have accessed infertility services (n.p.). At this time, the number of cis females seeking alternative (nontraditional) treatments alone or alongside traditional fertility treatments is unknown. However, given the increasing presence on social media (e.g., Facebook, blogs, Twitter, Instagram) of alternative methodologies, treatments, and supplements, and the explosive growth of eCourses (Mind, 2017; Naturally, 2017; Unlock, 2017) as well as the increasing use of alternative therapies within reproductive endocrinology and infertility (REI) practices, "alternative users" likely number in the thousands or tens of thousands (ASRM, 2015; Blasi, 2017; Integrative, 2017; Manheimer et al., 2008; NCCIH, 2008; Organic, 2017; Sharf, Geist-Martin, Cosgriff-Hernández, & Moore, 2012; Thomas, 2017; see also Derkatch, 2016).

Regardless of technical medical definitions, individuals may conceptualize infertility as a journey, a challenge, a condition, a disease, or even a social construct (Barnes, 2014; Johnson, Quinlan, & Marsh, 2018; Sandelowski, 1993). Some individuals who experience repeated early miscarriage identify as infertile (Anonymous personal communication, 2017), while others do not. Definitions of infertility are bound by time and social context and shaped by individual identities, shifting cultural constructs, and intersectional systems of oppression (Bell, 2010; Breitkopf & Rubin, 2015; Jensen, 2016; Johnson, 2016; May, 2007). Therefore, the term "infertility," its meanings, and its implications for individuals and social groups remain contested. In this chapter, we define infertility in the widest terms, including the traditional—though heteronormative—definition of 12 or more months of unprotected sex in a cis gender, heterosexual partnership (Chandra, Copen, & Stephen, 2014; WHO, 2017). We also include secondary infertility (the inability to become pregnant for 12 months after having carried at least one pregnancy to term) (RESOLVE, 2017; WHO, 2017). LBGTQ+ (an acronym which seeks an inclusive representation of a full range of identities and lived experiences) couples and/or individuals who may not have diagnosed fertility issues have unique conception needs and often require assisted reproductive technologies (ARTs) to become pregnant. Therefore, some use the (potentially ableist) term "impaired fecundity" to describe individuals seeking a gamete for conception (Chandra, Copen, & Stephen, 2014; Johnson, Quinlan, & Marsh, 2018). Given the emotional, social, physical, and financial challenges that accompany fertility issues, we understand delayed conception, diagnosis, and treatment as a crisis for those desiring children. Not all cis females desire to participate in this "rite of womanhood" (e.g., motherhood); nor must womanhood and motherhood be linked for any individual of any gender. And yet, the inability to conceive is still problematically framed as a female failure in a society where female value is linked to reproduction and women are assumed to be "natural mothers" (Solinger, 2007, p. 12; Vandenberg-Daves, 2014; see also Koeber, 2018).

Historically, the blame for infertility fell on female patients, as the "failure" of the cis female body became institutionalized in the absence of medical knowledge (Breslaw, 2012; Ehrenreich & English, 1978; Janik, 2014; Leavitt, 1995; Vandenberg-Daves, 2014; Weiner & Hough, 2012). The ongoing taboo on discussions of infertility adds to the stress faced by cis females receiving the messages around infertility diagnosis and treatment many patients receive and/or internalize. Infertility is a personal crisis: depression, anger, frustration, uncertainty, marital instability, and even anxiety-related sexual dysfunction have all been documented among people seeking fertility care (May, 1997; Mazor, 1984; Sandelowski, 1993; Thorn, 2009; Wirtberg et al., 2007). In fact, the social and emotional challenges faced by contemporary cis female patients are eerily similar to those of more than a century ago—even if treatment outcomes are far superior.

We briefly examine historical constructions of infertility and fertility treatments, starting with Dr. J. Marion Sims's work at the Woman's Hospital in New York City in the 1850s. We trace broad trends in treatments and play close attention to "psychogenic infertility" in the 1940s and 1950s, to assist us in making comparisons to expertise on social media today. Historically, women sought home remedies and/or spiritual healing and sustenance for their inability to conceive, and by the mid- to late 1800s, gynecologists became the most common source of medical treatment (Marsh & Ronner, 1996). Before the mid-1800s fertility experts were midwives, who are often considered experts today (see chapter 4)—the lay-technical expertise divide has been and continues to be imprecise. For the contemporary context, our conceptualization of traditional fertility treatment focuses primarily on individuals or couples seeking ARTs with REI specialists and reflects the overarching biomedicalization (increasing technological complexity and market-driven nature) of infertility diagnosis and treatment in post–World War II America (Breitkopf & Rubin, 2015; Clarke, Mamo, Fosket, Fishman, & Shim, 2010; Johnson, Quinlan, & Marsh, 2018).

At the turn of the twentieth century, the legitimized medical treatment for infertility was handled by gynecologists, traditional/technical experts interested in gaining market share from midwives, and other practitioners previously tasked with treating women's reproductive health. Medical practice became both wider (e.g., more techniques) and more specific (e.g., increasing specialization), so we include reproductive endocrinologists, embryologists, and urologists in our discussion. Today, these providers request and analyze some diagnostic tests, perform some treatment regimens, prescribe medications, and, in the case of REIs, perform higher-level diagnosis and treatments, such as intrauterine insemination (IUI), in vitro fertilization (IVF) or IVF with intracytoplasmic sperm injection (ICSI) and laparoscopic examinations, removal of endometrial tissue, and other adnexal surgeries (operations on organs "next to" the uterus, including the ovaries and the fallopian tubes) (ASRM, 2012; Johnson, Quinlan, & Marsh, 2018).[1] Again, historically, technical experts were doctors, particularly gynecologists who engaged in surgical treatment, but also legal eclectic practitioners like Dr. Melendy (1904) who focused on dietary changes and homeopathic treatments.

In the context of this chapter, "lay experts" include patients and practitioners outside of the more traditional technical sphere. We include patients, supportive communities, community advocates in groups such as RESOLVE and Fertility for Colored Girls (FFCG), online support communities, and bloggers and

social media users who draw attention to fertility and infertility issues. Historical "lay experts" included friends, family, and spiritual healers and companies marketing patent medicines direct to those seeking conception (Cramp,
1921). Currently, the "lay expert" label includes alternative or nontraditional
practitioners, such as yoga instructors, acupuncturists, naturopaths, counsel-
ors, faith leaders and spiritual healers, and journalists, many of whom produced what Tomes (2002) called "proto-science journalism," which provides
medical information in lay publications for private citizens. At the same time,
we acknowledge that an increasing number of traditional practitioners support or utilize alternative therapies, such as dietary changes, endocrine system
"flushing," targeted yoga practice, fertility acupuncture, and herbal supplementation (Anonymous personal communication, 2017; Blasi, 2017; Inner
Peace, 2017; Integrative, 2017; Manheimer et al., 2008) and/or work with alternative therapists and practitioners alongside traditional treatment protocols
(Manheimer et al., 2008; NCCIH, 2008; Sharf, Geist-Martin, Cosgriff-
Hernández, & Moore, 2012).

The "lay expert" sphere in this chapter is unique because no matter the range
of information they might seek or the methods they may try, many REI patients
find it necessary to gain a more expert-level knowledge about their reproductive health, the ins and outs of complicated protocols and treatments, insurance
coverage, and alternative therapies (deLacey, 2002; Johnson, 2016; Johnson,
Quinlan, & Myers, 2017; May, 2007). We find that REI patients also seek advice
and emotional support as well as medical information (Johnson, 2016; Johnson,
Quinlan, & Marsh, 2018; Johnson, Quinlan, & Myers, 2017; see also "How," 2015).

Even given these expanding definitions, the technical/lay binary presents a
false dichotomy, particularly for users seeking medical expertise on social media
platforms. In this chapter, we include the conclusions of trained dieticians, journalists who translate scientific publications for the public, bloggers with no
technical training, and experts like Tasha Blasi. Blasi (2017), a former science
teacher who today operates online as a fertility consultant and popular vlogger,
draws on various medical traditions, and uses lay and technical expertise interchangeably, resulting in a unique expert perspective without a clear category.
Some of the eCourses we address use technical expertise from the nineteenth
century but reframe it. As such, it is difficult to clearly delineate two forms of
expertise or how these forms of expertise are expressed distinctly in various
social media settings.

To be clear, we make no claims about the efficacy of any treatment or methodology or the likelihood of any treatment outcome, nor do we compare the fee
structures of technical, lay, or other experts. Rather, our research with nearly
200 individuals confirms scholarly findings of the long-standing tension between
body- and mind-centered approaches in both technical and lay contexts.[2] As an
REI practitioner informed us, patients are looking for increasingly integrated

(traditional and alternative) protocols and that trend will continue as millennials seek infertility treatment (Teaff, 2014). Furthermore, we know that some of today's popular alternative approaches (e.g., dietary changes, exercise, positive thinking fostering structural neurological changes) also appear in the history of traditional research and treatment. Exploring historical conceptualizations of infertility and its causes provides a framework for understanding present-day approaches and treatments, notably the resurgence of the mind-body connection among lay (and some technical) experts on social media.

Despite assumptions that traditional and alternative medicine and practice are distinct systems, we found evidence of overlapping and interconnected systems from nineteenth-century gynecologists, mid-twentieth-century psychoanalysts, and present-day traditional and lay experts. The boundaries between approaches and beliefs about fertility have been and continue to be permeable, and this can create real tension for fertility patients, amounting to contradictory or confusing messages about what treatments or methodologies to pursue. A number of our interviewees expressed frustration with the diagnosis "unexplained" (Sandelowski, 1993). The lack of a concrete diagnosis can increase frustration and feelings of powerlessness and anxiety. Once given this nebulous diagnosis, patients may seek additional expertise to obtain answers to a difficult question: My doctor says I am healthy. What can't I conceive?

A HISTORY OF FAILURE: THE STRUGGLE FOR
EFFECTIVE FERTILITY TREATMENTS

Taken together, the research by Jensen (2016), Marsh and Ronner (1996, 2010), and May (1997) on the history of infertility composes the most comprehensive medical history on infertility and infertility treatment to date. They conclude that accurate understandings of the causes of infertility as well as successful treatments have progressed slowly and language describing the bodies of those seeking treatment has been and often continues to be confusing or disempowering. Jensen (2016) investigated the intellectual history of infertility, tracing the linguistic transformation of terms such as "barren," "sterile," and "fecund" to the medically defined binaries, "fertile" and "infertile." This metamorphosis paralleled shifting conceptions of the body within medicine and American society (Jensen, 2016). Marsh and Ronner (1996, 2010) studied the progression of available treatments, experiments, and trends in gynecology, and eventually reproductive endocrinology, from the mid-nineteenth century through the 1990s, when REI practices became the mainstream approach to fertility issues in the United States. Jensen (2016) and Marsh and Ronner (1996, 2010) addressed the lack of effective treatment protocols available until the late twentieth century, noting how the dearth of basic reproductive knowledge about when and how ovulation occurs significantly delayed progress.[3] Tests to ascertain the presence of blockages in the fallopian tubes and other structural anomalies were not reliable until the early 1920s, while estrogen and progesterone were not discovered until the 1930s and not available in synthetic form until the 1940s. Ovulatory drugs were not available until the 1960s. And early on, drugs (particularly Pergonal) prompted too many high-order (multiples) births and other complications (Culliton, 1966; Marsh & Ronner, 1996).

Today, patients and practitioners have access to a wide array of tests to uncover structural and hormonal issues. Treatment options now include reparative and exploratory surgeries, ovulation drugs, intrauterine insemination (IUI), and IVF (Johnson, Quinlan, & Marsh, 2018; Marsh & Ronner, 2010). Recent innovations represent one of the first marked leaps forward in biomedical fertility treatments since the arrival of IVF in the late 1970s and 1980s (Jensen, 2016; Marsh & Ronner, 1996, 2010). The first IVF baby born in the United States, Elizabeth Jordan Carr, arrived on December 1981. Before that, patients faced low treatment success rates (Jensen, 2016; Marsh & Ronner, 1996, 2010; Reedy, 2007; Rongy, 1911).[4] For example, in the late nineteenth century, doctors helped fewer than 5% of patients conceive (Marsh & Ronner, 1996); early artificial insemination (AI) worked less than 1% of the time (Sims, 1866). By 2014, the Society for Assisted Reproductive Technology (SART) reported the national average outcome for IVF cycles for health patients under 35 as 41.2%. The highest reported IVF success rates (per cycle, by agency) for this same cohort range from 44% to 54%.[5] Traditional scientific research continues to push the limits of what is possible, including the potential for (temporary) uterine transplants (Cleveland Clinic, 2017), 3-D printed ovaries for transplant (Raja, 2017), and IVF with genetic material from three individuals (Amato, Tachibana, Sparman, & Mitalipov, 2014).

Those familiar with IVF and increasingly technical ARTs may assume the past two decades represent the most interventionist period in reproductive medicine. However, the late nineteenth century marked the first major era of technical medical expertise in treatment for infertility, or as it was then termed "sterility" or "barrenness" (Jensen, 2016; Marsh & Ronner, 1996), and the level of high-risk intervention in the burgeoning field of gynecology was quite significant. The focus on categorizing, treating, and curing sterility among late nineteenth-century physicians reflected a particular cultural context in America—namely, the cult of (white) motherhood, fears about nonwhite fertility alongside declining fertility rates among white, middle-class mothers, and related fears of women's increasing participation in higher education, as well as a growing interest in specialist medicine and the emergence of new or improved medical instruments that allowed obstetricians and gynecologists a less obstructed view of internal reproductive organs (Blackwood, 1878; Kline, 2001; Marsh & Ronner, 1997; Sims, 1866). Physicians approached sterility in females as a medical disorder best cured by surgical intervention (Jensen, 2016; Marsh & Ronner, 1996; May, 1997).

One of the "star" doctors from this period, often called the father of modern gynecology, was Dr. J. Marion Sims, whose brutal, likely nonconsensual experiments on enslaved women launched his career as a gynecologist and infertility specialist (Marsh & Ronner, 1996; Washington, 2006). Sims forced enslaved women on "loan" or purchased from their owners to endure (in some cases) dozens of surgeries on the perineum without pain medicine and dosed them with opioids afterward, forcing these patients into a horrific cycle of withdrawal and further surgeries to earn another dose of opioids (Washington, 2006). Following a positive response to his "research," Sims moved from Alabama to New York City and between 1853 and 1855 began the Woman's Hospital of the State of New York (Jensen, 2016; Sims, 1866), where he used his previous experience in perineal surgery to launch a career in the surgical treatment of sterility.

Sims's focus on sterility as structural (bodily) represented a shift from previous rhetoric around infertility, which held women morally and spiritually responsible for their inability to become pregnant or carry to term (Jensen, 2016). His theories on sterility and treatment eschewed appeals to spirituality (e.g., prayers and supplication to a Christian God) (Jensen, 2016). Sims viewed women's bodies as machines that required a machinist to correct malfunction and "framed women as largely blameless for their condition" (Jensen, 2016, p. 34). However, Sims's view of the gynecologist as an omniscient reproductive machinist simultaneously disempowered female patients by framing them as powerless in the face of sterility (Jensen, 2016).

Sims's descriptions of preferred surgical interventions suggest that his procedures were not gentle, even with consenting patients. He attacked the offending organs and forced cervixes open (Jensen, 2016; Marsh & Ronner, 2016; Sims, 1866). Still, his methods reflected a typical approach of gynecologists in the second half of the nineteenth century, many of whom favored "probing, scarifying, stretching, dilating, incising, cauterizing, and amputating" (Blackwood, 1878, p. 1) to treat gynecological issues, including sterility. In this "machinist" period of fertility medicine, practitioners favored highly invasive, likely very painful treatment. For example, Sims favored "cervical incision" or sometimes "amputation," whenever he found a "conoid" cervix (today categorized as normal) (Marsh & Ronner, 1996, p. 59; Sims, 1866).

Some practitioners asserted that women were also responsible for protecting and/or maintaining the machinery of their reproductive system (Jensen, 2016; May, 1997). For example, once physicians discovered gonorrhea caused pelvic inflammation and blocked fallopian tubes, doctors suggested women with these conditions were either promiscuous or the naïve victims of their husband's premarital dalliances (Jensen, 2016). However, the women most at fault were those who used contraceptives or had abortions, since these choices reflected depraved attempts to thwart the natural order of reproduction, which destroyed reproductive function (Jensen, 2016).

Nineteenth-century technical and lay experts also popularized the theory of sapped reproductive energy as the cause of sterility (Jensen, 2016; Smith-Rosenberg, 1985). At the time, medical theory asserted that the reproductive organs require a specific amount of mental and physical energy to develop properly, specifically during adolescence (Campbell, 1888; Jensen, 2016; Smith-Rosenberg, 1985). As a result, many practitioners argued against secondary and higher education for females to protect fecundity (Bigelow, 1883; "Books," 1946; Campbell, 1888; Engelmann, 1901; Jacobsen, 1946; Jensen, 2016; Macomber, 1924; Smith-Rosenberg, 1985); variations of this argument persisted for nearly a century. The notion that participating in educational or other cognitive pursuits saps energy from physical development is a derivation of the "woman as machine" conception of sterility, although in this version, women maintain their own machinery through the willing sacrifice of intellectual pursuits (Jensen, 2016; Kerber, Kesslar-Harris, & Sklar, 1995; Smith-Rosenberg, 1985). Despite the popularity of the reproductive-energy theory, some doctors—including many female doctors—fervently disagreed (Jacobi, 1886; see also Engelmann, 1901). Dr. Mary Putnam Jacobi conducted a quantitative study complete with statistical tables and concluded there was no correlation between academic study and sterility (Jensen, 2016; Morantz-Sanchez, 2000). Jacobi (1886) parted with energy theorists by suggesting that women frequently contributed energy to the reproductive system. However, like Sims, she favored a surgical approach (Jensen, 2016). Surgeries were nearly universally performed on female patients, as were the vast majority of nonsurgical lay treatments.

Alternative practitioners or lay experts, also called medical sectarians and eclectics in the nineteenth century (Breslaw, 2012; Hoffert, 1989; Janik, 2014; Starr, 1982), prescribed various treatments for infertility, including teas and tonics made from ingredients such as black cohosh or "squaw vine" (Marsh & Ronner, 1996).[6] Homeopathic physician Dr. Melendy (1904) recommended sex right after menstruation, camping in the woods for a summer, and "balm palmetto capsules" (p. 374). Hydropaths advised alternating hot and cold body wraps (Marsh & Ronner, 1996) and, along with other practitioners (Foote, 1898; Kellogg, 1891), counseled "barren" women to avoid alcohol, tea, and coffee. Hydropaths were particularly suspicious of invasive treatments (Janik, 2014) and felt that if water therapy did not work, women should accept childlessness (Marsh & Ronner, 1996). Thomsonian practitioners, who followed the medical ideology of Samuel Thomson, also advised noninvasive therapies, including sweating out impurities (Janik, 2014; Weiner & Hough, 2012) and root-based tonics (Marsh & Ronner, 1996). Meanwhile, even allopathic (traditional) practitioners such as Dr. Gardner counseled patients to follow a balanced diet and maintain an exercise regimen (Marsh & Ronner, 1996). Dr. Blackwood (1878) noted that practitioners ordered a "change of air and scene . . . with tonics and diet" at home (p. 1). Dr. Campbell (1888) advised nutritious food, regular exercise and "tonic remedies such as iron, quinine and strychnine" (p. 449). Allopathically trained Dr. Foote (1898) preferred a low-level electric current applied to the reproductive organs with his invention, the "Magnetic-stool" as well as his "impregnating speculum" and "No. 10 Soluble sanitary Tampons," though how these would cure infertility is unclear (pp. 484, 512, 911–912). Hence, the fluidity between what today we call "alternative" and "traditional" medical approaches is also reflected in the practices of some nineteenth-century practitioners.

The public also purchased products sold by "hucksters" or "quacks," in stores and through mail order, to cure sterility. Across the country, newspaper advertisements with product endorsements encouraged "barren" women to try supplements and tonics like Lydia E. Pinkham's Vegetable Compound, to which one "Mrs. Cora Gilson" credited her recent pregnancy ("A story," 1899). Many of these products came under attack by the American Medical Association after a large-scale investigation of these patent medicines and their contents (Cramp, 1921). Forensic research revealed that many tonics and supplements were composed of alcohol, sugar, opioids, and ingredients such as carbolic acid, an antimicrobial that can be both extremely volatile and, in the wrong concentration, deadly ("Use," 1878).

The most provocative allopathic infertility treatment in the late nineteenth century later became known as artificial insemination (AI), or today IUI. Sims admitted to experimenting with "artificial fertilization" (Sims, 1866, p. 364). Six patients endured more than 50 inseminations over two years; one became pregnant and miscarried (Marsh & Ronner, 1996; Sims, 1866). Few other physicians publicly supported the procedure, although the aforementioned Dr. Foote (1898) felt that if "medicines or electricity or both" failed to improve male sperm, "the artificial injection of healthy male spermatic fluids may be made so as to induce impregnation" (p. 515).

Through the end of the nineteenth century and into the early twentieth, treatment options included surgery and cervical dilation, prayer and religious devotion, avoiding contraceptives and abortion, avoiding higher education or mental taxation, and following a balanced diet while getting proper exercise. Patients also pursued treatments with eclectic practitioners such as homeopaths and hydrotherapists (Janik, 2014; Jensen, 2016; Marsh & Ronner, 1996). By the early twentieth century, "sterility" yielded to "infertility" as a descriptor for the inability to conceive. However, the options for patients remained largely the same. The focus on energy preservation and an ongoing fear of falling birthrates among Anglo-Saxon women, whom many believed were inappropriately expending their energy outside the home (Engelmann, 1901; Gregg, 1905), continued apace with rising nationalism in America and Europe (Bederman, 1995; Dennett Papers, 1874–1945; Jensen, 2016; Meaker, 1934; "We," 1946). In fact, claims of ever-increasing infertility in America or the larger Western world date back to the mid-nineteenth century. For over a century, physicians, community experts, and others regularly raised the specter of increasing infertility, though nearly all cited the identical "new" infertility/sterility rate between 10% and 15% (Aral & Cates, 1983; Curtis, 1924; Engelmann, 1901; Gregg, 1905; Hale, 1878; Kroger & Freed, 1950; Macomber, 1924; Meaker, 1934; "We," 1946; "Why," 2016).[7]

In the early twentieth century, AI improved and became more common, especially as researchers developed a more accurate understanding of human ovulation. As the Planned Parenthood Federation (1944) brochure "To Those Denied a Child" stated, AI was an exciting new option, but "if examination reveals that the male cells of the husband are wholly inadequate it will be futile to use the husband's sperm" (p. 14). Dr. Sophia Kleegman (1963), one of the few female gynecologists who specialized in sterility in the early twentieth century, maintained a private practice and clinic in New York City for decades (Dickinson, 1883–1950; Marsh & Ronner, 1996).

Beyond AI, the few new theories that emerged in the first half of the twentieth century focused on the chemical compounds and eventually the role of hormones in reproductive health (Jensen, 2016; Marsh & Ronner, 1996).[8] The rise of reproductive endocrinology began in the mid-1920s. At the outset, researchers and practitioners in this field thought that healthy reproductive cycles were evidence of nerves working in harmony with chemical hormones (Jensen, 2016; Marsh & Ronner, 1996). In 1933, Dr. Robert L. Dickinson founded the Committee on Maternal Health, which researched infertility and the role of endocrinology in both infertility issues and contraception (Dickinson, 1883–1950; Jensen, 2016). In the 1930s and early 1940s, notions of internal chemistry and hormones embellished and extended earlier claims about diet, stress, and energy conservation, making way for the twentieth-century concept of "psychogenic infertility," which we discuss in greater detail below. Practitioners suggested that a restricted diet, "nervous strain," too much education, and other constitutional concerns impacted internal chemical function or prevented conception altogether (Engelmann, 1901; Jacobsen, 1946; Jensen, 1996; Marsh & Ronner, 1996; Planned Parenthood Federation, 1944). Doctors also tried dietary therapy to balance hormones, including the use of calcium; numerous studies between 1920 and 1950 examined the efficacy of vitamins A and E and even the existence of "a hitherto unrecognized dietary factor essential for reproduction," referred to elsewhere as "Vitamin X" (Abere & Corner, 1953, p. 153; Evans & Burr, 1925; Marsh & Ronner, 1996; "We," 1946).

A few important tests came out of this period as well. In 1921, I. C. Rubin invented "tubal insufflation" (also called "the air test") to determine the health and capacity of the fallopian tubes (Marsh & Ronner, 1996, 2010). Also notable was the creation of the hysterosalpingogram (HSG), using radiology to trace fluid (rather than gas or air in Rubin's test) through the uterus and into the fallopian tubes, revealing uterine polyps or fibroids as well as tubal issues. Recently, online journalist Tim Newman (2017) mistakenly claimed this same procedure "offers new hope," apparently unaware that the HSG is a routine procedure for patients at nearly all REI practices in the United States and has been for many decades.[9] His lack of knowledge of the history of fertility treatment could offer lay readers false hope here. Even today, full tubal blockage requires surgery. Early on, tubal insufflation and HSG helped between 6% and 25% of women to conceive, depending on the level of tubal patency, although practitioners like Dr. Frances Seymour claimed much higher success rates with repeated HSG use (Marsh & Ronner, 2010).

Considering these new studies, tests, and treatments and improvements in AI, it is surprising that treatment results (pregnancies) remained unimpressive (May, 1997). Well-known fertility experts in the late 1910s and 1920s reported success rates of 16% to 20% (Marsh & Ronner, 1996, p. 144; Rongy, 1911; see also May, 1997). By the 1930s, 28% of patients in treatment with a gynecologist became pregnant (Marsh & Ronner, 1996, pp. 144–145; Reedy, 2007), and by 1944 Planned Parenthood cited a success rate of 30% (p. 15). The first half of the twentieth century saw an enormous amount of diagnostic and treatment development, but a disappointingly small increase in success rates.

Between the 1940s and 1970s, Dr. John Rock and biologist Miriam Menkin (and others) continued their research into human embryo fertilization (Rodriguez, 2015). Menkin fertilized her first human embryo in vitro in 1944, but it took decades to turn this success into a viable treatment for infertility (Rodriguez, 2015). The result, well documented in Marsh and Ronner's *The Fertility Doctor*, is the recent explosion of individuals seeking ARTs and IVF in particular (Christensen, 2014), even though infertility rates remain largely static (Marsh & Ronner, 1996). Breitkopf and Rubin (2015) referred to the ART industry in the United States as the "Wild West" (p. 46). In this multibillion-dollar market, insurance coverage, when offered at all, is problematic and extends only to traditional or biomedical ARTs, excluding alternative treatments (Mamo, 2010). This might drive individuals to seek treatment with an REI specialist before they have exhausted other options.

In the 1980s, IVF revolutionized treatment for infertility and offered the chance of conception to individuals previously denied a chance at pregnancy. But Breitkopf and Rubin (2015) reported the enormous profitability of the procedure and pointed to the increasing importance of the Internet in expanding the global marketplace for ARTs. As the Internet and social media are expanding the global marketplace for medical treatments of all kinds, individuals may struggle to wade through the "traditional" and "natural" options in such an unregulated environment. The explosion of resources and options available online for infertile individuals also complicates the process of making an informed choice. When procedures are peddled for profit in this context, how can a consumer know what programs/methods/techniques are "good"?

Social media (e.g., Twitter, FB, Instagram, YouTube) are further complicating the contemporary commercialization of infertility by drawing attention to both traditional and alternative fertility modalities and expanding the global infertility market. By 2017, one could find hundreds of Twitter accounts for REI practices and thousands of accounts focusing on "natural" or alternative infertility treatments (Andrews, n.d.; Anna, 2017; Organic, 2017; Thomas, 2017). As we discuss next, social media today echo historical patterns, as they offer up a host of lay experts providing services and products aimed to give patients a mental path through and out of their infertility.

It Isn't You—It's You: A Closer Look at Psychogenic Sterility

We find the evidence offers some support to the thesis that a woman's life experiences, and the conflicts arising therefrom, may, and do, make themselves evident in the form of impaired fertility. (Kelly, 1942, p. 220)

While the search for structural cures for infertility continued, a great deal of mid-twentieth-century medical thought focused on women's minds. In the early 1940s, Dr. Edith Jacobsen (1946) recounted the cure of a patient with infertility named Sylvia for the readers of the *Psychoanalytic Quarterly*. After years of menstrual and ovulatory difficulties, Sylvia sought specialist intervention, including endocrine and hormonal treatments and biopsies. As Dr. Jacobsen triumphantly recounted, "What the clinicians failed to accomplish, analysis achieved. After several months of treatment . . . her breasts grew larger, the inverted nipples became normal . . . in the eighth month of her analysis Sylvia became pregnant without having previously menstruated" (pp. 332–333). Jacobsen (1946) cataloged Sylvia's childhood ambition at home and school, and as an adult in her career. Sylvia's "masculine strivings . . . though essentially hysteria" also illustrated the diversion of reproductive energy to intellectual pursuits (pp. 342–346). According to Jacobsen, psychoanalysis saved Sylvia from her masculine proclivities, restored her femininity, and removed the mental blocks to ovulation and conception.

If this material seems familiar, it is. From the mid-nineteenth century up to the present day, cis female fertility patients have been counseled to manage their energy stores by pursuing feminine endeavors, to have a positive, sunny outlook, and to remain cognizant of stress, anxiety, and nervous strain (Jensen, 2016; Marsh & Ronner, 1996; May, 1997; Reedy, 2007). Patients continue to hear from friends, family, medical practitioners, and partners to relax, to not worry, and to manage or mitigate work stress. In our contemporary qualitative and survey studies, individuals attempted to control or handle their stress around pregnancy by going to therapists, attaining massages, receiving acupuncture, ingesting fertility supplements (herbs), avoiding toxins, practicing fertility yoga, joining fertility support groups, and going on vacations. Patients also sought stress mitigation through the Internet, including private FB groups (e.g., Broken Brown Egg, Secondary Infertility) and fertility hypnosis (Syna, 2017).[10]

In 1883, Dr. Bigelow insisted that "woman is, in every particular able to keep pace" (p. 12) with men, yet he feared that *acting* on this equality would draw energy away from the reproductive system: "We are still confronted with the problem of her physiological ability to assume such callings of mental activity" (p. 12). Bigelow (1883) claimed that "mental rest is absolutely necessary in many women to perfect ovulation" (p. 15), while Campbell (1888) maintained that reproductive organs are malformed without sufficient energy, and then ineffective (p. 436).

More than a century later, individuals in our qualitative and survey studies reported feeling chastised for expending too much mental energy on becoming pregnant. They heard statements such as "Don't overthink it" (Trixie) and "You're thinking about it too much" (Shawn). In the history of cultural language about infertility, the reproductive energy economy changes over time—which systems and which activities dominate as "enervators" shift. Still, the emphasis remains: in a limited energy economy, one can easily shut down reproductive capacity by spending/using energy incorrectly or by inadvertently directing energy toward the wrong bodily system, through the wrong tasks, insinuating a lack of appropriate femininity.

Regarding systemic interaction and involvement, these contemporary views differ from but yet also reflect older, traditional medical assumptions in America (see also Koerber, 2018). Engelmann (1901) suggested that impaired digestive activity could be present alongside sterility issues, while Campbell (1888) detailed "genital ganglia," from which there is a "vast predominance of the ganglia and plexuses of the nutritive or vaso-motor system over the cerebro-spinal element" (p. 435). Kelly (1942) referred to the "peripheral autonomic system" and its nucleic linkage to the "generative organs" (p. 217). The terms differ but the goal is the same; each author took pains to demonstrate a literal mind-body connection in sterility. In 1920, Bandler directly connected endocrine activity and emotions and cited "hypothyroidism" as the underlying cause of "nervous conditions" sometimes called "hysteria" or "neurasthenia" (pp. 387–388). Jacobsen (1946) connected Sylvia's "endocrine deficiency" with her sterility and blamed emotional issues for the endocrine dysfunction. Kelly (1942) noted the "psychic control of fertility via the endocrines" (p. 219). Hence, the notion of emotional (nervous) exhaustion causing systemic dysfunction within bodily systems, prompting sterility or fertility issues, continued to appear in the medical literature, even as knowledge of the structural causes of infertility increased. These claims reflect a long-standing medical tradition of a mind-body connection, one promulgated by technical experts into the mid-twentieth century and now amplified by lay experts, particularly on social media. Some technical and lay practitioners have posited and continue to suggest that if our minds are powerful arbiters of reproductive health, controlling emotions and mental perspective could be vital to conception.

Another continuity in the medical literature is the idea of policing of femininity as a way to protect fertility. There is the continuous suggestion that women cannot handle too much "nervous strain" (late nineteenth century), "masculine strivings" (mid-twentieth century), and "stress" (twenty-first century)—especially strain and stress caused by extrafamilial activities—without impacting their reproductive potential and capacity. By the 1940s, the impact of the mind and emotions on fertility held particular significance as "psychogenic sterility" came to the fore, dovetailing with a midcentury obsession with women's potential rejection of or ambivalence about their required "feminine" roles. "Psychogenic" refers to impaired health or bodily dysfunction, which occurs "without clearly defined physical cause or structural change in the brain" (APA, 1952, p. 5; see also Jensen, 2016; Marsh & Ronner, 1996; May, 1997). Again, the notion of nonstructural sterility was not new—previous practitioners referred to this phenomenon as "nulliparous sterility" (Campbell, 1888 p. 450), "artificial sterility" (Engelmann, 1901, p. 895), "constitutional sterility" (Macomber, 1924, p. 681), and "functional sterility" (Kanman, 1946). As Kanman (1946) asserted, "An idea can be converted into a symptom . . . that emotional conflicts can result in . . . dysfunction in the generative organs . . . seems inevitable" (p. 1215).

However, unlike previous forms of mental exhaustion and strain, psychogenic sterility was framed as subconscious—patients were not even aware their minds were preventing fertility, despite their deep longing for conception and children. Like other physicians influenced by Freudian psychology, Kelly (1942) counseled that unfilled longing for children could rupture the ova prematurely, tragically thwarting an inherently feminine desire (see also "We," 1946). Kanman (1946) and Jacobsen (1946) offered that "resistance against accepting [a] mature feminine role" must be cleared before ovulation and conception were possible (p. 345; see also Kroger, 1952; Kroger & Freed, 1950). Kroger and Freed (1950) outlined the connection between psychogenic factors and infertility most succinctly: "The fact that many sterile women are consciously eager to get pregnant and are bitterly disappointed by their inability to do so does not rule out the hypothesis that in some women their unconscious wishes against pregnancy predominate" (p. 870). Elsewhere Kroger (1952) posited that some women unconsciously avoid intercourse during ovulation and cautioned practitioners that helping an emotionally unstable woman to become pregnant was a "hollow triumph" (p. 550). Hence, even the deepest desire for children could be thwarted by subconscious immaturity, aggression, or resentment. Even subconsciously, the patient had only herself to blame.

In the mid-twentieth century, gynecologists and psychoanalysts directed patients to overcome psychogenic blocks through psychoanalysis, by reducing stress, fostering a positive outlook, and/or quitting work (Kanman, 1946; Kroger, 1952; "We," 1946). As detailed in 1946 in *Ladies' Home Journal*, an author and self-proclaimed "career girl" ("We," p. 28) suffered through years of failed treatment; after consultations with multiple doctors, she "considered quitting her job" (p. 29). In desperation, she planned a six-month leave from her job and discovered she was pregnant. She credited the end of her professional striving for her conception and asserted that gynecologists "found a relation between a happy, placid contented frame of mind and fertility" ("We," 1946, p. 29).

A version of these ideas continues today. In 2014, our study participant Valentina remembered hearing, "Maybe your job is too stressful." On CNN, Senthilingam (2017) reported that heavy lifting and shift work could harm women's fertility, while Walton (2011) referenced Dr. Nicole Noyes of New York University's Fertility Center, who "tell[s] her patients who have very stressful jobs to try to work less while they are trying to conceive." The difference is that practitioners seeking stress-reduction measures could ask patients to consider their work (should economic circumstances allow), but women aren't being asked to leave the workplace altogether to adopt the "proper" feminine roles needed for conception.

Another midcentury treatment for psychogenic sterility was adoption, presumably forcing a cessation of masculine professional striving when the woman left work to care for the adopted child and this allowed the yearning for a child to cease (Kanman, 1946; Kelly, 1942). In response, the body could reorient mental energy from "wishing" to normalizing ovulation (Kanman, 1946; Kroger & Freed, 1950). It is possible these common yet outdated medical claims resulted in the long-standing myth that adoption prompts conception (Johnson, 2016; Kroger, 1952). Unfortunately, women continue to hear vestiges of this technical expertise today through friends, family, or peers, such as "Why don't you just give up and adopt?" or "At the office: You should just adopt!" (Johnson, 2016, p. 84).

While many treatments focusing on the body have come and gone, an emphasis on psychogenic factors continually resurfaces: in 1984, Mazor concluded that physicians cited psychogenic factors as the cause of fertility issues in 30% to 40% of cases over the preceding[20] years (p. 23). As late as 2008, Dr. Berga of Emory University claimed that "much of what we view as disease may reflect reproductive alignment in the face of reversible metabolic or psychogenic challenge" (p. 537).[11] In 1952, Kroger claimed that "chronic worriers" suffer from spasms of the fallopian tubes. Fast-forward to 2014, when a study participant with a diagnosis of occluded tubes underwent a tubal ligation. When the surgeon reviewed the results (both tubes were fully functional), he suggested worry and trauma could be causing tubal spasm.

Your Psychogenic Fertility, Now in an eCourse

Examining social media today, we find a similar focus among lay experts and alternative practitioners on clearing mental blockages, remaining positive, "relaxing," and meditating on conception and pregnancy. For example, Brockmyer (2017) offers eCourse students "a step-by-step guided emotional healing process to stay positive throughout your fertility journey." A participant with secondary infertility was told that changing her thought process would allow her to become pregnant again. She said, "I have been told to subscribe to . . . behavioral thought patterns in order to bring me baby number two" (Anonymous personal communication, 2017). Another participant revealed her deep hurt when her sister (who gives "tough love") and a therapist encouraged her to read *The Secret* by Rhonda Byrne (2013), suggesting she needed to put "positive thoughts out there so that positive things would happen to me."

Multiple eCourses to help individuals find the cause of their infertility are available in the expanding market of fertility support and alternative treatment modalities. Individuals who launch the infertility eCourses vary in expertise from a biology teacher who went through IVF ten times (Blasi, 2017) to a certified holistic nutrition coach/functional diagnostic nutrition practitioner (Unlock, 2017). Methods are advertised in multiple social media locations such as Instagram and YouTube. Many alternative courses of treatment focus on mindfulness and other methods of stress reduction and mitigation, including changes to diet, exercise, and overall lifestyle (Blasi, 2017; Brockmyer, 2017; Mind, 2017; Mindful Fertility, 2017; Naturally, 2017; Raupp, 2017; Unlock, 2017).

Many eCourses use medical concepts with roots in traditional nineteenth-century sterility treatments (Bigelow, 1883; Campbell, 1888; Engelmann, 1901; Jacobsen, 1946; Macomber, 1924; Melendy, 1904). For example, Brockmyer's (2017, emphasis added) eCourse descriptions relied on an updated energy reserve ideology: "Digestive health is the foundation of fertility and is absolutely crucial for improving fertility. A poorly functioning digestive system *steals energy away from your reproductive system* and can cause systemic inflammation." A number of our study interviewees and survey participants relayed messages from family members and friends around the theme of "relaxing." Verna lamented, "I hated when people told me to relax during sex and it would happen." Joy's mother told her, "Relax, you will have a baby, be positive." Participants found these comments hurtful and felt these remarks placed blame for unsuccessful treatments and failure to conceive on the patient in treatment. Other participants were told to relax by becoming more passive—the "don't try" method. Shelby lamented hearing, "I know this one couple who couldn't get pregnant, tried for years, and then when they stopped trying, they got pregnant!" Someone told Elisa, "Just stop trying! It'll happen if you relax!" For participants, "do not try" may be interpreted as a condemnation of their efforts to conceive. As UptownMama12 (2017) said in a BabyCenter forum, "While I understand the reason behind all the advice, I refuse to dismiss what I know is true. I haven't failed because of 'trying too hard' or 'wanting it too badly.'"

Today medical research attempts to zero in on the impact of stress resulting from lack of conception and infertility diagnosis and treatment as well as how stress impacts conception (Johnson, 2010; Louis et al., 2011).[12] The results are inconclusive. After all, individuals in distress continue to become pregnant. But traditional and lay practitioners agree: stress can negatively impact treatment experience and outcomes. In online communities composed of infertile cis females on blogs, FB, Instagram, Twitter, and even Pinterest, there are hundreds of links, conversation threads, and memes highlighting frustration around the "just" claims. "Just adopt!" "Just relax!" Recent online editorials continue to draw attention to the complications of this advice, with titles like "Stop saying 'just relax' to people with infertility. Everyone experiencing infertility has heard it, but no one has been helped by it" (Zoll, 2017; see also Campbell, 2017; Purtell, 2015).

Despite resistance to these messages, there is evidence that cis female patients have internalized these messages. Cori (2017), a blogger, acknowledged the connection between stress over conception and difficulties conceiving: "When you've been trying for a baby . . . it can be easy to fall into a pattern of frantic trying, followed by periods of stress and finally disappointment . . . it is also likely to be contributing to the problem. It is much easier to conceive if you are as relaxed and stress-free as possible." Another blogger, Samantha, found this linkage defeating: "Is your anxiety and depression a behavioral thing? Do you just need to relax and not think about it? Just stop thinking about it—it'll happen. I hear it a lot." Individuals we interviewed internalized the idea that stress may have impacted their ability to conceive, particularly after hearing repeated directives to "relax" or "de-stress." Despite their hurt and anger over unsolicited advice to "fix" their mental state, patients actively sought stress reduction. In an interview, Arlene recounted her efforts to integrate relaxing music and infertility treatment: "I remember [a nurse] . . . laughing because . . . I played some theme music during [an IUI]. . . . I just felt like that was going like to put me in a positive head space and I was trying to . . . do some positive thinking stuff."

Figure 1, taken from Instagram, is a jarring visual representation of the intersection of technical and lay expertise, of traditional and alternative fertility methods, and at the center of it all, the command to relax—to master the mind. Shots or "superfoods," pills or coconut oil, the message is the same—if it doesn't work, just relax.

This cornucopia of products raises the question of who is profiting from the distress of cis females who struggle with infertility. Technical experts are often characterized as profit seekers, while lay or alternative experts (and their meth-

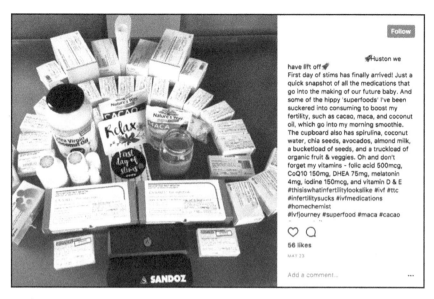

Figure 1. RELAX. Instagram.

ods) tend to be viewed as value neutral or likely to take a patient-centered, empathic approach. Investing $47 (Unlock, 2017) or $1,172 (Raupp, 2017) for eCourses compared to $1,000 or $10,000 and up for IVF cycles (Johnson, 2016) figures into people's decisions about which path to take (e.g., alternative and/or traditional treatment routes). Online courses may be more affordable, attracting individuals who cannot easily access biomedical models, but there is still an economic and then emotional cost when and if these methods do not lead to conception. If the courses encourage the purchase of more products, such as expensive special food and supplements, the costs can quickly get out of control.

Breitkopf and Rubin (2015) examined the ways people without race and class privileges struggle to access the traditional, biomedical ART market, sometimes foregoing treatment. But their work did not address the remaking of these hierarchies within lay expertise, particularly in social media contexts. When online and social-media-based lay websites and experts such as John Thomas (2017) encourage "overcoming infertility naturally without drugs," these alternative experts are inherently labeling any traditional approach as unnatural and therefore, lesser. The "Unlock your Fertility" (2017) eCourse proposes to help students "get their mind-set right," which is not a value-neutral statement (n.p.). What if a patient tries the "natural" way without success? What if the meditation and mindfulness don't bring about conception? What if a patient has "failed" even after "taking charge" of her health and "listening to [her] body?" Here messages of empowerment are complicated and potentially traumatic when conception does not occur. Alternately, when traditional practitioners say that alternative therapies (e.g., acupuncture) are a "complete waste of money," as one of Bethany's REI doctors told her, they are invalidating the patient's desire to practice agency and to seek out any and all roads to success.

LAYERS AND INTERSECTIONS

Despite a commonly held understanding of lay expertise as an open, democratic, and empowering form of medical knowledge, technical and lay expertise reproduce similar, top-down power hierarchies, and both biomedical and alternative patients may suffer for it. Consider that throughout this history, medicine, and thus infertility diagnosis and treatment, has been classed, raced, and gendered. Other structural forms of injustice add layers to the already sexist concept of the female body (e.g., a binary understanding of female biology as being inherently weak and flawed), which guided research and treatment well into the twentieth century. For example, Sims treated his patients differently (and in different locations) based on their class status (Marsh & Ronner, 1996; Vandenberg-Daves, 2014), and racialized conceptions of the body remained common across medical disciplines well into the late twentieth century (Hoberman, 2012; Washington, 2006). Explicit statements of racial or class differences may be less common in medical writings today. Yet racial and ethnic minorities experience higher rates of infertility and receive fewer diagnoses and treatments (Inhorn, Ceballo, & Nachtigall, 2012).

The expense of biomedical treatments and a frequent lack of insurance coverage tend to create overwhelming challenges for low-income families. Inhorn, Ceballo, and Nachtigall (2012) argued that since IVF fees compose 25% or more of average per capita income, "ARTs are used mainly for white elites who have the money to pay for them" (p. 183). They also note the difficulties faced by immigrants with language barriers. In a study of 234 individuals from less privileged ethnic and class backgrounds, all participants reported immense stress related to fertility treatment. Inhorn, Ceballo, and Nachtigall (2012) concluded that minorities are "despised as reproducers" in a society characterized by structural injustice (p. 194). In the nineteenth and twentieth centuries, practitioners used racist claims to define infertility as a primarily white, middle- and upper-class disease (Campbell, 1888; Hoberman, 2012; Inhorn, Ceballo, & Nachtigall, 2012; Kline, 2001). Long-standing racial stereotypes about the hypersexuality and hyperfertility of African American women also impact diagnosis and treatment. Because they were considered by white medical theorists to be too "hardy" from "out-door" work (i.e., slavery; Campbell, 1888; Kline, 2001) to become infertile and too uncivilized for mental infertility, structural issues impacting African American women were overlooked (Hoberman, 2012). Until 1966 endometriosis was thought to be a "white woman's" disease, and as late as 1997 gynecologists diagnosed African American women with pelvic inflammatory disease instead of endometriosis; many were sterilized as a result of this misdiagnosis (Hoberman, 2012). These stereotypes continue to result in traumatic experiences. Racism in medical practice also creates a particular kind of erasure, in which women of color struggle to see themselves represented in promotional materials and find support groups for fertility challenges (Inhorn, Ceballo, & Nachtigall, 2012).

On the Internet and across social media platforms, organizations like Fertility for Colored Girls (FFCG) and online personalities like GloZell aim to combat this erasure. GloZell's (2016) video on infertility is particularly fascinating in that it addresses every part of this chapter, including the cost of care and treatment, the use of alternative and traditional treatments and therapies, and emotional advice. Before going to an REI doctor, she tried wheatgrass, organic food, vaginal steaming, and yoni eggs: "It's a crystal that's shaped like an egg. And you insert it, and then you're right where the issue is. . . . I'm trying not to be graphic" (GloZell, 2016). People gave her advice like "oh yeah you need to do that for energy" and "all you need to do is pray." Eventually, she visited two specialists, who said they "couldn't help her"; the third identified severe endometriosis and suggested IVF cycles and a surrogate (GloZell, 2016). After six IVF cycles, GloZell (2016) was open about the financial challenges: "Fertility is very expensive. . . . Like I've got a payment plan." She says she posted the video to "break the wall down" to help others with similar stories. Like many individuals with structural infertility, for GloZell alternative methods might not be sufficient, even though her interest in alternative methods guided her fertility journey at the outset.

For individuals who identify as trans and nonbinary, fertility has a different kind of complexity, although other members of the LBGTQ+ community may feel like "despised reproducers" (Inhorn, Ceballo, & Nachtigall, 2012), especially in a society where many of their rights are under attack (e.g., movements against gay marriage, North Carolina's HB2 "bathroom legislation").[13] Overall, there is a marked lack of trans-specific health communication and training about trans and nonbinary issues in the REI field (Teaff, 2014) as well as in medicine as a whole (World Professional Association for Transgender Health [WPATH], 2017). Today, there is little available research on trans and nonbinary pregnancy and few statistics on female-to-male (FTM) individuals seeking medical help to get pregnant or simply attempting it on their own (Hempel, 2016). For example, when journalist Jessi Hempel's brother, a trans man named Evan, sought care during pregnancy in 2013, his pregnancy was the first of its kind at the Fenway Institute (Hempel, 2016). There is little in the way of support for trans and nonbinary individuals struggling with infertility, from technical or lay experts, in either traditional or alternative settings. Trans and nonbinary individuals report the added burden of educating their medical professionals—thus, they are forced into a kind of medical expertise to receive care with less trauma (e.g., sex insensitivity, forced or denied care, verbal abuse) (Hempel, 2016; Kosenko, Rintamaki, Raney, & Maness, 2013).

Self-identified FTM individuals (FTM stands for "female-to-male"; individuals may also identify as DFAB, designated female at birth, or AFAB, assigned female at birth) can consider stopping their testosterone (T) and taking estrogen or other drugs to resume ovulation (Hempel, 2016).[14] However, accidental pregnancy while on T can and does happen (Hempel, 2016). There are also questions about kids and teens taking hormones to delay puberty or transition because hormone supplementation can impact the development of sperm and ova. Even in our research with cis women, we found that individuals going into early menopause also face challenges around the preservation of their fertility. Amy (2014) wanted to "bank her eggs" at 15 but couldn't find a doctor willing to do it since she was "too young" to make the decision. Dr. Juno Obedin-Maliver of San Francisco also discussed cryopreservation (egg freezing) with her adult patients before they begin hormone replacement therapy, though eggs can still be viable after T therapy (Hempel, 2016).

Some trans and nonbinary individuals became parents before they transitioned and acknowledged the added complexity of pregnancy post-transition. In an interview, Chase Hayes (2017) discussed the idea of pregnancy after his transition. Hayes had his child before he transitioned and has since had a hysterectomy because he knew he wanted only one child. During his pregnancy with his daughter, he said, "The belly and stretch marks didn't really bother me that much. I was very dysphoric about my breasts, though at that time, I didn't know why I was so dysphoric about them." Hayes acknowledged the difficulties he might feel if he chose to pursue pregnancy after transition: "If I had transitioned and still wanted to carry a child, I think I would have hated every change that happened to my body. Just seeing something so feminine happen to someone who wanted to be very masculine looking would have been very hard even though I really wanted a child. . . . I would hide it as long as I could have them just become very reclusive the rest of the pregnancy." Dylan Myrick (2017) told us that he "never had an urge to have children . . . I've always seen myself as a father or male figure in someone's life." He acknowledged that other trans men don't feel the same way: "I think some would still see themselves [as] the birthing father." Each situation and story is unique. For example, Trystan Reese identifies as a "man with a uterus." When Reese announced that he was pregnant, he said, "I feel like it's a gift to have been born with the body that I did, and I made the necessary changes so that I could keep living in it, both through hormones and through other body modifications" ("My," 2017, n.p.). Reese and his partner Biff Chaplow worked closely with a medical team, pursuing a process that was "as healthy and safe as possible" ("My," 2017, n.p.), which for Reese included managing the emotions and stress of body dysphoria, particularly around his growing belly. Luckily, the medical team working with Reese and Chaplow received training to meet Reese's needs.

For emotional and social support, particularly for dealing with body dysp-morphia and finding informed, trans-inclusive medical providers (technical experts), social media offer an opportunity to hear about similar experiences and connect with others. For individuals trying to decide if, when, and how to pursue hormonal and other fertility treatments for pregnancy, there are a few Internet resources available, including a website with a list of trans-friendly fer-tility and prenatal medical providers from around the country. In this list, tra-ditional and alternative methods are not divided into categories and technical and lay experts are listed together (Trans Birth, 2017). The World Professional Association for Transgender Health (WPATH, 2017) offers a host of resources for trans and nonbinary individuals but does not focus on fertility or pregnancy issues. There are also public and private FB groups, with names such as Fertil-ity, Conception, Pregnancy and Childbirth for Queer and Trans Families, that aim to create safe and inclusive spaces for individuals to ask questions, gather resources, and support one another.

The various psychological, social, and emotional pressures of nonbinary preg-nancy can be challenging, requiring new ways of understanding fertility, gen-der, and practitioner-patient communication. As Evan's brother acknowledged, "Pregnancies like Evan's . . . will stretch our cultural perceptions of gender norms even further. . . . What if you are born into a female body, know you are a man, and still want to participate in the traditionally exclusive rite of womanhood?" (Hempel, 2016, n.p.). At the same time, our exploration suggests some trans and nonbinary men would not say they were born into a female body, arguing instead that they were born in a body that society does not view as male. Our society's limited understandings of gender and gender fluidity are problematic in much the same way as our society's limited conceptualizations of what defines both mothers and experts. Therefore, we are reticent to draw overarching conclusions about trans and nonbinary fertility or make any claims about the experiences trans and nonbinary individuals may have while managing their fertility. Uni-versal claims regarding the psychological impact of fertility treatment on trans and nonbinary folks do not hold up against our limited interviewing. The chal-lenge is making sure all fertility patients (regardless of class, race, sex, ability, gender, etc.) receive adequate, appropriate support, without holding patients solely responsible for the success of traditional, alternative, or integrated treat-ments and without asking them to discipline their minds to achieve conception.

REI patients from a wide range of economic backgrounds, with diverse racial, ethnic, and gender identities, seek advice and emotional support during REI treatment (Inhorn, Ceballo, & Nachtigall, 2012; Johnson, Quinlan, & Marsh, 2018; Johnson, Quinlan, & Myers, 2017; Teaff, 2014). While the particular needs of these communities differ, the desire to connect with others may lead individu-als to social media. Historically, technical experts struggled to find effective treatment for infertility and many believed unseen processes had a marked impact on fertility, such as outlook and the economy of mental energy. In the present, REI patients looking for support, a definable source of infertility (e.g., dietary issues), and/or a less invasive treatment for infertility might actually find a continuation of historical trends.

Throughout the history we've recounted here, a few things remain ever present, including the vulnerability of females (including nonbinary and trans individuals), seeking treatment from a wide range of experts, and engaging in expensive, cascading testing and intervention with uncertain outcomes and the potential for serious self-blame if pregnancy does not occur. When infertility is the question, one answer is frustratingly consistent across time. Infertile? Maybe it's just your state of mind.

PART II

PREGNANCY AND BIRTH

CHAPTER 3

RED UNDERWEAR, GENES, AND MONSTROSITY

PREGNANCY AND SOCIAL MEDIA SURVEILLANCE

What sacrifices would a true mother not make to give to her dearly loved invalid child the single blessing of health. . . . But she often makes the task needlessly hard by deferring it. The time to bestow all priceless gifts on the little one is before its advent into the visible world.

—*Melendy (1904, p. 345)*

On August 21, 2017, Melissa Medina, five months pregnant, lay on a bed with blackout shades drawn, wearing red underwear with a safety pin attached. Like millions of other Americans in the path of eclipse "totality," she planned to watch the rare event with safety-approved glasses. However, with a history of miscarriage and difficult pregnancies and due to the influence of nervous friends and family members' "wives' tales," Melissa followed ancient expert advice to protect her unborn child. She found it comical but also limiting and aggravating, adding, "I don't believe any of it, but now they [her family] got me all stressed out about it," and later she said she was "flabbergasted" and "couldn't believe what [she] was hearing" at her family's urging (Medina, 2017). She even tried to cajole her familial lay experts with religion: "I told them we are Catholics and we don't believe in superstitions." Her sister responded, "Don't test it" since she knew Melissa's pregnancies were high risk (Medina, 2017). Family admonishments via email or through text message came paired with articles such as "Pregnant during the Eclipse? Superstitions Say It Could Harm Baby" (2017). Precautions included not using knives, praying, fasting, bathing, and avoiding magnets (Mack, 2017; "Pregnant," 2017). "Before the eclipse reached its peak I went to the hallway where I don't have any windows and all doors were shut around. I stayed in the hallway about 15 minutes" (Medina, 2017). Despite the extreme precautions taken, Melissa "kept thinking this is silly" but simultaneously doubted herself for "not believing what [family and friends] believed" (Medina, 2017).

Curious to know how pervasive these precautions and theories were, we posted in a private Facebook (FB) group of academics with children, many working within the United States. We received well over 100 comments—dozens within 30 minutes. Leah recounted the precaution against walking outside during a lunar eclipse to prevent "a cleft lip/palate or aural atresia (malformation of the ear)" common in the Latinx population (Medina, 2017; Private FB Group, 2017). However, fears of ecliptic activity are certainly not limited to one cultural background—another member of the group, Sydney, said she was "physically yanked away" from a full moon to prevent a "stain/large birthmark on baby's face." Others heard babies are more likely to be born during a full moon.

We did not find any research that strongly correlated lunar events with pregnancy outcomes, but the notion of a connection reflects long-standing cultural traditions, folklore, and beliefs from early religious traditions (Derham, 1708; Mack; 2017; Park & Daston, 1981; "Pregnant," 2017; see also Das et al., 2005; Law, 1986). Historically, the idea that viewing the moon or eclipse rays would lead to physical or personal calamity (Derham, 1708; Goldman, 1940) including monstrous birth (Derham, 1708; Park & Daston, 1981) was common. In the seventeenth, eighteenth, and nineteenth centuries, "monstrosity" reflected "aberrations in the natural order" (Armitage, 1917; Park & Daston, 1981, p. 22; see also Weiner & Hough, 2012), but under Baconian influence in Western Europe and the United States, monstrosity became a medical concern by the mid-nineteenth century (Armitage, 1917; Ballantyne, 1914; Park & Daston, 1981). Medical experts then turned their attention to behavioral choices to avoid monstrosity and to ensure the future health of the unborn. We found that choices women made (or were made for them) during pregnancy may have resulted from a more medicalized (crisis-based) view of pregnancy.

When we started reviewing pregnancy expertise by experts, past and present, we found three major categories: what to eat/what not to eat, what to do physically/what to avoid, and how to feel/how not to feel. Expert advice ranged from overarching suggestions for eating a healthy, sufficient diet (Ballantyne, 1914; Harms, Johnson, & Murry, 2004; Kellogg, 1891; Melendy, 1904; Murkoff & Mazel, 2016) to detailed missives such as refraining from drinking tap water to avoid arsenic (Private FB Group, 2017).

What follows is a comparison between collected and coded pregnancy behavior recommendations from FB outreach and historical pregnancy manuals by technical and lay experts.[1] After gathering 156 comments in less than 12 hours, we noticed some familiar themes and repetitions. We specifically asked for the "wildest" directives individuals received during pregnancy, and many commenters mentioned which kinds of experts doled out prescriptive expertise. Next, we reviewed historical documents, including magazines and newspapers, to see when and how this expertise emerged in the pregnancy behavior compendium. We rarely found behavioral directives for pregnancy in these publications, so we turned to expert manuals that covered sex, women's health and reproduction, and feminine behavior in marriage ("wifely duties"). We studied manuals by (male and female) allopathic and eclectic physicians (technical experts) as well as lay experts (e.g., mothers) and found that most of today's expert advice has roots in the late nineteenth and early twentieth centuries.

As we discussed in chapter 2 on infertility, experts across the spectrum connect emotions and mentality to reproductive health outcomes for cis women and trans and nonbinary individuals.[2] Therefore, some experts (technical, lay, and everything in between) link personal choices to pregnancy outcomes and reproductive health issues such as gestational diabetes, which can complicate pregnancy and birth. The linkage between personal responsibility and pregnancy health and outcomes also spans the expertise spectrum. When writer and blogger Heather Kirn Lanier's (2017) daughter was born with a genetic difference, the perfection of her pregnancy behavior underscored her shock at the outcome ("I took superfoods. I took reiki"). Lanier's association of pregnant women's behavior with babies' health had deep roots. Weiner and Hough (2012) reported doctors' willingness to blame women for poor outcomes in the antebellum South, even as they celebrated feminine strength and power to create. Dr. John W. Ballantyne's popular 1914 book continued to blame poor pregnancy health and outcomes on the lack of prenatal knowledge among pregnant women.

In this chapter, we examine the historical and contemporary pathologization of pregnancy, how this process extends and deepens on social media platforms, and how this disempowers pregnant bodies. While some women do experience particular health crises during pregnancy (e.g., gestational diabetes, preeclampsia, cervical issues), we find that the focus on pathology historically and socially frames all of pregnancy as a crisis. We explore how social media platforms intersect with tenuous new findings in the field of epigenetics to maintain the pathologization of pregnancy in American medicine as well as the wider culture. We examine the desire for "just a healthy baby," reflecting digitized expertise as well as lay expert folklore and reproducing unacknowledged ableism in our deepest desires.

Second, we explore the continuity of some pregnancy behavior expertise across time and across forms of expertise. For centuries, pregnant individuals in America chose to follow prenatal expertise that reflects their embodied experiences, their lifestyle, and their familial, cultural, and religious practice (Barker, 1998; Leavitt, 1999; Leavitt & Numbers, 1997; Private FB Group, 2017; Sargent & Davis-Floyd, 1996).

In our research, individuals viewed technical experts as obstetricians, midwives, nurses, ultrasound technicians, acupuncturists, and other medical practitioners, due to their job-specific or medical training. This category also includes partners, family members, and friends working in these capacities. Individuals conceptualized lay experts as friends, family members, partners, colleagues, shopkeepers, security guards, librarians, and strangers of unknown employment who did not appear to have medical training. In the past and in the present, texts and advice manuals (by experts of all types) have played an important role in directing prenatal behaviors (see Curry, 1999; Ehrenreich & English, 1978, 2005; Grant, 2012). And yet there are widely varying perspectives on expertise among pregnant individuals, including those who follow current expertise, ignore it, and/ or adopt information that runs counter to technical expertise but comes from other trusted sources (e.g., lay experts like other mothers) (Browner & Press, 1996).

Pathology for All: Pregnancy as Health Crisis

As the whole of American medicine traveled toward professionalization (late nineteenth century and early twentieth), allopathic doctors sought increasing cultural authority and more stages of life came to be defined and understood through a medical lens and through the interpretation of credentialed medical experts (Starr, 1982). In the twentieth century the specializations of obstetrics and pediatrics emerged, and medicine moved away from general practice (Barker, 1998; Breslaw, 2012; Foucault, 1975; Starr, 1982). As such, prenatal care was a twentieth-century addition even for obstetricians (Barker, 1998). Prenatal data were not collected until 1972, when 38 states were collecting data (Barker, 1998). Barker (1998) estimated that between 1900 and 1920, fewer than 5% of American women had contact with an allopathic physician before delivery (p. 1068). This does not mean women didn't discuss their pregnancies with lay practitioners, midwives, family members, friends, and pregnant peers. The U.S. Children's Bureau received thousands of letters with questions about pregnancy behavior and the care of infants and young children; lay and technical experts penned response letters with information and encouragement and included pamphlets, which the Bureau also distributed freely around the country (Ladd-Taylor, 1986). In fact, the similarity between early twentieth-century and modern-day pregnancy behavior admonitions (by technical and lay experts) is suggestive of both the dissemination of technical expertise to lay experts as well as the influence of lay expertise (particularly folklore) on early prenatal practice. At the same time, the medicalization and pathologization of pregnancy occurred primarily in the first half of the twentieth century (Barker, 1998) and continues today.

Technical experts defined pregnancy as a time of grave responsibility well before the mainstream establishment of prenatal care in the mid-twentieth century (Barker, 1998). Dr. John H. Kellogg (1891) (creator of Kellogg's Corn Flakes) urged mothers to remember that their behavior during pregnancy impacted "the physical, mental, and even moral well-being of her child" (p. 402).

Before the late nineteenth century, physicians struggled even to confirm pregnancy (vs. "womb congestion") until well into the second trimester (Ulrich, 1990; Weiner & Hough, 2012). As such, early pregnancy was an ambiguous period, positioning pregnant women as ideal subjects of technical expertise (Barker, 1998; Weiner & Hough, 2012). When the power to ascertain pregnancy (diagnosis of pregnancy) shifted from patient to expert, pregnancy itself became an illness, requiring guidance and medical intervention (Barker, 1998; Weiner & Hough, 2012; Wertz & Wertz, 1977).

The aforementioned movement away from understanding monstrosity as a religious curse and instead as a complex medical phenomenon preceded the rise of prenatal care. Yet this shift reflects a "biomedical rhetoric of pregnancy" in that it also rejects folklore as ignorant and potentially dangerous (Barker, 1998). But as with so many social and cultural processes, change was uneven and, as the example that started this chapter reminds us, perhaps never fully complete. Historically, there is overlap between the view of pregnancy as a nonmedical process (e.g., early nineteenth century and before) and the biomedical view of pregnancy (Barker, 1998). Pregnant individuals continued to perceive themselves outside of medical models and resisted the categorization of "patient" into the early twentieth century (Barker, 1998). As Apple (2006) recounted, the medicalization and pathologization of pregnancy paralleled the movement of birth into hospitals and related physician oversight of pregnant bodies, which we discuss in chapter 4.

Prenatal Care (PC), an early publication of the Children's Bureau, is demonstrative of the shift in medical authority from patient to allopathic doctor and the shifting categorization of pregnancy from life event to illness or biomedical process (West & U.S. Labor Department, 1913; see also Barker, 1998; Wertz & Wertz, 1977). These shifts are most apparent between the first version of PC, by Mary Mills West and the U.S. Department of Labor in 1913, and versions from the 1930s (Barker, 1998; Brown & Parker, 1996). Between 1900 and 1930, more than 20 million women received copies of PC, which described pregnancy as both natural and pathological (Barker, 1998). These guides constructed pregnancy as a dangerous, medically acute period, necessitating technical medical expertise, while they perpetuated a white, middle- and upper-class version of pregnancy and encouraged a corresponding set of behaviors and practices (e.g., male physicians, not midwives, who could be immigrants or, in the South, people of color). By 1935, instead of guiding pregnant individuals (here, only women) in proper hygiene and preventative measures to ensure prenatal health, the text continually directed women to technical medical experts (Barker, 1998). Importantly, PC neglected to mention midwives or nonallopathic practitioners, undermining all other prenatal experts and expertise. By the nineteenth century, physicians and midwives embraced varying recommendations; often two practitioners or two midwives offered oppositional or contradictory information (Private FB Group, 2017; Sargent & Davis-Floyd, 1996; Tiran, 2006). Moreover, as we discuss in chapter 4, despite the ascendancy of technical expertise (e.g., OBGYNs), midwifery and other "alternative" birth methodologies experienced a resurgence in the 1970s, and today there are more options available on the spectrum between technical (physician) and lay (midwife, doula) prenatal and birthing care in the United States (Barker, 1998; Wolf, 2009).

A similar process is apparent in *What to Expect When You're Expecting* (*WTEWYE*), one of the most popular pregnancy advice manuals of the late twentieth and early twenty-first centuries (Donadio, 2006; Lancaster, 2017; *USA Today*, 2011; see also Seigel, 2014). In the 1984 version, the authors, including Mary Mills West, a lay expert, encouraged women to advocate for themselves and to ask practitioners questions when they felt confused or disagreed (Lancaster, 2017; Wolf, 2009). Recent versions of the book continually direct pregnant folks back to a doctor, while suggestions to self-advocate have been dropped (Lancaster, 2017; Murkhoff & Mazel, 2015). In the fifth edition, Murkhoff and Mazel (2016) repeat allopathic physicians' expertise regarding herbal tea consumption during pregnancy. Ultimately, *WTEWYE* encourages patients to submit to intense medical surveillance before making a wide range of decisions (see also Seigel, 2014). The text specifically sites "social media" as a source of medical misinformation and says "Dr. Google's" expertise must come second to that of your medical expert (Murkhoff & Mazel, 2016, p. 11).

Like women in the late nineteenth and early twentieth centuries, today's pregnant individuals are buffeted by a wide range of experts and informational resources. An important difference is that social media platforms (e.g., blogs, FB, Instagram) on technologies such as smartphones, e-readers with Wi-Fi, and smartwatches offer a far more expansive range of possibilities and of claims to expertise and authority. Present-day prenatal expertise is certainly deeply influenced by the success of the medicalization and pathologization of pregnancy in the twentieth century. But in the age of social media, how do individuals perceive and choose reliable experts? Technological advancements, such as testing urine for ketones, can prevent serious complications and disease, and medical science has contributed significantly to prenatal health and vastly improved outcomes for mothers and babies. Scholars examining American motherhood point to a link between the rise of "scientific motherhood" in the late nineteenth and early twentieth centuries and the precipitous decline of infant mortality (Apple, 2006; Foss, 2010; Vandenberg-Daves, 2014). However, there are compelling reasons for pregnant individuals to avoid total submission to surveillance. First, submission to surveillance as patients opens individuals to an enormous amount of conflicting and sometimes contradictory information on what to eat, do, and even feel during pregnancy. Second, individuals lacking structural privilege (e.g., those with low economic status, people of color, and undocumented or nonbinary individuals) become particularly vulnerable to abuses of power and internalized shame around their identity as abnormal pregnant individuals (Abbasi-Lemon, 2016; Ayala & Freeman, 2017).

EXPERTISE CONTINUITY: FEAR EVERYTHING

The continuity and popularity of pregnancy guides suggest that in periods of uncertainty or crisis, individuals continue to seek expertise as a form of precaution, even in the more contemporary period when infant and maternal mortality present a much less acute threat. If we understand pregnancy directives from technical and lay experts in terms of embedded gender expectations, constructing one form of performativity expected of cis women during their childbearing years, the continuity of expert advice becomes more logical. In this context, experts are explaining how to perform pregnancy, not necessarily providing accurate health information. Despite enormous success in lowering infant and early childhood mortality in the twentieth century and the integration of germ theory, bacteriology, and virology, lay expertise and some technical expertise on pregnancy behavior remained static for much of the twentieth century, with some notable exceptions. Today, smoking and heavy drinking during pregnancy are discouraged, while earlier in the century many pregnant women smoked and imbibed alcohol regularly (Private FB Group, 2017; Sargent & Davis-Floyd, 1996). As we suggest in our introduction, "being a good mother" begins potentially before pregnancy, during "preconception," and the expected outcome for performed self-denial, vigilance, and right behavior during preconception and pregnancy is an able-bodied, attractive, "normal" child.

While some scholars point to the shifting nature of knowledge on prenatal health from both technical and lay experts (Brown & Parker, 1996; Ehrenreich & English, 2005; Sargent & Davis-Floyd, 1996), it was surprising to find nearly the entirety of the information our contemporary commenters had to offer in some of the popular home and female health advice manuals from the late nineteenth and early twentieth centuries, including Dr. Robert Armitage's (1917) *Private Sex Advice to Women*, Ballantyne's (1914) *Expectant Motherhood*, Drake's (1908) *What a Young Wife Ought to Know*, Guttmacher's (1962) *Pregnancy and Birth*, Melendy's (1904) *Vivilore*, Kellogg's (1891) *Ladies' Guide to Health and Disease*, and West and the U.S. Department of Labor's (1913) *Prenatal Care*. These texts span the period, represent both male and female medical practitioners, and include both technical (e.g., Dr. Emma F. A. Drake, Dr. Ballantyne) and lay (Mary Mills West) experts as well as practitioners of alternative forms of medicine, such as Dr. Mary Reiss Melendy and Dr. Kellogg, who worked in public health and focused on nutrition. The appearance of an identical or similar prescriptive in these manuals does not suggest these experts were the first or only to give out the information. In fact, it is difficult to tell which of these originated in folklore and influenced early prenatal medicine.

Pregnant individuals today receive dietary recommendations similar to those that practitioners doled out 100 years ago. Some of the expertise seems ageless in its overarching theme—eat a healthy, nutritious, varied diet, which assumes mothers have access to healthy and varied foods (Armitage, 1917; Guttmacher, 1962; Kellogg, 1891; Murkoff & Mazel, 2016). In the what to eat/what not to eat category, what *not* to eat played a much more significant role, again heightening the notion of pregnancy as a crisis itself. The continuing suggestion is that so much of what we take in could be toxic or unhealthy for the fetus. The foods and substances our contemporary participants were instructed to avoid include caffeine, cold water, tap water, Diet Coke, soda, eggs/undercooked eggs/runny eggs, hot sauce, peanut butter, anything "unhealthy," pickle juice, soft cheeses, sushi, lettuce/salad, and sesame seeds (Private FB Group, 2017). At the turn of the twentieth century, Kellogg (1891) insisted that drinking tea and coffee created children with "weak will-power" (p. 424), while Dr. Melendy (1904) reported that women of "nervous temperament" ought to avoid the indulgence of nighttime tea and coffee (p. 382). West and the U.S. Department of Labor (1913) advised against tea and coffee in *PC*. Alternatively, Dr. Drake (1908) recommended a "cup of coffee taken in the morning before rising" to help settle the stomach (p. 149). Ballantyne (1914) counseled his patients to drink tea and coffee in moderation. While experts encouraged drinking water, they often encouraged warm over cold (Kellogg, 1891; Melendy, 1904), except in early pregnancy when attempting to avoid miscarriage (Melendy, 1904). Ballantyne (1914) noted that hot or cold water in the morning or before bed could temper nausea and discomfort. As far as eggs are concerned, Drake (1908) advised patients to be sure they could stomach fish first, while Melendy (1904) and Kellogg (1891) warned against eating excessively rich food (considered unhealthy and agitating for the digestive system) and advised avoiding "animal foods" (Kellogg, 1891, p. 405). Kellogg (1891) also feared hot sauce as it "engenders a love for stimulants in the disposition of the infant" (p. 424). Kellogg (1891), Melendy (1904), and West and the U.S. Department of Labor (1913) classed alcohol as a harmful stimulant, while Ballantyne (1914) feared women would overindulge to settle their stomachs (p. 185). Whether or not the suggestions are correct or effective misses the point. In each case, the individual adopting the practice or limiting the behavior fulfills the individual responsibility mandate of American pregnancy; the person has "done something" to ensure a good outcome in the form of a healthy baby.

Similar to a long-standing recommendation in historical manuals given by experts, we witnessed FB commenters relaying stories of family members urging them to drink more milk (Ballantyne, 1914; West & the U.S. Department of Labor, 1913). The U.S. dairy endorsement in the twentieth century most likely resulted from consumer response to prodairy marketing and medical experts pushing bovine dairy as part of dietary trends of the time (Foss, 2010; Vandenberg-Daves, 2014). In 1962, Guttmacher suggested drinking a full quart a day. Perhaps seeking to ease anxiety over the volume required, he included, "You get equal credit for the milk you drink and pour over cereal and the milk you use in the preparations of custards, pudding, cocoa and milk soup" (pp. 92–93). Of course, many of the directives available today are reflexive of the evolution of the American diet and palate—peanut butter, sushi, some soft cheeses, and Diet Coke don't emerge from the historical manuals examined because most Americans were not yet eating these foods, so they remained outside the purview of prenatal expertise. Likewise, few (if any) manuals and websites today offer "milk soup" as a way to meet the required calcium intake (Guttmacher, 1962, p. 92).

Both lay and technical expertise tracked on FB occasionally strayed into the bizarre: one grandmother informed her granddaughter not to drink pickle juice, exclaiming, "That shit is like razorblades. It will cut that baby right out of you" (Private FB Group, 2017). Another person heard that *knitting* would tangle the baby's cord around the neck. Reflecting contemporary concerns about absorption of chemicals and food allergies, others heard not to swim in chlorinated pools for fear of infection (Private FB Group, 2017), and one physician advised against eating peanut butter or the baby could "develop peanut allergies in utero"; someone else heard this from a mother-in-law (Private FB Group, 2017). Recent research is mixed, and some studies have found a correlation (Sicherer et al., 2010), while Boston Children's Hospital advised, "Pregnant Women Need Not Avoid Peanuts" (Boston, 2013; see also Baïz et al., 2017). Thus, some recommendations are always in flux, even as others appear stable over long periods.

Perhaps the most extreme (and limiting) recommendations covered physical activity. Expert directives encompassed obvious restrictions, such as on heavy lifting (Private FB Group, 2017), which Ballantyne (1914) also advised against. However, lay experts also advised against low-impact physical activity, climbing stairs, walking up hills, working, walking, standing, or even any activity whatsoever. Some family members recommended watching TV on the sofa because everything else might endanger the health of the baby (Private FB Group, 2017). Many demanded that pregnant individuals stop working altogether. Sharon found the owner of a diner wouldn't seat her in a booth because she would "squish the baby" (Private FB Group, 2017). Many individuals, despite a history of running, heard from friends, family, and strangers that they must stop. Technical experts also advised against running, one saying it is "like a goldfish in a bag," while a nurse worried that running could jostle the baby (Private FB Group, 2017). While at the gym, a stranger approached Barbara to ask if her "husband let [her] exercise while pregnant," demonstrating that some think pregnant bodies are public property. Historically, enslaved pregnant bodies were literal property, and for much of the nineteenth century, men had legal rights to their wives' bodies and their offspring through the common law status of women (Feinman, 1992; Kukla, 2005; O'Connor, 2001; Salmon, 1983). Today, people disperse their knowledge and sometimes touch the belly of strangers, crossing boundaries that remain firm in other social interactions (see Chavkin, 1992; Grosz, 2011; Longhurst, 2001).

Historically, physicians also advised the curtailment of physical activity. Practitioners from the late nineteenth century to the mid-twentieth century urged caution during the first trimester to prevent early miscarriage (Ballantyne, 1914; Drake, 1908; Guttmacher, 1962), and Guttmacher (1962) even advised an hour's bed rest "in a darkened room each afternoon" for this purpose (p. 84). Technical/ professional experts also told pregnant individuals at all stages of pregnancy to avoid overstrenuous exercise. A century ago, Dr. Ballantyne (1914) specifically mentioned bicycling (then a new activity) and dancing as "violent kind[s]" of exercise "unsuitable for pregnant women" (p. 194; see also Browner & Press, 1996). Dr. Ballantyne advised walking as the best kind of exercise, as did Kellogg (1891). In 2017, Gloria heard her baby could be born "chubby" if she avoided daily walks (Private FB Group). The call for regular exercise during pregnancy from technical experts has been consistent for more than a century: Dr. Drake (1908) urged pregnant women to exercise daily, "as a religious duty" (p. 108), while Kellogg (1891) said it was hard to overstate the "advantages to be derived from the taking of regular, systematic exercise" (p. 410). In 2016, Nancy's doctor advised against bicycling, even at six weeks, while Anna was directed to stop going to Zumba classes. Yet most doctors today encourage exercise, so long as it is well tolerated outside of pregnancy.

Among lay experts, the most common directive (by far) for expecting women focused on how to avoid wrapping the umbilical cord around the baby's neck. Social media commenters heard many variants of "don't lift your arms over your head" to avoid this. One person noted that many people shared this piece of expertise, but no one could explain where it came from or what it meant (Private FB Group, 2017). Another shared that her mother-in-law, a doctor, offered the same information. She added, "She did retract though after she thought about it a sec" (Private FB Group, 2017). Interestingly, while this information might be the most pervasive, we found no discussion of it in the historical manuals we analyzed, even though maternity casebooks from the Boston Lying-In Hospital outpatient programs and the New England Hospital for Women and Children cited ample cord wrapping with and without consequences (Boston Lying-In, 1832–1981; New England Hospital, 1885–1900). Today, a "nuchal cord" (meaning around the neck) is considered common, though is not always safe for the fetus (Clapp et al., 2003; Peesay, 2012). These long-standing myths might simply reflect the commonness of nuchal cord across time and a sincere desire for prevention. Still, the information pregnant individuals receive from friends, family, acquaintances, and strangers resurfaces and in some cases reproduces the same or similar myths across time.

Today, 20% to 56% of expert advice directed at pregnant women comes from family members or media sources and is often "inconsistent with [medical] recommendations" (Eisenberg et al., 2015, p. 1). But as we've seen, the recommendations are often inconsistent within and outside social-media-based sources (see also Ayala & Freeman, 2016). Mothers today face more experts warning of an ever-growing list of toxins, threats, and potential hurdles—the 2016 version of *WTEWYE* includes a much more comprehensive list of risk factors than the 1984 version, potentially causing more anxiety and fear for pregnant and non-pregnant readers alike (Abbasi-Lemmon, 2016; Lancaster, 2017). Similar to late nineteenth- and early twentieth-century expert advice manuals, texts such as *WTEWYE* list risks and dangers and recommend consulting medical experts of some type but ultimately place the responsibility for managing these risks on the mother alone (Abbasi-Lemmon, 2016; Ayala & Freeman, 2016; Lancaster, 2017; Wetterberg, 2004).

No matter how wealthy, well connected, or powerful, mothers cannot eradicate all toxins from their environment (e.g., air pollution), and so the notion of personal responsibility reflects a "fatal combination of responsibility and powerlessness" (Frye, 1983, p. 9; see also Ayala & Freeman, 2016). Structural change is the most effective answer for eradicating BPA and air pollution and creating a risk-free environment for pregnancy, for example, through EPA or FDA regulations or well-funded public campaigns. While individuals and communities can and do effect change, most expertise on pregnancy behavior locates the activities and the consequences at the level of the individual, thus shifting attention from the most meaningful forms of prevention (Ayala & Freeman, 2016; Richardson et al., 2014). In manuals such as *WTEWYE* as well as in protoscience journalism, the focus on individual responsibility for pregnancy outcomes increases the policing of pregnant bodies (Ayala & Freeman, 2016; Lancaster, 2017), particularly during the life cycle of early motherhood.

Currently, protective behaviors for the health of the not-yet-conceived extend back into the teen years, long before many individuals have decided on the future of their maternal life (Ayala & Freeman, 2016). As we discussed in chapter 1, this elongates the life cycle of early motherhood drastically and increases the likelihood that both conception and pregnancy are imbued with greater personal responsibility. Furthermore, technical and lay experts in the nineteenth century questioned the impact of pubescent education and activity (e.g., outdoor exercise) on future fertility; the long preconception period seems to be resurfacing.

As with other issues impacting the mother-child dyad during the life cycle of early motherhood, social media platforms further complicate expertise directed at pregnant women. First, more technology may lead to increased surveillance by others (e.g., who can view your online pregnancy narrative and comment) and by yourself (e.g., through apps and eBook versions of pregnancy advice manuals). While 3-D and 4-D ultrasounds provide a more detailed, accurate landscape of pregnancy's interiority (Kroløkke, 2010), the external acts of pregnancy, including what to eat, how to comport one's self emotionally in public spaces, and how to engage with the physical world (e.g., getting out of cars, carrying bags and children, working out), also encourage scrutiny. Externally, as one's pregnancy becomes more visible, a larger number of lay (e.g., strangers who have been or are also pregnant) and technical (e.g., medical practitioners of any kind) experts feel free to hold forth on one's perceived behaviors and mood. Social media can mean solace from these prying eyes, as women commiserate online about the burdens of expertise. Yet users may not be able to selectively withdraw from the eyes of the Internet or the judgments leveled at pregnant women online; this can result in an impression of few off-ramps when the scrutiny feels overwhelming.

Social media also exponentially increase the volume of expert advice, while simultaneously offering ever more experts to proffer said expertise. Some information has emerged and circulated widely, throughout American history, accuracy aside (e.g., hands above the head strangles the baby). Other advice maintains popularity with technical experts and not lay experts (e.g., the importance of exercise). And other advice is context specific (e.g., eating sushi or milk soup). Therefore, how can individuals find accurate, helpful advice? How can pregnant individuals interact with social media in ways that do not heighten fear and anxiety, increase personal surveillance, and potentially produce shame? If we examine the availability of digitized/Internet-based expertise directed toward pregnant women, the types of expertise become harder to categorize with clear-cut, distinct groupings. As previously mentioned, when we conducted an informal online FB poll on pregnancy advice, the response was significant. Some called out family members and strangers, while some reported advice they ignored from obstetricians, nurses, and midwives. Even the act of public collection here can have varying impacts: positive in that individuals experience a sense of camaraderie and community and negative in that reading these accounts could prompt further fear, anxiety, and behavior modification in other readers. Our participants noted that some of the online comments caused them anxiety; some followed lay and/or technical advice despite their training. For example, Anuja noted that her "Indian grandma" advised against sesame seeds and she "listened to her . . . it felt like it would be bad luck not to" (Private FB Group, 2017).[3]

Popular advice manuals and books describing the adventures, annoyances, and stresses of pregnancy are now online as well. On the Internet-based commerce behemoth Amazon, the most popular pregnancy-related texts in August 2017 had some form of digital presence: *WTEWYE* and the Mayo Clinic's guide to pregnancy are available in a smartphone app as well as an eBook; Gaskin's (2003) *Ina May's Guide to Childbirth* (which discusses pregnancy) comes in a Kindle version; Karp's (2015) *The Happiest Baby on the Block* has an eBook version, an associated white noise app, and dozens of YouTube videos demonstrating the book's methods; McCarthy's (2014) *Belly Laughs* has eBook and Google audiobook versions. Mothers in the early twentieth century usually lacked access to full-length books like these, though many received pamphlets and free publications from the Children's Bureau. Caretakers today can carry all of these texts and thousands more on their personal devices for a nominal fee and even engage with social media sites linked to these publications, making expert directives far more accessible and voluminous. Gender scholar Sophia A. Johnson (2014) argued that these new technologies are a digitization of historical self-help or guidebooks and more knowledge may result in more physical and emotional labor during pregnancy and motherhood. On the other hand, for women whose bodies have been traditionally seen as leaky and out of control, the technologies may allow them control; selecting and following expert directives that speak to them can provide an empowering experience (e.g., diet, exercise, and gathering information) via technology.

Advice from lay experts regarding available expertise adds yet another layer to the contemporary context. For those still purchasing hard copies of expert advice manuals, Amazon offers a wealth of book reviews. Even in the comments section for Amazon book reviews, pregnancy and parenthood are performative— with commenters choosing to self-identify or remain anonymous and making claims that categorize them as friendly to or antagonistic toward medical models of pregnancy (see also Krto̷lo̷kke, 2011). These comments allow users and readers to situate themselves as lay experts with varying levels of experience. For example, one reviewer who disliked *Ina May Gaskin's Guide to Childbirth* recommended that anyone planning a hospital birth should avoid the book: "It makes you feel insecure about hospital practices" (Amazon Customer, 2017). Another reviewer left a glowing review: "Anyone of childbearing years, both men and women, would benefit . . . because it helps normalize what has become almost a disease to treat rather than an everyday . . . process" (Mommy Division, 2017). Many of the comments direct potential buyers to digital sources and/or social media. Regarding *Happiest Baby on the Block*, Jesse C (2015) identified as a lay expert: "As an expectant parent who wants to be well informed, I have a lot of books on my reading list." Next, Jesse C directed readers to the web: "If you're new/expecting parent, do yourself a favor and find this info for free on the Internet." Lisa W (2016) gave four starts to *The Pregnancy Countdown* (Magee &

Nakisbendi, 2012), but noted that she read it "along with using a couple different pregnancy apps." Erica (2013) offered that *Pregnancy Countdown* provided "more detail than online forums." Regarding the Mayo Clinic's *Guide to a Healthy Pregnancy* (Harms, Johnson, & Murry, 2004), Cathy G (2016) typed, "Nice to have a hard copy but in this day and age, apps are more comprehensive," while Beatrice (2014) found it to be "a good companion to other pregnancy books and apps." Reviewers of Murkoff and Mazel's (2016) *WTEWYE* (fifth ed.) occasionally claimed the book provided too much information. An Amazon Customer (2016) urged people to skip it: "Too many bad things in here that give mothers-to-be anxiety and too much medical jargon . . . save yourself the money and download a free pregnancy app." Commenter rob (2017) was troubled by *WTEWYE*'s practice of noting when there was scant research on a topic or behavior. For him (2017) scientific findings are perceived as "political correctness" gone awry; instead, he wished for firmer advice and perhaps expertise with ironclad confidence. Even as these reviewers complained about or questioned jargon-laced technical advice, the majority spoke with decided confidence in their individual ability to choose accurate expertise.

Individuals can also track their pregnancies through a host of smartphone apps and listen to podcasts specific to their life stage such as "Birthful," "Pregnancy Podcast," "Preggie Pals," "Baby in Bloom," and "Pea in the Podcast" (Gillespie, 2017). They can read thousands of pregnancy-specific blogs and view online versions of magazines such as *Parenting* and *Mother and Child* (see also Apple, 2006). Beyond all this is the ubiquity of social media platforms such as FB, Instagram, and Twitter, all offering a constant stream of purported expertise. While these resources can ensure that pregnant individuals today are the most informed and prepared, the information can become overwhelming and intimidating and sometimes inaccurate or problematic, adding another layer of imposed vigilance to an already heavily monitored and directed experience. Moreover, heightened surveillance reaches ridiculous levels of minutia: in the fifth edition of *WTEWYE*, Murkoff and Mazel (2016) warned readers not to walk and use their cellphones at the same time, lest they lose their balance, fall, and risk injury. Instead, "park yourself on a park bench, stand against a wall in the mall"—a singsong, slightly saccharine warning about the dangers of smartphone technology (Murkoff & Mazel, 2016, p. 71).

Recently, scholars have started to address the performativity of pregnancy on social media platforms, analyzing pregnant selfies and pregnancy narratives on FB (Johnson, 2014; Massa & Simeoni, 2017; Zappavigna & Zhao, 2017). As more people turn to the Internet as their main source for news and information (Baker, Wagner, Singer, & Bundorf, 2003; Thon & Jucks, 2017), it is apparent that social media platforms play a role similar to that of newspapers at the end of the nineteenth century and into the early twentieth, when Americans began to expect information on new scientific/medical breakthroughs in their newspapers

(Tomes, 2012). At the turn of the twentieth century, Americans enjoyed reading about new birth methods (Johnson & Quinlan, 2015, 2017; Tracy & Boyd, 1914, 1915), tracking epidemics (Barry, 2005; Tomes, 2012), and the development of new medical techniques and experiments (Tomes, 2012). Today, with the 24-hour news cycle and the constant stream of information coming out on the Internet, news media continue to post links on various social media accounts (e.g., FB, Instagram, Twitter) to protoscience journalism pieces, but they also have dedicated spaces online for these pieces, including NPR's "Shots: Health News from NPR"; longtime newspaper giants such as the *New York Times* have sections called "Health," while the *Washington Post* has both "Health and Science" and "Wellness" sections. It is in this context that yet another layer of expertise disseminates through social media and directly to pregnant individuals with Internet access and/or smartphones. Given the speed at which information is posted, and the proclivity of news agencies of all kinds to use "click bait" titles or titles crafted to attract attention and draw traffic to the parent site, it is understandable that individuals would come across a posting with a title like "How a Pregnant Woman's Choices Could Shape a Child's Health" and be compelled to click.

Although some journalists receive training in scientific reporting, the vast majority of the reading public are not trained to properly contextualize scientific findings. The brevity of many social media posts may further misrepresent study findings. Consider, for example, the term "epigenetics," which author David Epstein (2013) defined broadly as "the study of how our actions and experiences can cause chemical 'marks' to attach to genes and turn the activity of the genes up or down" (n.p.). This is actually an incomplete definition since epigenetics is one part of the newer field of developmental origins of health and disease (DOHaD) (Richardson et al., 2014). Science journalist John Hamilton (2013) cited "growing evidence" that epigenetics provided a vital tool for determining the risk of problems like diabetes, despite the fact that most epigenetics research hasn't led to the capacity to predict these risks (Richardson et al., 2014). Hamilton (2013) included what are bound to be overly simplistic claims, such as "by switching certain genes on and off, some cells become heart cells while others become brain cells," but does report one researcher's conclusion that "a complete epigenetic explanation of autism or any other disease is a long way off" (n.p.). How long is "a long way off"? That is unknown. Problematically, the author and the interviewee also failed to acknowledge that autism is not universally understood or labeled as a disease. We maintain that epigenetic terminology preys on parental fear to draw attention to articles.

Thankfully, there is protoscience journalism available that attempts to debunk and/or critique these write-ups on epigenetic research. Epstein's (2013) book excerpt on famine and genetic alteration offers a more accurate representation of the English and Danish studies the article recounts for the website Gizmodo. Epstein is clear: "To say that the study of epigenetics is in its infancy would be to exaggerate how far along it is. At the moment, the questions vastly outnumber the answers" (n.p.). Still, media reports on recent findings related to epigenetics lead to mother blame, with headlines trumpeting that pregnancy diets alter DNA, 9/11 survivors "transmitted trauma to their children," and "pregnancy should be time to double-down on healthful eating . . . to avoid a lifetime of struggling with obesity" (Lombrozo, 2014, n.p.). On the whole, scientific findings recounted through protoscience journalism entrench the pregnant individual as the sole protector of the fetus and the only responsible party if something goes wrong. This responsibility reflects back on gestation itself, underscoring pregnancy as a health crisis in which genetic development can go awry without our knowledge.

Less frequently, journalists take the focus off of mothers themselves. For example, Lombrozo (2014) concluded that structural change (e.g., increasing access to healthy food and adequate medical care for all pregnant individuals) is most needed. Sarah Richardson and her colleagues (2014) addressed the growing worry over epigenetics among the general public, pointing to "the long history of society blaming mothers for the ill health of their children" (p. 113). She maintained that findings within DOHaD cannot (or must not) be used to lecture and police pregnant women and urged "scientists, educators and reporters to anticipate how DOHaD work is likely to be interpreted in popular discussions" (p. 132). However, this is precisely the issue. Despite some debunking and some critique, the click bait articles tend to have the farthest reach and therefore the potential for the most significant impact. Furthermore, the inability of both protoscience journalists and the reading public to correctly delineate between causality and correlation and to assess the import of scientific study outcomes also strengthens the pathologization of pregnancy (Ayala & Freeman, 2017; Lombrozo, 2014; Richardson, 2014).

Social media both extend and deepen maternal surveillance and perpetuate the notion that pregnancy itself is a crisis, regardless of the actual health of the pregnant individual (Leaver, 2017). Again, certain facets of social media platforms can provide solace and community for pregnant women, but even within private groups and private Instagram streams, users can continue to police those who do not perform pregnancy under the specific tenets of each social media subcommunity. Historically and today, individual mothers have been blamed for pregnancy outcomes in ways that reflect race, class, and gender expectations, even when the data are inconclusive (Ayala & Freeman, 2016). According to Kukla (2008), many women obsessively self-monitor their "diets, exercise regimes, emotional states, hair care product use, and just about every other aspect of daily life" to prove and perform "good" motherhood (p. 73), even though the advice they are receiving often at best reflects research showing slight correlation rather than causation.

Problematically, in the early twentieth century and today, on or off social media, the psychological ablutions and bodily rituals suggested by the full spectrum of experts are available primarily to those with race, class, gender, and ableist privilege. In some respects, mother blaming in nineteenth- and early twentieth-century advice from lay and technical experts is repackaged and reiterated in protoscience journalism on epigenetics. For example, what turns a gene on or off? The stakes are high, given the implications of intergenerational impact. Will drinking a Diet Coke impact your great-grandchildren? In the infancy of epigenetics, scientists are unclear what environmental impacts are intergenerational, meaning there is little dependable information on what constitutes an epigenetic risk. Reading pregnancy literature, whether historical or contemporary, an expectant person could assume that every choice, every action, every meal, every movement, every stress or discomfort has the opportunity to powerfully impact the health and well-being of the unborn. While the science may have come full circle, the blame never shifted: the fault lies with the mother.

Conclusions on Pregnancy and Performativity: Put on Your Dancing Genes

The female body and certainly all pregnant bodies continue to face ongoing and even increased medical scrutiny in the Internet age, by advisers from various backgrounds, perspectives, and levels of training, across the spectrum of expertise. Given the attention to personal responsibility in previous and present-day proclamations on pregnancy behavior, it is valuable to consider who this perfect pregnant person *is*, as constructed by available expertise. For over a century the ideal mother is a cis, white, middle- or upper-middle-class, educated, and able-bodied female. In West and the U.S. Department of Labor's (1913) *PC*, class, race, and ethnic differences tended to be erased and the advised subject became a "composite of woman under the guise of scientific universalism." As pregnancy became medicalized and increasingly understood as a pathological crisis, expertise around prenatal care coalesced and institutionalized an ever narrower conception of a "good" pregnancy, and with that "good" motherhood. As Lanier (2017) recounted, "I ate 100 grams of protein a day. I swallowed capsules of mercury-free DHA. I gave up wheat for reasons I forget. I kept my cell phone an arm's length away from my belly to avoid damaging my SuperBaby with electromagnetic waves. I did not own a microwave. I shopped at Whole Foods, bought all organic, sometimes racked up bills of $300 a week. I never let a kernel of GMO corn touch my estrogen-laden tongue" (n.p.). Here Lanier makes clear the class privilege inherent in the performance of pregnancy. How "good" is the food you eat? How "clean"? It should be noted that the policing of food for quality is not unique to technical experts—lay experts and nontraditional medical practitioners perpetuate this same practitioner–patient hierarchy, rooted in class-based notions of healthy eating and reflecting current interests in diet and consumption. A midwife told Evelyn she could shop only at Whole Foods during her pregnancy, an assumption that class privilege is shared by those who can (or are likely to) avail themselves of midwifery in Evelyn's community (Private FB Group, 2017).

The consequences of constructing desirable motherhood on this model (now 150 years strong) are that anyone who exists outside this narrative is automatically unfit and fails to find proper representation in the available discourse or is marked a "bad mother" from the beginning, increasing the likelihood of loneliness and isolation after giving birth (Flavin, 2009; Lancaster, 2017; Richardson et al., 2014; Woliver, 2002). Moreover, defining pregnancy as crisis removes personal agency, even as it increases personal responsibility, and this occurs within the unequal racial, class, gender, and able-bodied order in which we live. Next, we examine some specific forms of privilege and review how pregnancy as a crisis, as well as social media surveillance, is further complicated through various lenses of privilege.

In 1908, Dr. Drake (1908) thought every reader had a servant to bring her coffee in bed. Today's pregnancy manuals, apps, and online advice remain nearly as implicitly biased toward middle-class women as the advice manuals a century ago. Revealing an inadequate awareness of the limited choices working-class women have in the workplace, recent issues of *WTEWYE* urge working-class women to move to a quieter, less stressful environment and to "choose" a position that removes them from toxic substances, to consider taking an earlier maternity leave, and to engage other privileged accommodations (Lancaster, 2017; Murkhoff & Mazel, 2016). The assumption that women can just change much of anything about their workplace or drastically shorten their earning potential before adding the financial burden of a child to their home displays remarkable ignorance. Economics professor John Komlos (2017) starkly remarked, "Fetuses exposed to toxins or infections will be irreparably damaged" (n.p.). Later, Komlos pointed to the necessity of structural change for universal gains in health and wellness, a slight shift from the personal responsibility we've seen in other contexts. Still, contemporary fears of prenatal exposure to toxins are stoked by expert advice, but few reasonable paths to adequate protection are offered for those who lack economic resources.

If working-class families do not have disposable income with which to purchase apps or data plans that allow for the use of free apps, web surfing, posting in forums, posting in private FB groups, and other online interactions, does this mean their motherhood is less engaged or less committed? How does the inability to engage in heightened self-surveillance through social media now define the quality of one's motherhood? Leaver (2017) conjectured that the "device-ification" of pregnancy (Johnson, 2014) normalizes intimate surveillance and "unplugged parenting is likely to be increasingly positioned as both irresponsible and aberrant" (p. 8).

Like class, examining prenatal behavior framed by race adds layers of difficulty. Historically, the external ownership and control of the pregnant body reached the grotesque: women who were enslaved and pregnant had to dig holes in the ground before being whipped, to protect their unborn, also the property of their owners (Hicks, 1937; Roberts, 1999; Weiner & Hough, 2012). Further, the brutality of enslavement complicated the idea of monstrosity in that some believed that whipping during pregnancy left scarring on your unborn baby's body (Weiner & Hough, 2012). Again, though enslaved women were likely called to account for any "defects" in their babies and doctors blamed these women for the ill health of their newborns, they had little control over their pregnant bodies, despite efforts to protect and nourish their babies (Weiner & Hough, 2012). Schwartz (2006) noted that doctors preferred to blame personal behavior rather than overwork for miscarriage and preterm labor.

Between the ending of slavery (and therefore the end of total lack of ownership of one's body) and the overall health improvements brought about by immunization, antibiotics, and African Americans' own health advocacy, there have been marked improvements for all populations. While not a new development, the ongoing and entrenched additional challenges faced by African American women during birth and in the early postpartum period are drawing attention again (Dusenbery, 2018; Villarosa, 2018). In October 2017, Simmons recounted the renewed efforts of "black doulas, midwives and reproductive health advocates" to combat rising maternal deaths among African Americans. The entrenched disparity for both mothers and babies on the basis of race is well documented. Twenty years ago, Barker (1998) noted that despite increases in access to prenatal care, rates of low birthrates in predominately African American communities remained resistant to reduction, in large part because social, economic, and political justices were not improving apace with prenatal care (see also Ayala & Freeman, 2016). Komlos (2017) also pointed to entrenched prenatal health disparities on the basis of race: "African American babies are disadvantaged by the time they take their very first breath in the world" (n.p.).

Ableism also complicates the experience of pregnancy because women who are pregnant may be treated as if they are fragile or disabled, but this is not the same as living with a disability (see Young, 2005). Some view the pregnant body as ugly, and for some a discomfort remains regarding the public display of pregnant bodies (Grosz, 1994; Oliver, 1993; Young, 1990). If we view pregnancy as a crisis, this view encourages a linkage between pregnancy and disability (e.g., legally, maternity leave is disability leave) and impedes the understanding of the experiences of women with disabilities (pregnant or not) (Abbasi-Lemon, 2016). Pregnant individuals with disabilities remain largely ignored and sometimes stigmatized by expert directives that fail to reflect their needs and lived experience. Individual differences are often not acknowledged. For example, Olivia was advised by a wide range of experts not to ride her bike, yet for her walking provoked falls while biking never did (Private FB Group, 2017). Desiree was told directly "not to be around disabled people/not to let them touch my belly . . . that this would 'cause the baby to be born disabled' [Angry face emoticon]" (Private FB Group, 2017). These claims of expertise must be expressly painful for pregnant individuals with disabilities to overhear or hear about.

Furthermore, able-bodied individuals sometimes have babies with disabilities, and those experiences remain stigmatized. Until the mid-twentieth century at least, monstrosity and (infant) disability were often synonymous, meaning that disability was formally a type of monstrosity, thought to be brought upon by spiritual forces or unusual atmospheric events. Even after the discovery of genes and the human genome, genetic differences were thought to result from personal irresponsibility, an accident, or an unknown developmental error. In Guttmacher's (1962) manual, the following passage aims to relieve parental fears: "This is a difficult subject with lay readers, for each prospective parent has a secret dread that his or her child may not be normal. . . . A third source of comfort must be the realization that in this enlightened era few obstetricians are cruel enough to fan the spark of life in a hapless monster unless sincere religious conviction dictates such a conservative policy" (pp. 247–248). While this passage may be shocking to present-day readers, it reminds us that as late as 1962, American medicine exhibited little in the way of acceptance toward bodies with disabilities generally and thus disabled pregnancy more specifically.

In one sense, ableism provides the most consistent example of prejudice across the spectrum of expertise. Technical experts can be direct and crassly insulting about pregnant bodies and children with disabilities, genetic differences, and developmental issues, as Dr. Guttmacher was in 1962. Alternatively, some lay experts or alternative practitioners frame all pregnancies as "good," making it harder to tease out how this universally positive framing of pregnancy and pregnant bodies silences disabled and/or chronically ill individuals. For example, in her *Guide to Childbirth*, Ina May Gaskin (2003) questioned the pathologization of pregnancy, pushing back against the notion that pregnancy is a crisis or a form of sickness; on its surface, this is a necessary and empowering message. But problematically, Gaskin grounded the idea that pregnancy is a "normal" physiological process by framing "normal" or "natural" pregnancy and birth as able-bodied (Abbasi-Lemon, 2016). Her pregnancy and birth stories recounted the importance of an innate "woman-ness," underscoring that a cis female body is "beautiful and admirably designed to give birth" (Gaskin, 2003, p. 270).

Gaskin acknowledges variation in pregnancy and birth, and while her statements are likely meant to encourage and uplift, they simultaneously silence narratives of different, abnormal, or chronically ill bodies. Gaskin's language failed to acknowledge mothers with disabilities and questions whether or not certain chronic conditions exist. Shockingly, Gaskin (2003) claimed there is "no treatment for GD, either with diet or insulin, that improves the outcomes for mothers or their babies" (p. 196), though, like a traditional practitioner, she still recommends dietary changes and exercise to manage blood sugar. She admitted gestational diabetes in some pregnancies is a food tolerance issue, but this is still ableism in that it erases or questions the nature of a serious health condition. Her reframing of an endocrine disorder as food intolerance and her claim that dietary changes (which she herself has prescribed) do not improve outcomes help maintain the notion that all pregnancy is "natural" or "good" and therefore all bodies are designed for pregnancy and birth. But are individuals with gestational diabetes having a "good" pregnancy? If their body does not respond to dietary changes and requires insulin, do they have a "good" body or a "bad" one? Here too an expert's framing encourages self-surveillance and questions the very nature of individuals' bodily worth.

If people without structural privilege engage in more individual self-surveillance but don't have access to the right products and supports (e.g., organic food, perfect prenatal vitamins, meditation, prenatal yoga and massage, prenatal workouts, personalized prenatal health care), then increased access to information utilizing this framing of prenatal health and success will highlight their failure and fewer and fewer individuals will have an empowered pregnancy (see also Leaver, 2017). For those who can access these resources, do these performative acts, framed as prevention and protection, give a false sense of security? For writer Heather Lanier (2017) they did, and created, in her words, "the very best of my many failures to date." During her pregnancy, she remembered "the belief that I was entirely responsible for wellness . . . [that] expectant mothers . . . are supposed to become conduits of total safety" (n.p.). Lanier concluded that the danger of believing one has full control over their body leads to blaming individuals for their disability or their baby's, just as we now (largely) blame pregnant individuals for poor outcomes. In pregnancy, "poor outcome" generally means miscarriage, a pregnancy loss, preterm birth, and/or an ill child or a child with a profound and/or identifiable difference, an exhausting and counterproductive cycle of blame. In Lanier's (2017) case, her perfect pregnancy and her imperfect child broke her heart "and put it back together in a shape that is bigger than I knew was possible" (n.p.).

There is evidence that individuals are resisting the heightened surveillance of social media during pregnancy, particularly as expert advice (lay and technical) reaches overbearing proportions. In 2017 the Facebook group We Are Mothers reposted a Romper article in which a woman describes the "pregnancy police" and outlines the intrusive ways strangers in public attempted to direct her behavior, including admonitions to drink decaf coffee, not gain too much weight, and deliver vaginally ("10 things," 2017). We were fascinated by the lay experts in the comments section under this article on the We Are Mothers page, making overarching and/or blanket statements, out of context, and not backing said claims with any source or research. Of course, social media posts are not academic research and most posters do not cite their claims, but a number of posters confidently adopted an expert tone, generally to disagree with or shame the writer. Consider this example: "I'm ambivalent. A pregnant woman IS feeding the baby everything she eats and drinks. Her Doctor should have told her that caffeine is a chromosome repair inhibitor and to avoid it. The village is reminder [sic] her, though it is rude to say it" ("10 things," 2017). First, there is no well-known research citing caffeine as a chromosomal inhibitor, and as we've seen in this chapter, doctors offer varying caffeine intake limits and guidelines to pregnant individuals. Second, the phrasing here, using technical terminology, is given with ironclad confidence, yet without any representation of this poster's educational background or type of expertise. Another commenter noted she gave up both coffee and cigarettes, seemingly equating their risk, while another quipped, "It's perfectly safe to have some caffeine" ("10 things," 2017). If individuals are looking for well-researched advice, the comments section on a social media platform is not the place to find it, though research suggests individuals are spending more and more time gathering health information from social media platforms (Weaver, 2017).

Emily Oster, a professor of economics at Brown University, wrote *Expecting Better* (2014) to address the limits of expertise, both technical and lay, given as prenatal guidelines. As an economist trained to measure available data in order to weigh risks and benefits before making decisions, she found pregnancy advice varied in quality. Oster also found that technical and lay experts gave divergent, even contradictory directives. She particularly disliked the way pregnancy "seemed to be treated as a one-size-fits-all affair" and began to approach her own decisions by reviewing available studies, then considering which risks she felt comfortable taking (p. 4). For Oster, one way to move the target off pregnant bodies is to substantially widen the target, allowing individuals the space to come to different conclusions on topics lacking sufficient research (e.g., caffeine, types of exercise). While Oster and others with extensive education and particular training can read and understand this research, structural inequality impedes both access to this information and the ability to comprehend and integrate it. In many cases, social media might provide the quickest and most accessible source of information (e.g., asking for advice on pregnancy symptoms in a FB group) (Private FB Group, 2017). Problematically, the source of information is not always known and misinformation is abundant (Kata, 2010). We propose that this is an important historical moment, when the destabilization of authoritative knowledge and questioning of science is augmented by social media platforms, which are meant to allow for the widest possible range of perspective, information, and expertise.

While there are no easy answers here, it is clear that the warp of expertise changes (e.g., dissemination) while the weft remains the same (e.g., don't raise your arms over your head). Historically and today, technical and lay practitioners have failed to fully address systemic inequality as a cause for pregnancy health crises. Instead, individual action remains the model by which society judges pregnancy outcomes.

It is evident that social media platforms complicate the performativity of pregnancy, even as they offer new resources for support, information, and reassurance. Ultimately, our urgent work is mapping and increasing resistance to social media as a tool of heightened surveillance and personal responsibility—in essence removing some of the consequences while keeping the benefits. We must think together, with all kinds of experts, using every type of expertise, about how to move the target off of pregnant individuals and onto the social and environmental conditions that constrain and endanger all citizens. Moreover, we must consider how social media platforms can assist this effort. To begin, we have to be willing to expand our definition of expertise beyond the technical and lay—what role do social media users play in expert discourse? And how do we challenge or uphold historical patterns of power as they play out in medical expertise online?

CHAPTER 4

"YOU WOMEN WILL HAVE
TO FIGHT FOR IT"

TWILIGHT SLEEP AND TRANSACTIONAL CHILDBIRTH
EXPERTISE IN TWENTIETH-CENTURY AMERICA

In August 1915, Mrs. Francis X. Carmody, known to fellow Twilight Sleep Association (TSA) members and supporters as Charlotte, entered a Brooklyn, New York, hospital to give birth ("Mrs. Carmody not," 1915). She almost certainly did not arrive with a printed birth plan or an understanding of the benefits of a baby-friendly hospital setting, rooming-in, or wearing her own slippers. She did arrive with a pain management plan: Twilight Sleep (TS), an amnesia-inducing drug cocktail to erase the memory of the birth and thus any related pain. Like thousands of American women annually in the early twentieth century (Loudon, 1992; Morbidity, 1999), Charlotte Carmody died while giving birth (Loudon, 1992; "Mrs. Carmody not," 1915). We cannot know if death was on her mind as she approached the birth, but we might assume that she, like the majority of women, was sentient of the dangers of childbirth in her day.

Extensive newspaper coverage of Carmody's work as a TS advocate and lay expert and of her death illuminates the deep divide between technical and lay birth experts in early twentieth-century New York City and indeed in the country as a whole. Some New York doctors (reluctantly) provided the method as a result of Carmody's work with the TSA ("Transactions," 1914b). Before her untimely passing, Carmody established herself as an educated, well-connected lay expert through a host of public activities including her involvement with the TSA (Dennett Papers, 1874–1945) and her public seminars and appearances to educate women on TS, which included plans for a nationwide lecture tour ("Four 'Twilight' tots," 1915; "Mrs. Carmody tells," 1914). In an address at a public gathering, she urged the audience, "If you women want it you will have to fight for it, for the mass of doctors are opposed to it" ("Mothers discuss," 1914, p. 18). She willingly provided information on her first TS experience for public magazines as well as promoting a book about TS, published by fellow TSA members and lay experts Marguerite Tracy and Mary Boyd (1915). In the pages of her local newspaper, the *Brooklyn Eagle* (*TBE*), supporters insisted that TS was part of Charlotte's legacy; Carmody's widower referred to individuals tying TS to her death as "'incompetent' gossipers" ("Mrs. Carmody died," 1915, p. 1; see also "Mrs. Carmody not," 1915). Headlines announced, "Mrs. Carmody dies suddenly at local hospital," adding however that "new treatment in no way connected with her death" ("Mrs. Carmody not," 1915, p. 14).

As a campaign driven by lay experts that directly impacted technical expert practice in New York City, TS is a unique example of lay-to-technical expertise transmission (Johnson, 2010; Johnson & Quinlan, 2015, 2017). Perhaps the most provocative part of this history is the success of female lay experts in altering technical expertise and obstetric care in hospitals at a time when midwives faced heightened scrutiny and restrictions (Breslaw, 2012; Crowell, 1907). Throughout the debate, lay experts co-opted technical terminology to raise awareness about TS (Hairston, 1996) and in some instances had more detailed technical knowledge than did practitioners. The popularity of lay expertise underscores the impact of what Tomes (2002) referred to as "protoscience journalism," which provided lay populations with information on scientific developments and new medical treatments (p. 630). Moreover, the extensive newspaper coverage of the TS debates from 1914 to 1917 highlights the power of newspapers for expertise dissemination—both lay and technical.

In this chapter, we trace the potential for lay expertise to impact technical expertise on mothers' childbirth decisions by examining the campaign for TS in the early twentieth century and the rise of "baby-friendly" hospitals in the past decade. We define technical experts as medical practitioners—that is, doctors (more specifically obstetricians), nurses, and midwives. We define lay experts as informed citizens advocating for change in obstetric practice. The particular story of TS in New York City suggested that lay expertise can and does impact technical expertise and practice, regardless of whether technical experts acknowledge this relationship and the influence of "nonexperts" in their practice. We conclude by examining present-day "baby-friendly" hospital policies, which include midwifery practices extending back centuries (Ulrich, 1990) and then "reemerging" in America in response to lay expertise and activism in the 1960s and 1970s (Davis-Floyd & Davis, 1996; Hartocollis, 2010). The impacts of lay expertise on technical expertise and practice do not automatically translate into what is best for or even accessible to all mothers. This case study demonstrates that the traditional lay-expertise binary fails to represent the ways in which medical expertise circulates and thereby impacts people's lived experiences.

NINETEENTH- AND EARLY TWENTIETH-CENTURY CHILDBIRTH IN NEW YORK CITY: VYING FOR POWER

The formal entry of "male midwives" into the birthing room began as early as 1762, when a training program began in Philadelphia (Breslaw, 2014). However, the movement from female to male birth attendants and from home to hospital occurred slowly, particularly for those without wealth and social connections (Breslaw, 2014; Starr, 1984). The professionalization of obstetric medicine, characterized by a traditionally educated male acting as a technical expert on birth, was hampered by the particularities of the nineteenth century. This was an era of unregulated education and practice and little to no unified instruction, examination, or training (Janik, 2014; Shyrock, 1966; Wertz, 1996). New York City's College of Physicians and Surgeons began conducting entrance exams in 1888, though the school charter dates to 1807 (Dalton, 1888, pp. 1, 193). Doctors struggling for professional supremacy in the nineteenth and early twentieth centuries were primarily concerned with their main competitors: non–technical experts following "irregular" or "eclectic" methods of medical practice (e.g., homeopathy, hydrotherapy, hypnotherapy). Traditional physicians pushed for medical licensure of all legal practitioners, which irregular practitioners (many of whom were women) resisted (Breslaw, 2012; Janik, 2014; Starr, 1982). In the mid-nineteenth century, a populist movement against technical expertise and traditional medicine flourished, creating new systems of medicine and understandings of illness (e.g., homeopathic medicine; Breslaw, 2012; Janik, 2014). Irregular practitioners formed a well-established, organized part of American medicine from the mid-nineteenth century until the 1910s. In that decade, the Flexner Report, based on the European model of medical education, established a new rating of the efficacy of medical education in schools around the country (Bonner, 1990, 1995). After the issuance of the Flexner Report, most eclectic medical schools closed. The diversity of medical practice in the United States, including the number of female doctors, narrowed significantly for nearly six decades (Bonner, 1995; Morantz-Sanchez, 2000).

Also limiting the market reach of up-and-coming obstetricians was distrust of technical/traditional practitioners and a reliable network of experienced female caregivers, including midwives. The main competitors for patients in New York City were predominantly immigrant midwives without formal education, whose birth outcomes remained superior into the 1930s (Crowell, 1907; New York Academy of Medicine, 1933).[1] In New York City, with large numbers of immigrants arriving in the late nineteenth century and early twentieth, women who were unable to afford a private doctor chose a midwife and often included female family members, friends, or neighbors in the childbirth experience. Meanwhile, as the hospital started to become the dominion of "legitimate" physicians, obstetricians were anxious to achieve credibility among established doctors (Breslaw, 2012;

Johnson & Quinlan, 2015, 2017; Vandenberg-Daves, 2014). To achieve and maintain control of birthing in New York City, obstetricians successfully lobbied for legislation that ensured midwifery practice was almost entirely under their purview by early 1914 ("Bills at Albany," 1901; Bureau of Child Hygiene, 1907; Crowell, 1907; "Legislature's proceedings," 1901).[2]

Beyond legislative strategy, obstetricians sought and tested new pain relief options, which attracted new middle- and upper-class patients and eventually gave them a firm foothold over midwives in northern urban areas (Breslaw, 2012; Ulrich, 1990; Wolf, 2009). Regardless of the professional advantages for obstetrics and the near universal use of anesthesia in general surgery by 1910, obstetricians continued to disagree about the efficacy and safety of pain relief during birth (Caton, 1999). From 1840 to 1880, ether and chloroform emerged as anesthetics available to upper-class, "delicate" women, but physicians noted that ether caused intense nausea, chloroform was hazardous to the liver, and babies seemed affected by both (Breslaw, 2014; Caton, 1999). Moreover, ether and chloroform could lead to hemorrhage or protracted labor by decreasing contractions; the "muscle-suppressing action" of opiates could halt labor entirely (Leavitt, 1986, p. 125). Some doctors refused to use anesthesia because they felt women did not need or want pain relief. In the January 1915 edition of the *American Journal of Obstetrics and Diseases of Women and Children*, an editorial argued against the notion that women experienced any fear of the birth process: "It may be safely stated as a matter of fact that at the present time most women do not regard with dread their oncoming confinement . . . like other disagreeable experiences, [difficult labors] are very apt to be talked over among a limited circle of women and being duly exaggerated in the telling, such isolated cases are frequently accepted as standards by women who are of a nervous temperament or of an unstable mental equilibrium" ("Editorial," 1915, p. 167). Despite this author's views, accepting the fear of pain and suffering in childbirth was common among doctors by the early twentieth century (Breslaw, 2012; Caton, 1999; Leavitt, 1986; Wolf, 2009). Mary Ware Dennett (Dennett Papers, 1874–1945), the president of the TSA (TSA, 1914), and Charlotte Teller, TSA member, public TS lay expert, and TS patient (Teller, 1915), addressed this fear as a foregone conclusion. Lay experts linked fear of childbirth with poor birth outcomes, including mental strain and maternal death (Tracy & Boyd, 1915; Tracy & Leupp, 1914). In the early twentieth century, lay and technical experts imbued fears of childbirth with race and class implications. Dr. Kenneth Junor of Brooklyn suggested, "There seems little doubt that, in our highly nerve-strung and corset-wearing women . . . childbirth is no longer a natural function," so "nature has to receive aid" (Junor, 1915, p. 146).[3] This remark represented the alleged pathological or "unnatural" character of childbirth for upper- and upper-middle-class women, thought to be the most civilized in society (Bederman, 1994; Weiner & Hough, 2012), while "lower" races (nonwhite) and classes (not middle or upper class) were thought to experience less pain due to a lower sensitivity to external stimulation (Dennett Papers, 1874–1945; Pitcock & Clark, 1992).[4]

Drug usage varied according to individual opinions of drug-assisted birth, but in 1914 the medical community had not yet agreed on the effects the drugs had on the mother or child and experimentation was still common (Caton, 1999; Hamilton, 1914; Pitcock & Clark, 1992; "Transactions," 1914a, 1914b). By the late nineteenth century and early twentieth, doctors began to experiment with "bromethyl, chlorethyl, nitrous oxid[e], antipyrin, cocain[e]," and even spinal injection, a precursor to the epidural (Ver Beck, 1915, p. 3). In 1914, Dr. M. W. Kapp (1914) urged obstetricians to use his birth drug of choice: heroin (p. 844). The main disagreement among obstetricians in New York City regarding TS was over the Freiburg Method (FM) of TS and the use of the drug scopolamine, vital to the FM.

The FM of TS began during the first stage of labor when the patient received an injection (generally in the thigh), most often composed of scopolamine and morphine, the former being the drug unique to the TS method.[5] Once the first injection took effect, the patient experienced pain relief from the narcotic and amnesia from scopolamine (Tracy & Boyd, 1914, 1915). Periodically, the doctor administered a memory test by displaying an object and/or asking a simple question (e.g., the date) (Johnson & Quinlan, 2015; Van Hoosen, 1915). After 15 to 30 minutes, the doctor showed the object or asked the question; if the patient remembered the object or question, she received another injection of scopolamine. The "testing" recurred until the patient failed to remember, which confirmed amnesia (Leupp & Hendrick, 1915). Subsequent injections did not contain a narcotic and thus did not relieve pain. However, the amnestic nature of scopolamine prevented the majority of women from remembering the experience and their discomfort (Sandelowski, 1984; Wolf, 2009).

The goal of the FM of TS was to keep the patient in an amnestic state, which allowed sufficient cognizance for direction from the doctor (Johnson & Quinlan, 2015; Tracy & Boyd, 1915). In the ideal case, the patient slept off the final injection and woke to meet her child (Tracy & Boyd, 1915). In the "Frauenklinik" of Drs. Gauss and Krönig, patients who could pay for TS in the "first-class ward" (i.e., the FM of TS) had private rooms, personalized scopolamine dosage, and a nurse present throughout the birth (Johnson & Quinlan, 2015; Tracy & Boyd, 1914, 1915). Rare for this period, middle- and upper-class TS mothers claimed an easy convalescence—including the ability to sit up hours after birth, eat a full meal, and spend time with their new baby ("Mothers discuss," 1914; Tracy & Boyd, 1914). To achieve these results, the FM of TS required state-of-the-art facilities and ample, well-trained staff—major hurdles for the American obstetrician struggling for professional status at that time. These same requirements ensured the procedure would be inaccessible for anyone without the funds necessary for optimal treatment, something the TSA aimed to change (Dennett Papers, 1874–1945; Johnson, 2010).

It was not just the struggle for professionalization among obstetricians or questions about drug safety that made TS a source of contention among physicians. The disagreement seemed to stem from the difficulty of the FM itself. In New York City, many obstetricians and other practitioners found TS practitioner and supporter Dr. John O. Polak's "exceptional results" difficult to achieve. The contraindications of the procedure were numerous and included eclampsia, a prolonged second stage of labor, and halted labor. Dr. G. L. Broadhead noted that several patients needed nurses to keep them from jumping out of bed (Transactions, 1914b; see also Hellman, 1915; Pitcock & Clark, 1992). Historian Jacqueline H. Wolf (2009) noted the "uncontrollable delirium" that scopolamine caused and could provoke physical aggression, screaming, and more in some patients (p. 50).[6] One laboring woman climbed onto the windowsill of her room with the intention of leaping off the ledge. It took three hospital nurses to subdue her, and she gave birth in shackles (Wolf, 2009). To offset the possibility of a sensory-based reaction to the drug, the Jewish Maternity and Lebanon hospitals in New York City placed patients in darkened rooms, covered their eyes with smoked glasses or masks, and stuffed their ears with cotton soaked in oil, sometimes covering the women's entire face with a towel (Wolf, 2009). Ideally, women had no memory of shackles or restraints if they were under the influence of scopolamine, although the possibility of delirium explains why some doctors expressed more hesitation over TS than the women who experienced the method. Both technical and lay experts listed potential side effects to the baby as well, including difficulty or depressed breathing at birth and, in very rare cases, death (Hamilton, 1914; Harrar & McPherson, 1914; Leupp & Hendrick, 1915; Polak, 1915; Rongy, 1914; Ver Beck, 1915).[7]

Technical and lay experts in favor of TS claimed that contraindications for mother or baby were clear indications of malpractice, insufficient individualization of dosage, or failure to fully adhere to the FM (Hellman, 1915; Leupp & Hendrick, 1915; Polak, 1915; Rongy, 1914; Van Buren Thorne, 1914; Ver Beck, 1915).[8] Drs. Gauss and Krönig insisted that closely following the FM drastically reduced potential side effects.[9] Dr. William H. Knipe, a New York City obstetrician who supported TS, claimed that "the poor results . . . we had obtained previously with scopolamine-morphin [sic] were due to the fact that we did not follow the Freiburg rules" (Ver Beck, 1915, p. 333). In New York City, a public debate ensued when supporters advocating expanded access to the FM of TS argued with detractors, who countered that the FM could not overcome the dangers of scopolamine itself. Supporters included well-known and respected doctors Polak, Knipe, Rongy, Beard, McPherson, and Harrar as well as TSA members, female lay experts, and previous FM patients. Despite differences of opinion, TS devotees and detractors agreed on several things. First, the procedure was complicated and the skill required was so intensive that only trained obstetricians should attempt it. Second, scopolamine was similar to ether and chloroform in that it had inherent risks. Third, not every laboring woman was eligible for the procedure: healthy women in the first stage of childbirth were the ideal candidates for TS. Fourth, the procedure required ample staff, so births should take place in the hospital.[10]

In the TS debates, both lay and technical experts wielded detailed knowledge of birth-related terminology. However, the women who traveled to Germany and experienced the FM or saw it firsthand (generally with a relative) became outspoken advocates and, after a good deal of further research, lay experts who published protoscience journalism on TS (Tracy & Boyd, 1915; Tracy & Leupp, 1914; Ver Beck, 1915). The bedside experience provided enough technical knowledge for lay experts to meaningfully challenge obstetricians in publications (e.g., newspapers) and in public spaces (e.g., speaking events), using technical language. The resulting disagreement illustrates the ways that lay experience and expertise can and do impact both technical expertise and medical practice.

Activists versus Obstetricians: The TS "Furor" in Manhattan (1914–1916)

Enamored with TS and considering themselves "lay experts" in the FM, patients-turned-activists returned from Germany and launched an early twentieth-century media blitz through newspapers, women's magazines, and books. For example, *The Truth about Twilight Sleep* author Hanna Ver Beck recounted, "I am not telling you anything from hearsay; I have spent six months in preparation for this work," and noted her translation of over 200,000 words from FM of TS birth records (1915, n.p.). Constance Todd described the response to her paper with Marguerite Tracy and concluded, "The indifference with which this paper was received, coupled with our knowledge of what had been accomplished at Freiburg, drove Miss Tracy and myself to address women directly" (1936, p. 14). Lay experts such as Todd and Tracy also hosted social events all over New York City to educate interested individuals on this particular form of TS ("Carmody babe," 1914; Dennett Papers, 1874–1945; "Four 'Twilight' tots," 1915; "Mrs. Carmody tells," 1914). In 1914, to continue to advocate for the birth method, lay experts formed the Twilight Sleep Association (TSA), which met in the offices of *McClure's Magazine* in Manhattan (Dennett Papers, 1874–1945). In the years before Carmody's death, New York City became the unofficial epicenter of the national TS movement and sparked a heated debate. Lay experts and patients seeking TS lobbied for access, while many technical experts resisted the pressure they felt to provide the FM of TS. However, in multiple city boroughs, the medical community responded as service providers answering consumer demand. For example, Dr. Polak claimed that expanded TS practice was needed in wealthier areas of Brooklyn because "the women demand it and we have simply attempted to supply the demand" ("Transactions," 1914a, p. 1024). In Manhattan and Brooklyn, lay experts fomented public interest in the method, and hospitals all over the city began offering TS; newspapers reported a wide range of results and varying levels of support on the part of technical experts ("153," 1915; "Dr. Polak approves," 1914; "No," 1915; "Opposes," 1915; "'Twilight' reduces," 1915).

Notwithstanding enthusiasm among pregnant women for the method, the medical community remained in unanimous agreement regarding the role of lay experts in the debate: these women threatened their professional authority. Technical experts, both obstetricians and general physicians, insisted that lay experts had no business ever addressing medical topics, even as they followed lay expert advice to study and implement TS. Some local physicians and many others around the country discussed the published work of lay experts with withering condescension. As early as May 1914, the *Medical Record* referred to the upcoming article about TS in *McClure's Magazine* as "painful magazine exploitation" and asserted that there could be "nothing but condemnation of the unreal and one-sided portrayal . . . of a strictly medical subject" ("Painless childbirth," 1914, p. 986). In August 1914, the *Lancet—Clinic* claimed that lay expert articles were deeply flawed, declared that authors "bribed some underling at the Freiburg Clinic," and reported Dr. Krönig's horror at appearing in any article of the American popular press ("The Twilight Sleep and business," 1914, p. 117). One doctor who supported TS nonetheless referred to lay experts as "sensational" and said the medical community's inclination to "ridicule the whole matter as preposterous" was natural and appropriate (Harrar & McPherson, 1914, p. 621). In October 1914, at a meeting of the New York Obstetrical Society in Manhattan, Dr. E. B. Craigin argued that TS was not as "easy a matter as represented in lay magazines" (Transactions, 1914b, p. 1030). Other doctors referred to the work of TS lay experts as "twaddle" and "rigmarole" and found lay articles "amusing" (Bogart, 1916, p. 40).

The challenge posed by female lay experts fomenting public demand continually resurfaced in technical medical publications from 1914 to 1916 (November 1914, January 1915, October 1916, and July 1916) ("Editorial," 1915; Hamilton, 1914; Hellman, 1915; Putnam, 1916; "Twilight Sleep again," 1916). As such, the so-called sensationalist press and the lay experts producing and disseminating this information to the wider public were of particular importance to the medical community. Articles on TS in women's magazines prompted inquiries by thousands of women. Most alarming for physicians and obstetricians was that these articles also suggested that women take their business elsewhere if doctors rejected the method. Some women did, so the loss of revenue was a real possibility ("Mothers discuss," 1914; Tracy & Boyd, 1914; Tracy & Leupp, 1914). While that lay expertise challenge to obstetric practice had social and economic implications, such as loss of stature and revenue, resistance from technical experts hindered women's attempts to increased access to pain relief methods.

It is understandable that the methods of lay supporters confounded the scientific rigor demanded by technical experts. For example, on May 28, 1914, the *New York Times* published a poem penned by Ethel Wolff (1914) praising the TS method and titled "The Bridge of Dreams." She wrote,

> In all the corners of the earth pale women hear . . . the river's roar sounds closer and more terrible. With faltering feet they near the bridge's gate—when, lo! Upon them falls the Twilight Sleep of rest, a peace of floating cloud and Summer Sea, a world where Care is not, and Pain unknown. . . . Oh Twilight Sleep! White magic of a master mind, whose sympathy for Woman wrought this priceless boon . . . to those most blessed ones whose children first draw breath, the while their mothers wander through a golden haze—a sleep that leads from hope to utter happiness! (n.p.)

Poetry aside, lay experts and FM supporters Marguerite Tracy and Constance Leupp (1914) appealed to the public's support for scientific findings in mass publications like women's magazines. In their *McClure's Magazine* article "Painless Childbirth," the authors stated that out of 3,600 FM birth records, a "great mass of homogenous statistical material" demonstrated the safety and efficacy of the method (p. 39). In fact, some female lay experts demonstrated a better understanding of the FM than many American obstetricians at that time (Shannon & Truitt, 1919). For example, lay expert, FM enthusiast, and author Hanna Rion Ver Beck (1915) studied and translated thousands of pages of German medical records for *The Truth about Twilight Sleep*. She described the FM of TS cocktail as "*separate* solutions prepared by a pharmaceutical chemist .03 per cent solution of crystal scopolamine hydrobromic in sterilized distilled water and one per cent morphin muriaticum solution" (p. 81). Yet doctors continued to lack this knowledge—in the journal *Surgery, Gynecology and Obstetrics*, doctors requested this exact information (proper solution and dosage) (Lynch et al., 1914, p. 654). Apparently, some physicians remained uncertain about these details, which were written up by lay experts and published for lay readers in women's magazines.

Still, some lay experts made inaccurate claims in publications discussing TS (Johnson & Quinlan, 2015). Tracy and Leupp (1914) argued that "the birth period is not appreciably lengthened" with the FM of TS (p. 42). In a follow-up article, Tracy and Boyd (1914) claimed "the only person inconvenienced by a deliberately lengthened birth is the attending practitioner" (p. 69), directly contradicting Tracy and Leupp's original assertion. Tracy and Leupp's (1914) claim that TS allowed for "painless childbirth" is also inaccurate—although they stipulated that TS amounted to "*clouded consciousness*, in which there was complete *forgetfulness*" (p. 41), "painless" was the chosen term (Dennett Papers, 1874–1945; Tracy & Boyd, 1914). The TSA pamphlet (1914) described TS more accurately as "a condition . . . actually the same as complete insensibility to pain" (n.p.).

TS in Brooklyn: Lay Success and Mother-Friendly Hospitals

The interest in TS in Brooklyn was particularly intense, and the activities of lay experts there directly impacted the practice of some obstetricians in Brooklyn, including Drs. Polak and Dickinson (Johnson & Quinlan, 2017). Similar to the situation in Manhattan, the lay impact on technical expertise is apparent in the pages of the popular newspaper the *Brooklyn Eagle*; different from Manhattan, however, was the extent of the impact. In Brooklyn, at the height of the "furor," TS became part of the borough's identity ("Borough," 1916). Initially, *TBE* reported resistance from technical experts to TS, while following the efforts of lay experts to bring the FM of TS to women in Brooklyn. If local doctors (technical experts) did not favor TS, how did lay experts use newspapers and public opinion to impact hospital practice? In the protoscience journalistic coverage of TS, *TBE* highlighted technologically state-of-the-art hospitals and hospitals, adding TS wards to make TS possible in their facilities (Johnson & Quinlan, 2015; "'Twilight Sleep' ward," 1914). Lay experts on TS became a fixture in *TBE* for years, and newspaper coverage of their work to bring the FM of TS into hospitals did not ebb after Charlotte Carmody's death (Johnson & Quinlan, 2017). Reflecting the particular perspective of *TBE*, the articles focused on the activities of white socialites fomenting public interest in TS and wealthy and/or famous individuals who gave birth using the method in the borough (Johnson & Quinlan, 2017).

In July 1914, *TBE* reported that practitioners in Brooklyn "frowned on the new treatment and severely condemned the widespread currency given to its alleged wonders as misleading and harmful in the extreme" ("Painless," 1914, p. 3). Drs. Dickinson and Polak planned to investigate the method further—not two weeks later, *TBE* reported on Dr. Polak's continued reservations on the FM ("Dr. Polak to study," 1914). In December 1914, Brooklyn-based Dr. Delano announced his concerns about TS at a local Medical Society meeting, during which he accused newspapers and magazines of "doing a great deal of harm, because most women who are about to become mothers are calling for [TS]" ("Say," 1914, p. 8). Brooklyn's doctors had their anxieties greatly alleviated, though, through a series of trips to Germany.

On August 17, 1914, three weeks after *TBE* reported Dr. Polak's resistance to TS, the paper reported, "Dr. Polak approves 'Twilight Sleep' after the visit to Freiburg, where he studied the new method. Difficulties to overcome. Treatment is limited by many requirements, but results are good." This "new" method is the same FM of Manhattan fame. Despite Dr. Polak's initial reservations, a second visit to the clinic in Freiburg in August 1914 prompted him to claim that "a woman can have a comparatively painless childbirth. . . . It is possible for us to obtain the same results from the treatment [TS] here in America" ("Dr. Polak approves," 1914, p. 9). Later that week, *TBE* reported that the Jewish Maternity Hospital in Manhattan had used TS in 125 successful cases ("'Twilight Sleep' here?," 1914, p. 13). On August 29, 1914, *TBE* declared Dr. Ralph Beach's "absolute success [with] the 'Twilight Sleep' method." Dr. Polak even went so far as to offer monetary support for women seeking TS who lacked funds ("Twilight Sleep now at," 1914).

In November 1915, German physician and FM expert Dr. Schlussingk, who arrived to train Brooklyn doctors in the method, said that "the intelligent American woman confidently expects to die every time she has a child" ("Dr. Schlussingk," 1915, p. 22) and offered TS as a reliable method to reduce fears around childbirth. Dr. Schlussingk framed TS as a necessity—and his views reflected those of lay experts active throughout the area such as Charlotte Carmody, Marguerite Tracy, Mary Boyd, and others.

The newspaper also highlighted lay experiences with the birth method, and reporters interviewed patients who delivered under the FM of TS and published their positive experience and enthusiastic support for the method ("'Twilight Sleep' here?," 1914). After her first TS birth, Carmody's experience prompted two *TBE* articles that suggested that Mrs. Carmody's birth experience in Freiburg led to Dr. Polak's trip in 1914 to observe the method ("Carmody babe," 1914; "Carmodys," 1914). *TBE* tracked Mrs. Carmody's work with the TSA, reported on her talk to over 1,000 women at Gimbel Brothers' Department Store, and mentioned other social events in which Carmody highlighted TS friendly hospitals and the benefits to mothers of TS hospital birth ("Mrs. Carmody tells," 1914; "Ready," 1915; see also Johnson & Quinlan, 2015). *TBE* published information on local TS births ("Births," 1915; "'Twilight Sleep' baby," 1914). Mrs. George McCann gave birth to the first twins born under TS in Brooklyn ("'Twilight Sleep' twins," 1915), and the wife of beloved national hero Jack Binns gave birth under TS with Dr. Polak at Long Island College Hospital ("Jack," 1915).

In early twentieth-century New York City, rising technical experts on birth were obstetricians, struggling to be taken seriously within traditional medicine. Nurses were secondary to doctors, and midwives were under attack (Crowell, 1907; Wolf, 2009). The lay experts who wrote nearly all of the books available to the public were women, most of them active in the suffrage movement, self-identified as feminists, white, and educated. Condemned (sometimes quite publicly) by the vast majority of the medical community, lay experts such as Carmody and her privileged peers of the TSA sought to bring mother-friendly births from the home to the hospital. Meanwhile, TS remained inaccessible to rural women, many immigrant women, women of color, and the vast majority of poor women. Even though a tiny minority of women experienced TS in its heyday, the TS movement served as an important catalyst in the decades-long trend of bringing birth into the hospital and increased the use and popularity of pain relief. If the FM of TS was a necessity for a fear-free, mother-friendly birth and hospital wards were best suited to provide the FM, then mothers needed to give birth in hospitals, with specially trained medical staff (Dennett Papers, 1874–1945).

Despite their critique of the obstetric method, their insistence on the FM of TS as the only viable birth method, and their privileged status, TS lay experts believed that all women deserved access to the method and that their expertise could educate the public and transform American childbirth. For a time, particularly in New York City, their work had a marked impact by extending the reach of technical expertise and encouraging middle- and upper-class women to birth in hospitals. Additionally, TS did not disappear, even though the particular drug cocktail changed (Dennett Papers, 1874–1945; Johnson & Quinlan, 2015, 2017; Todd, 1936; Wolf, 2009). As late as 1936, lay writer Constance Todd continued her public support for TS and sought to correct inaccurate information that she (somehow) found at the Kansas City meeting of the American Medical Association. Her letter to the editor appeared in the *New York Times*, where she noted she was "one of a small group of women who have studied analgesia for twenty-three years" and claimed that she and Marguerite Tracy "introduced twilight sleep to the lay public in McClure's Magazine" in June 1914 (Todd, 1936, p. 14). She defended her article with Tracy, insisting their work was "not sensational" and "not irresponsible, but informed and accurate" (p. 14). Regardless of the pushback or censorship from technical experts, lay experts continued to recommend and defend analgesic pain relief, even decades after the American TS furor ended.

A PIVOT FROM MEDICATED BIRTH: LAY EXPERTISE IN THE MID-TWENTIETH CENTURY

As we have seen in the case of the New York City TS campaign, the early twentieth century witnessed a marked increase in hospital births among urban, wealthy white populations, a trend that would extend into the twenty-first century. According to the Centers for Disease Control and Prevention (CDC, 2014), in 1900 nearly all U.S. births occurred outside a hospital; however, the proportion of out-of-hospital births fell to 44% by 1940 and to 1% by 1969, where it remained through the 1980s. Generally, by the mid-1920s American women with economic and physical access could select from a range of pain relief methods and more births occurred in hospitals. By the early 1950s, the vast majority of middle- and upper-class white women birthed in a hospital, and drug cocktails, which could include scopolamine, kept women semiconscious during birth (Caton, 1997; Wertz, 1997; Wolf, 2009). Ultimately, the legacy of TS was control of birth, by technical experts (doctors), in the technical medical setting (hospitals). The consequences of this shift extended further than a location change. The campaign illustrates the potential for lay expertise and technical expertise to be transactional rather than simply oppositional. Moreover, the influence of lay expertise on technical expertise in the TS campaign emerges again in the history of lay advocacy for birth, particularly in the natural birth movement in the mid-twentieth century (Klassen, 2001; Leavitt, 1986).

The lay-driven birth movements that began several decades later contested these developments and critiqued patient-doctor power imbalances, particularly in the hospital delivering room. The lay experts of the 1960s and 1970s argued that laboring women lacked the ability to resist (now common) interventions, including pain relief (Sandelowski, 1984; Wolf, 2009). Historian Christa Craven (2010) outlined the particularities of the "natural childbirth" movement, which emerged in the 1950s and reflected new concerns about the consumer experience in the wake of improved maternal mortality outcomes. In the campaign for "natural" (nonmedicated) childbirth, there are similarities to the TS campaign worth noting. For example, Craven traced the emergence of the movement to "middle-class and affluent white women," who became "disillusioned with the promise of 'painless' childbirth under anesthesia and what was touted as 'vacations' to modern hospitals for childbirth" (Craven, 2010, p. 42; Leavitt, 1986; Wolf, 2009). This time around though, advocates argued in favor of less medication and less intervention. Also, similar to the TS campaign, which reasoned that women ought to have more options for how and where to give birth, some natural childbirth advocates rooted their goals in "feminist ideals of choice" (Craven, 2010, p. 43). Feminist scholars in the 1970s framed highly medicalized hospital birth practices (e.g., routine enemas, shaving, episiotomies, high doses of drugs) as particularly Western, subjective, and not necessarily superior to more "traditional" birth practices in other societies (see Kitzinger, 1980). As criticism of obstetrics mounted, some consumers protested predominant birth practices in American obstetrics by taking their business elsewhere (Sandelowski, 1984), a tactic the TSA also found effective.

Craven (2010) also detailed the particular methods activists and lay experts (mostly feminist scholars) used (e.g., finding out the C-section rates in specific hospitals). Lay activists lobbied hospitals and doctors to permit family members in the delivery room, to perform fewer medical interventions, and to encourage breastfeeding (Craven, 2010). Similar to the TS movement, lay activists and midwives in the 1950s to 1980s who advocated for rooming-in, skin-to-skin contact, and breastfeeding helped bring about the Baby-Friendly Hospital Initiative (BFHI). BFHI (2017) is a global program supported by the World Health Organization (WHO) and the United Nations Children's Fund to encourage and recognize hospitals and birthing centers offering optimal lactation environments. BFHI programs include correlative policies thought to increase the potential for a "successful" breastfeeding relationship, including skin-to-skin contact, "room-in," and rejection of pacifiers (BFHI, 2017; Merewood, Philipp, Chawla, & Cimo, 2003).

By the end of the 1970s, the wider natural childbirth movement began to wane, in part because hospitals were starting to shift their policy to reflect the desires of their consumer-patients and because the cost of "natural" childbirth services and products (e.g., breathing classes, doulas) prevented low-income women from utilizing methods similar to those of white, middle-class women, a clear limitation of the movement. Again, similar to TS, the demographic group that launched the grassroots campaign benefitted from their advocacy and expertise, but despite concerted efforts, cost hampered the possibility of widespread access, even in communities where women of color advocated for alternative birth options (Craven, 2010; Leavitt, 1986).

By the late 1980s and early 1990s, nurse-midwifery became the natural birth role within the hospital setting, which allowed for legitimacy within technical expertise. But as Craven (2010) found, this development led to accusations of selling out and co-option. "Lay" midwives, meanwhile, refused formal education based in obstetric science and avoided entanglement in medical hierarchies (p. 45). While nurse-midwives received training and maintained a precarious status within the established medical system, some practitioners rejected it entirely and built different models (e.g., midwife-assisted home birth), independent of the technical medical model (Craven, 2010). The exit of these advocates and a resurgence of antiestablishment lay expertise directed organizing focus toward new systems, achieved through a revival of midwifery training and networks and a burgeoning home birth movement (Craven, 2010; Davis-Floyd & Johnson, 2006). Some involved in the more radical arm of the natural birth movement became active after birth experiences in which physicians overrode or simply ignored women's demands (Craven, 2010; Leavitt, 1986), and many activists seeking "the natural" in their deliveries began to explore birth at home (Treichler, 1990, p. 121). By 1976, more than a dozen organizations to support home birth had emerged at both the national and regional levels (Craven, 2010). Supporters of home birth and what would be termed "unassisted birth" (birth at home without medical attendants) included countercultural activists and fundamentalist Christians, uneasy partners in the effort to reduce the primacy of technical expertise in the birthing room (Craven, 2010; Treichler, 1990). The unassisted and home birth arms of the natural childbirth movement remain peripheral today, though home births are on the rise again (Craven, 2010). One issue that sustains these campaigns might be the poor birth outcomes for mothers in the United States today (Kristof, 2017; Martin, Cillekens, & Freitas, 2017). Compared to other countries with advanced obstetric care (including both technical and lay expertise), the United States fares poorly; two or more U.S. women each day die in childbirth (Martin, Cillekens, & Freitas, 2017).

Another branch of the natural birth movement of the 1970s focused on creating alternative treatment centers to support pregnant and birthing women. In 1975, Ina May Gaskin's groundbreaking text *Spiritual Midwifery* represented the middle-class, countercultural perspective of the natural birth movement in the period; the text remains one of the most widely read of its genre (Craven, 2010). Gaskin's organization and groups like the feminist group National Organization for Women sought informed and conscious birthing practices, including home births with midwives in attendance, in contradistinction to the interventionist model popular in allopathic medicine (Gaskin, 2002, 2003; Treichler, 1990).[11] To this day, Gaskin's the Farm Midwifery Center (n.d.-b) boasts high rates of success with twin birth and vaginal birth after cesarean and no maternal deaths; Gaskin publishes widely in both lay and technical publications, and birth statistics from the Farm appear in technical literature (Duran, 1992; Gaskin, 2002, 2003, 2008). Today the Farm has a team of certified midwives for individuals seeking a birth outside of the hospital; certified (technical) midwives and nurse-midwives attend births.[12] Ironically, while Gaskin initially set out to work outside hospital systems, her success has led to formal publications and the widespread popularity of her work likely impacted the rise of BFHI and baby-friendly policies in hospital settings. The success of natural childbirth activists (nationally and regionally) and her work on the Farm reflect the transactional nature of expertise around birth. In the twentieth century, lay birth experts influenced technical expertise by rejecting it or embracing it and helping transform it in the process.

BFHI and Social Media: Translating or Circumventing Technical Expertise

Alice Callahan (2017), a trained research scientist with a doctorate in nutritional biology and fetal physiology, runs a blog called "Science of Mom: The Heart and Science of Parenting" and wrote the book *Science of Mom: A Research-Based Guide to Your Baby's First Year* (2015). Callahan uses her technical expertise to translate scientific study conclusions, related to the life cycle of early motherhood, for lay audiences. In a handful of blog posts, Callahan advocates for the continuation of natural childbirth and baby-friendly hospital practices, such as rooming-in (Callahan, 2015), skin-to-skin contact (Callahan, 2013), and breastfeeding for more than 12 months (Callahan, 2012). Her Facebook page (which also advertises her book and outlines new research) is an excellent example of ways in which lay audiences can interact with technical experts on the Internet. Callahan answers blog commenters directly in the comments section on her blog and FB page (Callahan, 2013), particularly to clarify research claims. For example, in October 2013, Callahan posted a piece titled "The Magic and Mystery of Skin to Skin." In the comments, a poster asked, "Did you find any research about skin-to-skin helping with temp regulation?" (Callahan, 2013, n.p.). In response, Callahan referenced statistical significance and concluded, "My take is that the mean probably doesn't tell the whole story" (Callahan, 2013, n.p.). At the end of the chain, in which a number of people shared their personal stories, she said, "Thank you all so much for telling your stories. They're really helping me frame the way I want to talk about this in the book" (Callahan, 2013, n.p.). This act of translation confounds the technical/lay binary. Is Callahan acting as a technical or lay expert on FB? Or both? On social media, it is hard to track exactly how language impacts practice, particularly since many of these conversations are happening in insular communities where members have access to a "private" group or have self-selected and arrived at a site like Callahan's because of their perspective and practices. Unlike TS, where lay activists co-opted the language and presented it to a wide-ranging audience in popular publications, social media provide expansive access alongside insulation and reciprocal dialogue.

Some individuals have critiqued BFHI for being unfriendly toward mothers (Grose, 2014). New mothers who struggle to breastfeed report feelings of guilt or shame during interactions with technical experts such as nurses and lactation consultants at baby-friendly (BF) hospitals (Howe-Heyman & Lutenbacher, 2016; Strauss, 2016; Tuteur, 2016). Some women may feel pressured into breastfeeding and/or shamed for deciding not to. Additionally, BFHI is critiqued for classist assumptions because women are not allowed to be alone and some have to pay for their support partner to be there while rooming-in with a baby in the hospital (Howe-Heyman & Lutenbacher, 2016; Strauss, 2016). A woman who is alone and fatigued from childbirth may be at risk for injury if left alone with an infant (Pearson, 2016). For example, Maggie (author) gave birth in a hospital a few months from receiving its BFHI certification. After staff left Maggie and her daughter to initiate breastfeeding unattended, her daughter had a spontaneous breathing lapse and ended up in the NICU for observation.

BFHI policies (e.g., rooming-in) also prompt pushback. In an online article for parenting source sheknows.com, Ashley Austrew (2016) remembered her birth in a baby-friendly hospital: "By the time I got home from the hospital, my nipples were so cracked and damaged they'd bleed every time I tried to feed my daughter. I hadn't truly slept in days, and I was so overwhelmed by how little help I'd gotten in the hospital that I had a complete breakdown. Instead of encouraging loving attachment, my hospital experience actually just left me feeling drained and resentful" (n.p.). Austrew reviewed BFHI practices and took particular issue with rooming-in. She found her options limited and noted that she had no choice about the practice. Similar to other online publications and social media platforms, the conversation in the comments section for Austrew's article revealed public perceptions of expertise, and as expected, commenters did not seek to soften their delivery: "What's really disconcerting about this is that medical 'experts' (using that term loosely here) are the very people who are supposed to know . . . and yet this sounds like some new-age-holistic-homeopathic-woo-woo-Dr. Oz s**t. . . . It's appalling" (n.p.). Alternatively, some commenters never felt forced, pressured, or denied: "So I had the opposite experience . . . it was lovely" (Austrew, 2016, n.p.). Another commenter said after her births she sent her babies to the nursery and took a sleeping pill, to which an online critic responded, referring to the need for the baby to eat: "What would you have done if there weren't nurses and hospitals . . . what kind of mother are you?" As in other circumstances related to the life cycle of early motherhood, people go online seeking to vent or get support when they feel let down by technical experts, but in consulting lay experts, they take the risk of anonymous judgment.

Interestingly, a number of technical experts addressed other online commenters, giving their position and length of service, such as "I am a labor and delivery and nursery nurse for 22 years," before offering their views and opinions on BFHI (Austrew, 2016, n.p.). Many expressed frustration over BFHI practices, lamenting that "there is no size fits all" and "I think this whole baby-friendly theme has been a successful way for hospitals to cut costs" (Austrew, 2016, n.p.). Other technical experts expressed dismay over the pushback, sought to clarify policies and expectations, and suggested that readers view these policies on a case-by-case basis: "I think it depends on the hospital and I work in a baby friendly hospital . . . we do utilize rooming in. . . . It makes me sad to hear things like this. We are a baby friendly hospital and . . . we do not do these things. . . . Not all hospitals that are baby friendly are like this" (Austrew, 2016, n.p.). Here technical experts both agreed and disagreed with lay perspectives, but largely supported BFHI in their institutions.

Online articles are not the only locations where technical experts enter "lay" spaces on social media and offer advice. As new mothers, we joined several "closed" or "private" Facebook groups (unlike Callahan's, which is public) for mothers as we tried to navigate the lay-expert spectrum in our parenting and on behalf of our children. In these "private" spaces, Bethany viewed a conversation in which group members strategized how to circumvent baby-friendly hospital practices, specifically resistance to the use of formula and pacifiers.

> I have a friend who is a mother-baby nurse at a "baby friendly" hospital. . . . If you go in from the beginning saying you are formula feeding . . . you shouldn't get too much pressure. The stats the hospital has to get for BF only count those who come in saying they are BF or "going to try." . . . If you go in from the beginning saying you are formula, you're not counted towards the percentage of the hospital has to have who go home BF (80% I believe). . . . My friend told me to be sure to state from the beginning . . . I understand my decision and am educated on it . . . I am not going to be happy if anyone gives me crap about it either. Also—they should not have any pacifiers at baby friendly hospitals, be sure to bring your own. (Facebook, 2016)

In the course of this conversation, a technical expert offered advice about how to circumvent BFHI policies: "I'm a mother/baby nurse at [name of hospital] and we will give you formula if you request!:) like many have said bc we are a baby friendly hospital we have to encourage exclusive breastfeeding but we will abso-lutely give you formula if you want it! don't worry about bringing your own!" (Facebook, 2016). Facebook is unique in that it allows technical and lay experts to interact directly, outside of traditional medical settings. This external contact can be helpful or confusing, especially when individuals are unsure or unaware of what BFHI entails. Given that a technical expert (labor and delivery nurse) pro-vides a lay expert (birthing mother) with specific strategies to circumvent BFHI hospital policies, how is expertise "working" here? Again, these exchanges and interactions complicate the notion that lay prowess and technical expertise act mainly in opposition to each other or are siloed by context (Klassen, 2001).

Even though the policies and practices of BF hospitals grew out of grassroots activist efforts to depathologize hospital birth, BF hospitals can also create a cli-mate in which some mothers feel pressured to have a birth and recovery experi-ence they do not desire or cannot attain. In fact, all health choices individuals make that impact the mother-child dyad are complicated and contested, and available information continues to alter promulgated expertise, policies, and individual choices. BFHI patient policies are designed for a very specific mother, one who is in good health and able to understand and utilize BFHI-specific infor-mation and who has a supportive partner and/or family/community network as well as extensive access to supports outside of the hospital, including lactation experts. Accessing these experts requires a phone or reliable Internet and a com-puter or smartphone and insurance or funds to pay for support or transporta-tion to receive free support at a La Leche League meeting. These particulars narrow the pool of individuals "suited" to BFHI policies and procedures. It is unfortunate and counterproductive to their efforts that BFHI hospitals do not include specific provisions for white working-class or African American women or members of other minority groups who breastfeed at lower rates than white middle-class women (Blum, 1999). Barriers to breastfeeding, skin-to-skin con-tact time, and rooming-in include maternal-child issues that impact people of all races and classes, ranging from an HIV/AIDS diagnosis to drug or alcohol addiction, use of certain medications including antithyroid medication, use of mood-altering drugs, medical conditions such as severe eating disorders, untreated tuberculosis, or severe anemia, breast reduction or augmentation, and breast cancer and/or mastectomies (Li, Fein, Chen, & Gummer-Strawn, 2008). Some caretakers struggle to read materials in English or for religious reasons have restrictions on baring a breast in public places. Given our inadequate health-care system and the stark deficiencies in our leave policy for employed parents, uninsured mothers and those without maternity, paternity, or caretaker leave cannot access or have very limited access to the resources they need. How does BFHI engage adoptive and foster parents taking home newborns? It doesn't. Problematically, universal access to a particular birth method or policy is not the best solution for everyone.

A century of advocacy continues to broaden options available to birthing women, though structural hurdles, such as class-based access to birth centers, remain. The rise of birth centers with hospital-admitting privileges reflects the transactional nature of the dialogue between lay and technical experts throughout the twentieth century and the increase of options between home birth and hospital. Birth centers may be more economical than hospitals as well—since anesthesia (e.g., epidurals) and doctors are not a part of these births and patients go home hours instead of days later, the final bill is much lower than that for a hospital birth (Galewitz, 2015; Woo, Milstein, & Platchek, 2016). As Craven (2010) discovered, access to birth centers and other natural childbirth modalities is limited geographically; there are fewer in rural and high-poverty urban areas. Despite access issues, there is now an American Association of Birth Centers, and studies on birth center outcomes appear in publications such as *Journal of Midwifery and Women's Health* (Galewitz, 2015); national organizations advocating for birth centers and this journal exemplify the success of extant expertise impacting mainstream technical medical practice.

Importantly, the campaigns for both TS in the early twentieth century and natural childbirth in the mid-twentieth century show how individuals who reject dominant social structures influence technical experts. Here, the introduction of BFHI in the technical medical setting and the rise of birth centers illustrate the potential for antiestablishment lay expertise to impact technical expertise and practice. Today, discussions around birth options in legislative bodies (Craven, 2010), in individual practices (e.g., obstetric and midwifery), among professionals and/or patients, and on social media continue to complicate categories of expertise. How might one categorize a technical expert (e.g., a labor and delivery nurse) in a lay social media space (e.g., FB, Twitter, blogs) providing advice on circumventing current technical expertise? Does this represent the pinnacle of advocacy and activism, fostered by social media? The dominant, virtually unquestioned technical/lay expertise binary fails to represent the complex lives of female-identified individuals today—in part because it cannot contend with the intersectionality of oppressions faced by so many new mothers.

The idea that lay expertise is, by definition, grassroots and intuitively based belies the notion that lay expertise can claim to ascertain what is best for all female-identified individuals at all times and in all places. No expertise can do this. Furthermore, characterizing all lay expertise as grassroots ignores the ways that lay and technical expertise was and continues to be transactional, particularly for lay experts who work within available power structures. What is certain is that health systems must still assess the short- and long-term impacts of their employees disseminating "an expert opinion" on social media. For now, we have yet to see what this means for choice in health care, inside and outside the delivery room.

PART III

THE POSTPARTUM PERIOD

THE "FOURTH TRIMESTER"

CHAPTER 5

"ONE OF THE MOST CURIOUS CHARITIES IN THE WORLD"

INFANT INCUBATION AS SIDESHOW AND/OR MEDICAL SPECIALTY

I felt like an outsider who didn't belong. . . . For the majority of the first two months of Lidia's stay, I simply sat beside [her] incubator, watching the wavy lines dance on the monitor, waiting for the next opportunity to hold her.
—Michalik (2017)

In 2012, 21-year-old Madeleine Michalik and her spouse Mariusz welcomed their daughter, Lidia. Born at the gestational age of 25 weeks and four days, Lidia was 13.5 inches long and weighed exactly two pounds (Michalik, 2017). Later, Madeleine received a diagnosis of "incompetent cervix," which helped explain Lidia's early arrival (see Goldstein & Wolff, 1964, for an earlier use of "incompetent cervix"). Madeleine recalled Lidia's vulnerability the first time she touched her daughter after the birth: "As we pulled up to her plastic house, Lidia's nurse . . . lifted the blanket that was shielding Lidia from the bright fluorescent hospital lighting . . . she encouraged me to place my finger in her hand after showing me how to open the incubator door, and [her] small hand latched on tight" (Michalik, 2017). While Madeleine struggled to bond with and learn to care for her daughter, she participated in practices and rituals established more than a century before at late nineteenth- and early twentieth-century fairs, exhibitions, and sideshows focused on sharing new technologies for premature babies. These events showcased the power and lifesaving potential of applications such as electric lighting to warm premature babies. Incubation technology emerged first in French maternity wards, but then became a fixture at World's Fair exhibitions and Coney Island sideshows. Today neonatal intensive care units (NICUs), which focus on

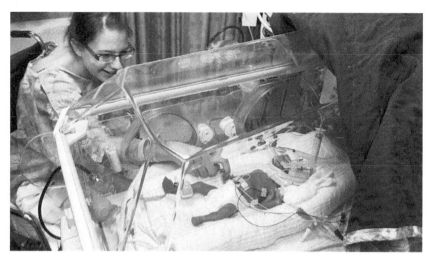

Figure 2. Lidia and Maddy in the NICU.

the care and growth of premature infants or "preemies," are found in the more privatized setting of the hospital, not the sideshow. NICUs reveal the vulnerability of premature babies and highlight concerns around mothers caring for babies with intricate care needs and delicate health (see Figure 2). Unlike today, mothers in the first half of the twentieth century were deliberately sidelined; far from being seen by technical experts as potential collaborative lay experts who would become primary caretakers, they were construed as incompetent and even to blame for having had a premature baby.

In the first three months of Lidia's stay (see Figure 2), Madeleine paid nearly $100 to park her car and view, hold, and care for her daughter (Michalik, 2017); between 1901 and 1940, audiences paid to view babies in the exhibit run by "Incubator Doctor" Martin Couney, the putative "father of neonatology" (Brick, 2005; "How," 2016; Liebling, 1939, "Life under," 2016; "Martin, A.," 1950; Silverman, 1979). In the first weeks after Lidia's birth, Madeleine observed as nurses performed the bulk of her daughter's care, while neonatologists dropped in for weekly checkups and evaluations. In 1906, parents could visit their children for free at Couney's exhibit, observe their children through incubator walls and/or glass panes, and view nurses performing the bulk of their care ("Baby incubators," 1901; "The dangers," 1898; Dorman, 1929; "Hints," 1903; Liebling, 1939; "Life under," 2016; "Ranson," 1933; Silverman, 1979).[1]

When we began this research, we wondered, who actually "mothers" NICU babies? Is this a technical/lay expert partnership? Is the technology taking the place of human interaction in meaningful, yet necessary ways? How does technology disrupt the traditional nursing care in these units (Sandelowski, 2000)? Is the NICU what Parks (2010) referred to as "cyborg mothering," with its ventilators, peripherally inserted central catheter (PICC) lines, and monitors? Throughout this portion of our project, our questions and definitions became more complicated and more perplexing and finally collapsed entirely. What are the implications for mothers, and for maternal and neonatal care, when expertise extends beyond the traditional medical care team and into a glass box on the boardwalk? What if, in the early twentieth century, an apparently uncredentialled showman at Coney Island, a lay expert, sold himself as a doctor and in the process he and his team kept thousands of premature babies from death? What difference would this make for how we discuss the care of preemies today?

In this chapter, we explore the complicated story of Martin A. Couney and his infant incubator exhibits, the complicated history of medical practitioners and incubator use among medical practitioners, and the modern-day NICU. Today's NICU is entirely technological yet imbued with explicit emotional and behavioral expectations, particularly for those labeled "mother," and also integrated with both technical and lay-based support systems. Our focus on Couney stemmed from a recent resurgence of interest in his story on social media, which mythologized his contributions to neonatal care. These social media narratives of Couney's work raise a number of questions about contemporary views of expertise in the life cycle of early motherhood. Between 1904 and the early 1940s, Couney's sideshow approach to neonatal care shocked and wooed a public newly interested in medical issues and excited about medical technology. Therefore, our focus on his history within neonatology is twofold: we examine how discourses surrounding Couney infiltrated that of neonatology as well as the ongoing perpetuation of Couney as a maverick operating outside of traditional power structure of medicine to save lives (see also Breslaw, 2012; Janik, 2014). Although Internet publications today guide the focus back to Couney as the singular hero at the heart of the effort, the nursing staff and parents who raised the babies he worked with rarely receive their due. We aim to bring lay expertise back into the story by highlighting the role that parents play in the lives of premature babies (preemies), by examining the contributions of NICU nurses as technical experts, and by wrestling with what type of expert Couney was—lay, technical, or something else altogether—and how his story connects to today's neonatal care.

For the purposes of this chapter, technical experts are defined as the individuals interacting directly with lifesaving or life-supportive technologies, including nurses, doctors, hospital technicians, occupational therapists, and other practitioners trained to help preemies adapt to and survive in the world. As babies grow and transition toward "graduation," parents step into this technical expertise as well, learning the specificities of feeding, bathing, and other kinds of care specific to preemies (e.g., preventing unnecessary germ exposure, monitoring PICC lines).[2] Lay experts include parents, friends and family members, and online community groups and contacts supporting the parents and their child through their journey from the NICU to the transition home. This form of expertise also includes activists and advocates of NICU families offering support through online communities (e.g., babycenter.com, Facebook [FB]), foundations (e.g., Graham's Foundation [GF]), in-hospital programming (e.g., NICU parents dinners and purple butterfly programs), and Kangaroo care volunteers.

As with other topics in this book, the history of incubation on Coney Island highlights the often blurry line between technical and lay expertise—Couney, a man who may not have had any technical or even formal training, became a noted and celebrated (for some) leader in neonatal medicine in the early twentieth century. Moreover, we might not know of Couney today if it weren't for social media, which continues to highlight "medical mavericks" in a time when confidence in technical expertise and traditional health care is tenuous and conflicted.

A Brief History of Machine-Based Incubation

As historian Jeffrey Baker (2000) argued, the development of the incubator was the catalyst for a "three-way contest" between obstetricians, pediatricians, and mothers (p. 321; see also Baker, 1993, 1996). Between 1880 and 1950, interest in the incubator and its use in American medicine shifted as many hospitals established neonatal units with incubators to support premature babies (then called "weaklings"; Budin, 1907). Before obstetricians and then pediatricians became the technical experts who monitor and guide the life cycle of early motherhood, midwives and mothers often focused on maintaining warmth (e.g., with laundry baskets and hot water bottles) and providing breast milk for babies born early or "on time" (Baker, 2000; "Exhibit," 1901; Liebling, 1939; Oppenheimer, 1996; Ranson, 1933; Zahorsky, 1905). As discussed in chapter 3, midwives oversaw the vast majority of births in the early twentieth century; over time, pain relief and other amenities eventually attracted women with means to hospital birth.

Most scholars credit the first human incubator to obstetrician Dr. Stéphane Tarnier, who had an instrument maker from the city zoo install one at Paris's Maternité Hospital in 1880 (Baker, 1996, 2000; "Exhibit," 1901; Raju, 2011). In 1883, Dr. Credé of Leipzig claimed his double-walled model was superior to and predated the Tarnier model (Baker, 1996, 2000; "Exhibit," 1901). Tarnier's research and his impressive results had a direct impact on medical interest in incubation throughout Western Europe, even though the first "infant nurseries" in hospitals had a dismal survival rate, in part due to intake of preemies days rather than hours after birth (Baker, 1996, 2000; Silverman, 1979).[3]

From the 1890s and well into the twentieth century, various obstetricians and public health officials publicly questioned the benefit of attempting to save these "weaklings." In this and other health situations, the ideology of eugenics (connected to the idea of "race suicide" in the United States) impacted ideas among technical and lay experts of who should be saved in medical emergencies. In the first four decades of the twentieth century, physicians, public health officials, and even politicians, absorbing and promoting nativist and racist fears, expressed concern about the decline of the "native" white population of the United States in a context of high immigration and higher rates of reproduction in impoverished communities (Baker, 1993, 1996; Bederman, 1995; Kline, 2001). Eugenic methods included sterilization of the presumably "unfit," and in some cases prohibitive marital laws to prevent the reproduction of unwanted, inheritable characteristics such as blindness and lack of intelligence (Dennett Papers, 1874–1945; Kline, 2001; Reedy, 2000). There was widespread support for eugenics, and these prejudices and fears complicated the notion of saving premature babies. People wondered aloud if such babies represented hereditary "failure," nature's way of weeding out babies, and some argued that these babies should not be saved (Baker, 1996, 2000; Day, 2013; Reedy, 2000).

Nevertheless, after Dr. Tarnier, obstetrician Pierre Constant Budin took on the "weaklings'" cause (Baker, 1996, 2000; Reedy, 2000). Dr. Budin advocated for premature babies and their mothers to be treated together, moving small glass incubators next to the mother's bed and employing wet nurses to feed these babies until their mother's milk came in (Baker, 2000). He eventually published a textbook on the care of premature infants (Budin, 1907). While in Nice, France, Alexandre Lion created a much more technologically advanced (and expensive) incubator model, which he charged individuals to view, without live babies in them (Baker, 1996, 2000). According to Baker (1996, 2000), Lion ran a *Kinderbrutanstalt* or "child hatchery" (later attributed to Couney) at the Berlin Exposition in 1896. The show was such a success that incubator shows became a regular fixture at World's Fairs and expositions and medical publications took note, perhaps beginning to understand the public interest in medical technology and a growing acceptance of the public display of bodies ("Baby incubators," 1901; "The dangers," 1898; "Exhibit," 1901).

While Budin focused on the incubator as an extension of the mother, Couney and pediatricians viewed the technology as a form of "artificial mothering"— an actual replacement for the mother (Greene, 2010; "Life under," 2016; "Mechanical," 1931). The notion of technological substitutes for motherhood had significant implications for approaches to both maternal care and infant care with respect to cultural questioning of maternal competence (Greene, 2010). By 1931, *Scientific American* claimed that without an incubator, "life would vanish instantly" for preemies and their "life-blood will come to them from the machine in which they are scientifically nestled" ("Mechanical," 1931, pp. 100–101). This magazine reflects the assumed power of technology and technical expertise in the early twentieth century, both of which could potentially supersede and replace mothers' abilities to birth, nourish, and care for their babies and children (see also Vandenberg-Daves, 2014).

Baker's (1996) *The Machine in the Nursery* is a masterwork in the history of incubators and incubation. He argues that doctors did not simply "reject" incubation. Instead, the historical trend toward medical specialization, the particularities of the public health movement, swiftly changing technology, costs, and conceptual disagreement around prematurity all created significant roadblocks for the institutional adoption of incubators. For our purposes in this chapter, a closer look at Couney assists us in examining definitions of lay and technical expertise as well as the contested roles played by doctors, nurses, and parents or caretakers in the early twentieth-century history of incubation. Couney's exhibition of live babies at World's Fairs and on Coney Island presaged the neonatal units familiar today in that parents became lay experts, caretakers, and advocates for their premature infants.

Sometime in the late nineteenth century, Couney started exhibiting German incubators (Altmann, likely a version of Lion's), and when he brought the exhibit to Buffalo, New York, in 1901, he launched a stateside career spanning more than four decades (Baker, 1996; Butterfield et al., 1997). The descriptions of Couney's exhibits (Coney Island or others) between 1901 and 1943 are similar: the long row of metal boxes, standing on legs, with the air piped in from outside; the tiny babies inside, wrapped at the waist with bows, mostly sleeping, with occasional "flutterings" of movement ("Baby incubators," 1901; "How," 2016; see also "Hints," 1903). Guests, including the babies' mothers, looked from behind railings or panes of glass ("Exhibit," 1901; "Hints," 1903; "Mechanical," 1931). Couney's incubator wards were showplaces, massive buildings, often with a private suite for Couney, a private room for wet nurses, and a sanitary kitchen. Photographs of the incubator did not include images of mothers caring for or observing the care of their babies; unlike today, parents were rarely present in these units ("Exhibit," 1901). At the New York World's Fair (NYWF), the exhibit boasted a suite for Couney (including a living room, bathroom, and private garden), his daughter Hildegarde (a nurse), the head nurse Madam Recht, and his personal cook and chauffeur (Libeling, 1939). Local hospitals supplied the infants (parental permission to do so is not always clear) (Liebling, 1939; "Mechanical," 1931), and registered physicians were often hired; seven nurses worked in the Coney exhibits (Dorman, 1928) (see Figures 3 and 4).

The incubators received outside air, run through a filter for purity, and temperature was maintained by a Bunsen burner, thermostat, and hand-hammered copper piping ("Exhibit," 1901; "Mechanical," 1931) (see Figures 3 and 4). The babies were fed by wet nurses, bottles, or a "nasal spoon" ("Hints," 1903; Silverman, 1979) every two to three hours. Couney reportedly said, "They are taken out of the incubators every three hours, covered in towels, taken into the nursery where they are changed and fed. They must be fed mother's milk in order to

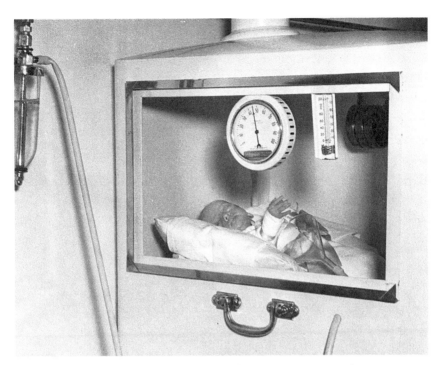

Figure 3. Infant in incubator. New York World's Fair 1939–1940 Records, Manuscripts and Archives Division, New York Public Library.

survive. Science has not succeeded in replacing the mother here" ("Mechanical," 1931, p. 180; see also "Exhibit," 1901). Still, Couney did not engage mothers in the feeding or other "cares"; his nurses performed the bulk of care for exhibit babies, which kept parents, and mothers in particular, at the periphery.

Eventually babies "graduated" to a nursery with bassinets and were fed from the bottle and/or breast before going home. Couney preferred his babies to weigh six pounds before releasing them ("Mechanical," 1931). Suggesting that the general public might have concerns about the public display of vulnerable babies, a reporter reassured readers regarding the seriousness of the exhibit: "Everywhere white tiling and nickel give not only the appearance but the reality of cleanliness. . . . The 'Q bator' is not an exhibit to appeal to the curious or vulgar . . . it is a sober, scientific exhibit, calculated to give valuable hints to mothers of children" ("Hints," 1903, p. 3). The reporter's description emphasized the remove of the mother from this pristine space. In exhibits, technology and technical expertise were designed to suggest the complete supplanting (or erasure) of the biological mother.

Despite the lavish surroundings and extensive staff, Couney and his team treated babies gratis, relying on entry fees to pay the bills in the early years. They

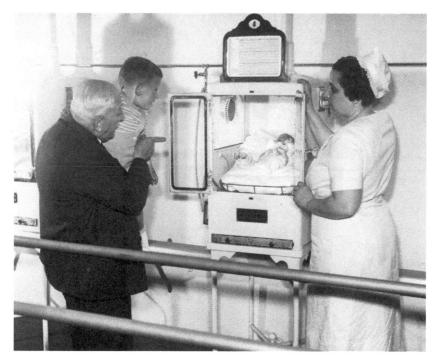

Figure 4. Infant incubator—Martin and Hildegarde Couney with boy looking at baby in incubator. New York World's Fair 1939–1940 Records, Manuscripts and Archives Division, New York Public Library.

nonetheless turned a handsome profit (Brick, 2005; "How," 2016; Liebling, 1939; Silverman, 1979). Dorman (1928) claimed that in 25 years of Coney Island exhibits, Couney's team cared for more than 6,000 preemies (p. 3; see also "Mechanical," 1931); an episode of PBS's *American Experience* reported that "of 8,000 infants brought to Dr. Couney over the years, 7,500 have survived" (Burns & Squires, 2006).

Mothering and Early Twentieth-Century Technical "Discipline" in Incubation Wards

Martin Couney remains one of the most positively portrayed and publicly beloved specialist practitioners in the past century. But his distrust of mothers of premature babies extended to the mothers' preconception and pregnancy behavior. He did not mince words about the behavior of pregnant women and the direct impact their choices had on premature birth. In a 1933 article, "Scolds Mothers of Babies Born Prematurely," he pitted "modern science" against "modern mothers" (p. 12). He wondered if improving technology made for more haphazard mothers, saying he had "mixed feelings about the chances" of seeing a normal, healthy child, noting the rate of premature births had "doubled" since 1893, though he provided no evidence for this claim ("Scolds," 1933, p. 12). He blamed the rise on women working (specifically overworking) and dancing, malnutrition due to the Great Depression, "hypernervousness" rooted in the "strain of modern life," eating lunch at delicatessens, and traffic accidents ("Scolds," 1933).[4] He therefore implicated a combination of poor personal choices and the environmental conditions shifting for American women in the first half of the twentieth century. Wondering what women could do about it, Couney argued that pregnant women could prevent premature births, but they would not because "you can't tell a girl today a thing . . . they won't listen . . . we can't do anything with them. But we can save their babies" ("Scolds," 1933, p. 12). Couney's paternalism, condescension, and mother blame were not unique. Doctors, public health workers, and progressive activists at this time expressed similar worry and judgments about "modern" women. Generally speaking, technical experts did not trust mothers (see also Kline, 2001).

Dr. Silverman (1979), also a neonatologist and an unofficial Couney biographer, noted that Couney was "hurt" by the fact that parents visited infrequently and were not easily persuaded to take their babies home when the time came (see also Day, 2013). While Couney is often depicted as a kind and sweet man, his views on contemporary mothers and parents were dour and no doubt influenced by the particular conditions in which he came to know parents: conditions of enforced separations in the early weeks and months of babies' lives (Astrinsky, 2007; Brown, 1994; Liebling, 1939; "Scolds," 1933; Silverman, 1979). Couney referred to the difficulties of transition from ward to home life, particularly the relationships of parents with their premature babies (Brown, 1994; Silverman, 1979); this theme repeatedly emerges in twentieth-century literature on neonatology and is echoed in contemporary experiences. For Couney baby Beth Allen's mother, this separation provoked fear and anxiety about her ability to care for Beth at home, something she was not eager to do (Allen, 2017). Similarly, in 2012, Madeleine reported that the transition home with Lidia was "filled with tension, stress, and doctors' appointments" (Michalik, 2017).

Not surprisingly, we also found that some mothers had no interest in bringing their babies to Coney Island, fearing their infants would end up in a "freak show" (Astrinsky, 2007; "Life under," 2016). In these cases, such as with Beth Allen and Lucille Horn, their fathers fought for their survival just after birth, while their mothers remained in recovery at the hospital. Horn's father, for example, wrapped her in blankets and brought her to the "incubator doctor" in a taxi (Allen, 2017; Astrinsky, 2007; "The freak," 2015). Silverman (1979) uncovered a 1915 picture of a father bringing his son home on what was termed "graduation day." Through a series of email communications, 76-year-old Beth Allen relayed to us that her father took the photographs she treasures at the Couney exhibit. Allen remembers her parents took her to visit Couney "on fathers' day" and attended his funeral in 1950 (Astrinsky, 2007). Couney viewed himself as a surrogate parent; on surviving baby Katherine's photograph, Couney wrote, "To my dear little Katherine from her foster father" ("Life under," 2016, n.p.).

Neonatal Nurses: Hidden Actors in the Couney Myth

At the Couney exhibits, a handful of nurses and wet nurses lived and worked around the clock (Astrinsky, 2007; Liebling, 1939; Silverman, 1979). For over 40 years, Madam Recht, lead nurse of early incubator adopter Dr. Budin, directed the nursing staff at Couney's exhibit (Gartner & Gartner, 1992; Liebling, 1939; "Life under," 2016; Silverman, 1979; "The Victorian," 1897). Famed *New Yorker* reporter A. J. Liebling (1939) documented that nurses in Couney's incubator exhibits felt that "making [a baby] grow is vicarious motherhood" (p. 24). Due to his focus on "mother's milk" and touch for the health of his preemies, Couney had exacting standards for both nurses and wet nurses. Dietary restrictions for wet nurses were unbending—if he found they ate a hot dog or indulged in an orange soda elsewhere at Coney Island, they were summarily fired (Liebling, 1939).[5] Nurse Lundeen, nursing director of Dr. Hess's "incubator station" at Sarah Lawrence Children's Hospital (Baker, 1993, p. 441; see also Baker, 1996, 2000; Gartner & Gartner, 1992; Silverman, 1979), worked directly with Couney at Chicago's Century of Progress Exposition from 1933 to 1934.[6] In an interview with renowned neonatologist Dr. William A. Silverman (1979), Lundeen expressed disgust over the "showmanship" aspects of Couney's exhibit (e.g., the small clothes, the diamond ring on babies' wrists for the audience), but had ample praise for Madam Recht's management of the unit as well as the overall standard of care for babies in the incubator. According to Dorman (1928), Couney said, "Of course, they require the best that science can give. But while my nurses are efficient, I wouldn't have a woman in the place who did not love children. That's something that's born in women—the mother heart—and I wouldn't have the best specialist who didn't really love babies. The babies respond to affection like flowers to the sun—they sense it, somehow" (p. 3). In Couney exhibits, nurses acted as secondary technical experts and their around-the-clock care of preemies created a kind of mother-expert hybrid, in which they "mothered" preemies in the most involved form of "scientific parenting" popular in the early twentieth century (Apple, 1995; Ehrenreich & English, 1978; Grant, 2012; Vandenberg-Daves, 2014).

Other nurses also engaged in mother-expert hybrid roles, but in formal medical settings. In Dr. Hess and Lundeen's incubator ward in Chicago, nurses were trained professionals who set up a program to transition preemies from hospital to home, and they encouraged parents to learn about proper care prior to discharge as early as the 1920s and 1930s (Reedy, 2000). Other wards were not as open to parental involvement. Instead, nurses limited or even banned parental visiting, fearing the spread of epidemic disease, such as influenza, measles, typhoid, and pertussis. For this same reason, wards regularly "aired and painted" rooms, though painting did little to remove germs (Reedy, 2000, p. 119).

It is unclear whether the neonatal hospital practice from the 1920s and 1930s resulted from the popularity of Couney's exhibits, although Hess and Couney did work together at the Chicago World's Fair, so it is possible that they informed one another's work. Despite Hess and Lundeen's focus on parental education, the environment in both Couney's exhibit and Hess's ward was not parent-friendly. They were built for medical technology and technical expertise. The increasingly technical prenatal space and the expanding need for specially trained professionals to care for both the preemie and incubator technology paralleled the movement of birth from home to hospital during this period, limiting the need for and relevance of lay experts in the birth and early life of infants.

Today, similar to Lundeen and Recht's day, NICU nurses perform the vast majority of day-to-day care and parent education. One nurse noted, "We have many, many pamphlets and educational materials we give parents when they first arrive on the unit and throughout their stay. We have a welcome packet, discharge guidelines, bottle feeding guidelines, etc. Before discharge, we require parents to take a 'Baby Care' class, and watch 'Safe Sleep' and 'Purple Cry' videos" (Masi, 2017). However, the learning curve and access to preemies for parents are vastly different even from the "liberal" policies in Lundeen's ward in Chicago. Madeleine visited Lidia around the clock, and her "kangaroo" skin-to-skin sessions had to be at least three hours long; Madeleine and her spouse took part in more and more of Lidia's "cares," including sponge baths, weight checks, and repositioning her body and some of her tracking devices, such as the "pulse ox" (Michalik, 2017). Elisa Miller Quinlan (2017) and her spouse engaged in care immediately as well: "The nurses encouraged me from day one to be involved with our baby's care such as taking her temperature, changing her diaper, feeding her, and doing kangaroo care," she said. Typically, nurses play a vital role in the early life of a premature baby, particularly in educating parents about safe techniques for "cares," but neither nurses nor the technology simply replaces or supplants the role of the parent in the incubation period. Instead, the nurse-parent relationship (technical-lay expert) is more symbiotic, constantly seeking to engage with parents and prepare them to bring their babies home.

COUNEY RECYCLED: SOCIAL MEDIA AND THE (LAY?) CHARLATAN IN A WHITE COAT

Martin Couney's story is debated both by scholars and by an ever-surfacing set of popular discussions and mythology. The inconsistencies, contradictions, and gaps in the story of Couney and his influence reverberate in today's social media, adding new layers to an attempt to understand the role of his expertise.

The mythos of Couney is revived anew each time a new scholar or journalist discovers his story (Brick, 2005; Brown, 1994; Darnell, Hampshire, & Orchard, 2016; Eltman, 2015; "Life under," 2016; Pascetta, 2014), one of his former patients dies after living into their 80s or 90s (Dwyer, 2017; Eltman, 2017; "The freak," 2015), or Hollywood becomes interested.[7] An upcoming film promises to show how Couney "was initially shunned by the medical community" and that medical professionals "sought to close down the exhibit," in yet another recapitulation of the simplified myths in Couney's record and role in American medical history (N'Duka, 2017, n.p.). Darnell, Hampshire, and Orchard (2016) reported that Couney earned his medical degree in Leipzig and studied with Budin. They also alleged that Couney included only white babies in the exhibits (Darnell, Hampshire, & Orchard, 2016). While we cannot show evidence proving nonwhite admissions (there is no surviving admissions paperwork), this assertion runs counter to other scholars' findings of racial and ethnic integration in Couney exhibits (Brown, 1994; Liebling, 1939; Prentice, 2016a; Ranson, 1933).[8]

Present-day social media depictions of Couney are almost universally positive, and many recount inaccuracies that surfaced over and over in the accounts of Couney written between 1900 and 1940. Some of the overarching narrative originated with Couney, and a significant portion of it remains uncertain at best, entirely unsubstantiated at worst. But what does this mean for the importance of Couney in the history of neonatology and as a technical or lay expert? As social media platforms (e.g., FB, Twitter) cut into television supremacy as *the* source of news and information, particularly for individuals under the age of 50 (Mitchell, Gottfried, Barthel, & Shearer, 2016), previously printed myths about Couney are diffuse. The myths resurface on Twitter, a powerful tool, although they are prone to misinformation in stories as nuanced as this, given the 280-character limit: "Inventor, Dr. Couney" (BabyWeConnect, 2017) and "#ConeyIsland sideshow saved more than 5k preemies" (Coney Island History, 2017) fail to uncover the inconsistencies in Couney's story and ultimately his impact on neonatal medicine. Digital news outlets can provide more information but often repeat unverifiable claims: "Dr. Martin Couney, a pioneer in the use of incubators . . . estimated he saved 7500 to 8500 babies" (Associated Press, 2015). Couney helped pioneer the use of incubators, but his professional status and the number of babies saved through his care are harder to prove. These claims entrench his status as a medical maverick, an identity that continues to play well with the American public.

As Janik (2014) demonstrated, popular interest in medical practitioners acting outside the bounds of "traditional" medicine has deep historical roots. In the antebellum South, interest in alternate traditions (particularly Thomsonism, with its "antielitist" approach; see also McMillen, 1990, p. 12) was, in part, a reaction to perceived northern claims of academic superiority as well as resistance to popular medical systems associated with abolition (such as homeopathy; Weiner & Hough, 2012). Hence, these alternative options also allowed individuals with particular political or social views to choose medical practices based on those alliances. Second, seeking out and utilizing alternative or "eclectic" medical systems in the unrestrained medical marketplace of the nineteenth century offered Americans an opportunity to avoid treatments often referred to as "heroic," which could be ineffective or even dangerous (e.g., Breslaw, 2012; Janik, 2014; McMillen, 1990; Starr, 1982; Weiner & Hough, 2012). This revived interest also reflects the tensions in our health care system today, including a resistance to power hierarchies and rising costs in traditional medicine, and helps explain the growing market for and interest in lay medical practice on social media, which we explored in our first chapter on fertility. On social media, lay practitioners offer individual empowerment and choice, even when their methods recycle previous technical expertise (e.g., nineteenth- and early twentieth-century methods) or are cost-prohibitive.

Today, the focus on Couney's "outsider" status highlights the long history of American fascination with antiestablishment medicine. Couney himself spent his life between categories. While he eschewed formal studies, scholarly publications, and, we suspect, actual medical licenses, he insisted on an ethical, sanitary, technologically advanced incubator exhibit and a highly trained, professional support staff of technical experts (see also Raju, 2011). In part, Couney's personal history and status are difficult to decipher because he repeatedly made a number of claims that remained unexamined for nearly 30 years after his death (Butterfield et al., 1997; Prentice, 2016a, 2016b; Silverman, 1979, 1980). Couney stated that "the incubator idea is very old. . . . After studying at Leipsig, Berlin, Paris, I developed and patented the one I use. . . . Of course, I did not originate the incubator idea. I have taken medals at all the world's fairs" (Dorman, 1928, p. 3; see also Eltman, 2015). In 1931, Couney said he had worked on the incubator in exhibits for "thirty-five years," beginning during his days "as an intern in the Hospital L'Enfant Jesus in Paris" ("Mechanical," p. 102). He asserted that he "ignored" hospital rules to improve incubators for preemies out of "pity" and that he developed his version with the Muencke brothers in Germany ("Mechanical," 1931, pp. 102–103). Regarding his survival rates, one reporter said, "Dr. M.A. Couney of Berlin" lost just "6 out of 56 infants at the Pan-American" exhibition, declared "4 out of 32 at Luna Park last year [1903], and but 3 out of 38 at Dreamland this year," making his stats better than the median of 85% other publications reported for Couney, such as the *Journal of American Medicine* ("Incubator graduates," 1904, p. 7; see also "Exhibit," 1901; "Incubator babies at," 1940; "Life under," 2016; "Mechanical," 1931; "Scolds," 1933).

The confirmable "truth" about Martin Couney is slippery. He is hard to categorize in part because he began his work in the age before extensive documentation of personal identification and he moved around Europe and the United States before settling in New York City. Combined with his background as a German Jewish man (Prentice, 2016a, 2016b; Silverman, 1979), the historical context helps explain the lack of a clear paper trail. Couney himself provided varying details about his educational and family background, his professional qualifications, the spelling of his name, and even his birthplace. For example, his birthplace is alternatively listed as Berlin or Germany ("Incubator graduates," 1904; "Martin A.," 1950), Breslau, Poland (Gartner & Gartner, 1992; Silverman, 1979; Snow, 1981), or Alsace, France (Brick, 2005; Brown, 1994; Gartner & Gartner, 1992; Silverman, 1979; Snow, 1981). After searching archival documents, journalist Claire Prentice (2016b) credits Krotoschen, Germany, and December 30, 1869, as his place and date of birth. On a 1904 American passport application, Couney reported his arrival to America on the *Gellert* in 1888. When Couney naturalized in Omaha in 1898, he stated continuous residence in Nebraska since 1888 (Prentice, 2016b, p. 57), though he later told reporter A. J. Liebling (1939) he saw Omaha during his first "visit" to the United States (p. 23). If the 1888 arrival date is accurate, it would have been difficult for Couney to complete the education and training he avowed before his initial arrival to the United States. His naturalization claims also call into question his attendance at exhibitions in Berlin in 1896 and London in 1897. There is ample evidence of a "Martin Coney" at Earl's Court, meaning his naturalization paperwork contains at least one falsehood.

Claims about Couney's status and success as a technical expert are also hard to prove. Neither the *Lancet* nor Couney himself alleged his technical expertise in medicine at the Earl's Court Exhibition in 1897. Couney fought for recognition as an ethical showman, nothing more. He did not refer to himself as a physician for the first 33 years of his work with premature babies. The first time he did so was on a U.S. census in 1930: previously he had called himself an "inventor," and on his 1903 marriage certificate he claimed he was in the profession of "surgical instruments," while in 1888 the *Gellert* listed Couney as a "merchant" (Prentice, 2016b, pp. 56–57). Even his given name is up for debate: Prentice notes that Couney's siblings preferred the spelling "Coney," which we see in his signature under the Earl's Court editorial (Schenkein & Coney, 1897). The previously noted success rate of 85% is also a problematic claim because Couney's statistics are difficult to confirm (Baker, 1996; Reedy, 2000). To our knowledge, the original records Couney refers to in articles and interviews did not survive (Dorman, 1928; "Incubator babies," 1940). However, Dr. Arnold Gesell, the author *The Embryology of Behavior* (1945), highlighted the research conducted (in part) with Couney and Nurse Recht at the NYWF. Gesell cited a survival rate of 89.6%, higher than even Couney claimed (p. 250).

While it is particularly easy to find misinformation and inaccuracy on social media, the inability of scholars to prove some of Couney's claims means that Internet-based articles and social media posts unintentionally perpetuate myths within the Couney narrative. The claim that the medical community (other technical experts) rejected Couney out of hand surfaces often (Brick, 2005; Brown, 1994; "Life under," 2016; NPR, 2015). According to a National Public Radio (NPR)

(2015) article, Martin Couney had "his" incubators "rejected by the medical community," even though there is evidence he partnered with doctors, including Dr. Fischel in Coney Island ("Incubator graduates," 1904; McCullough, 1957), Dr. Hess in Chicago (Hess, 1922), Dr. Edward Wallace Lee in Omaha ("Incubator graduates," 1904), and Dr. Gesell (1945) at the NYWF. After these exhibitions, Couney sometimes sold incubators to local institutions, such as the Children's Hospital of Buffalo after the Pan-American Exposition in 1901 (Silverman, 1979). If he had been universally panned by the medical field, it is unlikely doctors would have worked with him, publicly thanked him in their publications (e.g., Drs. Hess and Gesell), or purchased the incubators from his exhibits for use in hospital wards. In 1945, Gesell's praise for Couney, his well-trained nursing staff, and his outcomes was exuberant. He actually referred to the NYWF exhibit as a "hospital" and noted, "The small patients received superlative care. We could not have asked for more ideal arrangements . . . the mortality rate was remarkably low . . . the infants thrived" (Gesell, 1945, p. 250). The majority of the pictures in this book feature exhibit babies, and Madam Recht and her famous diamond ring also appear in the text (Gesell, 1945, p. 239; see also Silverman, 1979, p. 138).

NPR (2015) also claimed that Couney's efforts were largely unknown, when in fact his exhibits appeared at the most popular and widely publicized exhibitions of the day, including the Omaha Trans-Mississippi Exposition (1898), the Paris World Exposition (1900), the Pan-American Exposition in Buffalo, New York (1901), expos in Portland, Oregon (1906), Mexico City (1908), Rio de Janeiro (1910), and Denver (1913), the Panama Pacific International Exposition in San Francisco (1915), Chicago's Century of Progress Exposition (1933–1934), the New York World's Fair (Weglein, Scheir, Peterson, Malsbury, & Schwartz, 2008), and both Luna Park and Dreamland in Coney Island from the early 1900s through the early 1940s (Liebling, 1939; "Life under," 2016; McCullough, 1957; Raju, 2011; Silverman, 1979). An article referring to Couney as the "patron of preemies" appeared in the *New Yorker Magazine* (Liebling, 1939), and his work with incubators and infants continued to be discussed in New York City newspapers throughout the early twentieth century ("Article 8," 1916; "Babies in," 1911; Dorman, 1928; "Hints," 1903; "Incubator's," 1940; "Incubator babies," 1940; "Incubator graduates," 1904; "Invention saved," 1907; "Qbata," 1901; Ranson, 1933). In 1940, some of his statistics from the NYWF exhibit were published in the *Journal of the American Medical Association* ("Incubator babies," 1940). Oral histories confirm his fame: for the Coney Island History oral history archive, Elinoar Astrinsky (2007) interviewed Beth Allen. Allen referred to Couney as the "most prominent" person dealing with premature babies at the time of her birth in 1941 (Allen, 2017). She noted that he was famous "world-wide" (see also Allen, 2017; "Life under," 2016).

Online, the BBC trumpeted that Couney alone "saved a generation of babies," as a medical "pioneer" "shunned by the medical establishment" ("How," 2016, n.p.). Yet Dr. Silverman (1979) interviewed a number of physicians who met and/ or interacted with Couney during his career and recounted the "lavish" reception of physicians (e.g., private gourmet lunches and presentations) during the NYWF (1939–1940, p. 138). Finally, initial reactions from scientific journals supported Couney's efforts ("Baby incubators," 1901; "Exhibit," 1901; Raju, 2011; "The use," 1897). If Martin Couney was a showman and not a physician, do his ends justify his means? He never thought these babies were a waste of labor and resources; he worked for a lifetime to save them. The public paid for their care and observed these "tiny mites in a hothouse," in awe over their size and fight (Ranson, 1933). Still, these babies were far too young to consent to their presence in an exhibit, and the idea of premature infant care as a sideshow, with parents sidelined, raises many ethical questions.

Correctives to Couney narrative are unlikely to reach a wider public (Baker 1996, 2000; Butterfield et al., 1997; Prentice, 2016a, 2016b; Raju, 2011; Silverman, 1979, 1980). Prentice (2016a, 2016b) argued that there are insufficient records in the United States or Europe to confirm Couney's place of birth or his receipt of a medical education, degrees, or licenses of any kind in Germany, France, or the United States (see also Raju, 2011). Baker (1996) and Silverman (1979, 1980; see also Butterfield et al., 1997) pointed to the tenuous link between Budin and Couney. Nevertheless, recent online media sources continue to credit one "Dr." Couney with saving the babies in his unit (Astrinsky, 2007; Brick, 2005; Dwyer, 2017; Eltman, 2015, 2017; "The freak," 2015; "How," 2016; "Life under," 2016; N'Duka, 2017; NPR, 2015; Prentice, 2016a, 2016b).

What is true in recent online reports is that Couney's contemporaries did not unanimously support his work. Even after Couney established two permanent exhibits in Coney, there were professionals aghast at his willingness to display premature babies. For example, John D. Lindsay of the New York Society for the Prevention of Cruelty to Children said, "The society's investigation convinced me that the motive for the exhibit which was represented as 'charitable' was purely mercenary, violating every principle of medical or professional ethics. It was a side show advertised by the proprietors of the resort as one of the attractions with its Shoot the Chutes and Razzle Dazzle" ("Babies in," 1911, p. 4). Lindsay's rejection of the Coney Island exhibit as unethical was reflexive of the trends in American medicine in the late nineteenth and early twentieth centuries, which included the incorporation of medicine as a hard science, an altered medical school model (Bonner, 1995; Starr, 1982), the rise of the hospital as the center of treatment, training, and research, and the continuing isolation and rejection of nonallopathic medical practices (Bonner, 1995; Breslaw, 2012; Starr, 1982; Vandenberg-Daves, 2014). Even Couney's exhibit at Coney Island, with its cleanliness and rigorous treatment methods, was considered (by many physicians) beyond the pale of appropriate settings for the practice of medicine.

Recent attention to Couney's story on Twitter, FB, and blogs mimics early twentieth-century newspaper coverage in that it positions Couney at the center of the story, framing him as a lone actor. Moreover, social media platforms lend credibility to a historical actor who (likely) practiced without formal medical training, and often publicly blamed pregnant mothers for premature birth. And it is his story that we continue to tell, his expertise we continue to highlight. None of the conflicted details in the Couney narrative are sufficient to depict him solely as an unknown rebel operating entirely outside of the technical expertise of medicine. This notion is part fable, and it has had powerful implications for public perceptions of the history of medicine and the false binary of "technical" and "lay" expertise in which technical experts restrict the boundaries of respectable medicine for monetary gain and lay experts are altruistic heroes, acting outside the narrow bounds of traditional medicine. Meanwhile, a competing narrative suggests that formally trained doctors produce the only trustworthy methods or research and all lay experts or "alternative" practitioners are quacks and charlatans, looking to prey on the naïve who will pay top dollar for snake oil (see also Janik, 2014). The construction of medical expertise in American history is not this straightforward, and the tale of Couney the "incubator doctor" exemplifies the inefficiency of available terminology. Again, we find the expertise binary virtually useless for understanding the ways medical expertise is constructed, experienced, and narrated in our society.

Since expertise categories are social constructions that have material and corporeal consequences (Berger & Luckman, 1989; Searle, 1995), they can woo individuals into simplistic understandings of what expertise and knowledge are. These perceptions can cloud judgments of both capability and culpability. For example, while doctors initially thought "weaklings" weren't worth saving, they willingly sent premature babies to a well-compensated "physician," and many praised his results and eventually adopted his techniques. Yet Couney never worked in a hospital or published a book or formal study in a medical journal; his nurses performed the vast majority of actual medical care, and there is no documentation suggesting Couney performed surgeries or other medical procedures on babies in his exhibits (Prentice, 2016b). Doctors sent Couney babies for whom they did not have the technological support and referred babies to him knowing the strength of his facilities and the competence of his staff (Prentice, 2016b) not necessarily because he was a doctor.

What is clear is that Couney's nursing staff took excellent care of the babies in their charge, and many lived to an advanced age. Some are still living and talking about their unusual beginnings. Couney's incubator babies (lay experts) are universally positive about the exhibits, crediting Couney alone for their life: "I . . . felt indebted to Dr. Couney"; "if it wasn't for him a lot of us wouldn't be here"; "I wouldn't be here today so I think him"; "[Dr. Couney] gave me a wonderful life" ("Life under," 2016, n.p.). Neonatologists and scholars today understand the important impact Couney had on the field, including his emphasis on the value of breast milk, touch, and lower oxygen levels (Gartner & Gartner, 1992; Silverman, 1979, 1980). Without Couney, many people around the world might not have known about incubators. As Dr. Silverman (1979) noted, he was a pioneer of "preemie propaganda," a showman who kept the preemie cause alive for decades, while technical experts and hospitals slowly advanced various methods and technologies for neonatal care (see also Baker, 1996, 2000; "Mechanical," 1931; Reedy, 2007; Zahorsky, 1905). Regardless of Couney's actual place of birth, education, and/or training, his guise of technical expertise, his acumen as a showman, and his talented team of nurses (technical experts including his wife Annabelle Couney, his daughter Hildegarde Couney, and nursing director Madam Recht) ensured that thousands of premature babies lived, despite their class background, ethnicity, race, or gender (Brown, 1994; Liebling, 1939; Ranson, 1933).

MECHANICAL INCUBATION TODAY:
ON AND OFF THE SOCIALLY MEDIATED SIDESHOW

What does not explicitly emerge from the history of the Couney exhibits is the role of mothers, fathers, and other caretakers. And the definition of "mothering" is fluid here: once in Couney's exhibit, babies were kept warm and safe within incubators; they were fed, held, washed, and otherwise cared for entirely by nurses; and parents met their children at "graduation." In Couney exhibits, mothers were disciplined visitors—viewing their children behind a railing and unable to take part in their "cares." Meanwhile, Couney's language suggested that mothers were inefficient, incapable, or unnecessary (Brisbane, 1901; Greene, 2010; Reedy, 2000), raising questions about how they could be expected to trust themselves with their children.

While Couney blamed mothers (among other environmental factors) for premature birth, he enjoyed rounding up his "graduates" for public spectacles focusing on their long-term growth and development ("Incubator graduates," 1904; "Incubator's," 1940; Raju, 2011).

The mothers (see Figure 5), whose babies were part of the class of 1939 ("Incubator's," 1940), kept them alive and thriving without any pamphlets, at-home support, specialty doctors, eating, speech, or physical therapists, or, more than likely, the type of parental social support groups available today. It is unlikely that these mothers discussed the particularities of their experience in groups with other preemie parents.

Couney also noted parental hesitation but perceived all apprehension as laziness. When Beth Allen's mother expressed fear about taking over her daughter's care, Couney reminded her that she had just had a three-month vacation; Allen's

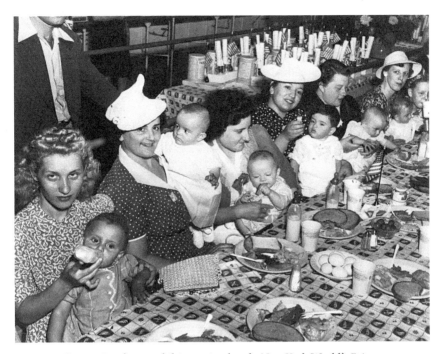

Figure 5. Couney incubator exhibit reunion lunch. New York World's Fair 1939–1940 Records, Manuscripts and Archives Division, New York Public Library.

mother remained so nervous that her father performed the first at-home bath (Astrinsky, 2007). Still, Beth Allen's parents visited her at the exhibit every day, though she shared that they never held or fed her and never spoke about the nurse-parent relationship regarding the transition home (Allen, 2017). Allen recalled the enormous struggle her parents had after her homecoming, even though they had ample intergenerational family support at hand (Allen, 2017). Deeply held cultural constructs around motherhood as women's most important work likely had a silencing effect for mothers and other caretakers who were struggling to connect with and care for their preemies. Couney's confident presence, beautiful and technologically advanced exhibits, and popularity with the public kept him center stage, while most of the nurses and parents faded into the background. Couney did not conduct any follow-up studies or track his babies, although he did boast about the wedding invitations and other letters he received, never from jail, he told Liebling (1939). One would think these babies married because of Couney; one could argue they lived long enough to marry, in part, as a result of their exhibition care.

Today, the transition from NICU to home begins early in the care journey, as NICU nurses and other medical providers attempt to make experts out of parents, and medical professionals are trained to help parents through this transition. This is the bind both caregivers and parents find themselves in today—NICU nurses want "parents that are highly involved but also trust the health care team to provide the best care to their baby" (Masi, 2017), a difficult line to walk for both parents and NICU care providers. Madeleine remembered: "Prior to Lidia's graduation to the special care unit, I was not able to pick her up unless the nurse gave approval, and in the first two months, I also required the nurse's assistance with removing her from the incubator. Of course, these rules were in place to protect Lidia, but the rules and restrictions did not facilitate bonding" (Michalik, 2017). Throughout this process, parents may struggle to take on the identity of "expert" as it relates to their child. Once home with Lidia, Madeleine continued to perform childcare as the NICU nurses had trained her: "I was afraid to vary from what I had observed because I felt the nurses would have the best techniques, and who was I to question them. As time passed, I was forced to make medical decisions for Lidia, and her doctors looked to me as the primary caregiver" (Michalik, 2017). Eventually, Madeleine became primary caregiver and decision maker—a fragile position given the beginning of Lidia's life.

The practices and procedures that link the Couney family, Dr. Hess and others, nurses Lundeen and Madam Recht, Beth Allen's and Lucille Horn's parents, and NICU parents and practitioners today are only part of the history of neonatal and pediatric health care in the United States. For example, Oppenheimer (1996) highlighted the role played by women's groups around the country in drawing public attention to infant mortality issues during the Progressive Era. Public health officials, sanitation experts, and even nonallopathic patent medicine companies attempted to respond to the interrelated issues of premature birth and infant mortality (Oppenheimer, 1996). Similarly, a wide range of voices and players are present in today's discussion and advocacy.

In the early twentieth century, "incubator mothers" might have traded stories or advice at a Couney graduation lunch. In the present, the stress and uncertainty common for NICU parents encourage individuals to seek one another out, in internal programs, such as NICU family dinners, with "graduate" NICU parent speakers, or on social media platforms, including online forums (Masi, 2017; Michalik, 2017; Miller Quinlan, 2017). Similar to other patterns of use of social media by mothers or people trying to conceive, social media can provide reassurance or create anxiety or both, as people seek information and resources about their situation. While Madeleine found comfort in online chat communities where she exchanged information and advice with other NICU parents, Elisa found it less helpful: "Reading about other's [sic] experiences didn't apply to my own and actually created stress by reading about babies coming home early (when we were delayed a few weeks beyond what we expected)" (Michalik, 2017; Miller Quinlan, 2017). However, smartphone technology did play a role for Elisa;

she and her partner used an app (GroupMe) through which friends and family could track their daughter's progress.

In 2009, Jennifer and Nick Hall started Graham's Foundation (GF) for Fighting Premature Babies, named in memory of their son (GF, 2017). This organization delivers support, advocacy, and research to improve outcomes for preemies and their families. They provide "preemie gear" and packages for NICU stays and transitioning home (GF, 2017). Additionally, they offer specific resources for parents such as a peer-mentoring program. Laura Martin (2015), a mother of twins born at 24 weeks and director of parent communication and engagement at GF, wrote a blog post, "Tips for Facing Doctors in the NICU," on the GF website. She is a lay advocate who trains parents to interact with technical experts, a role that did not exist before the late twentieth century. Parents on the site give advice such as the following: "Respect the doctor but also respect your instincts. You are a mother" and "It's your child and sometimes you just need to use your gut feeling on things if you disagree with a treatment, routine, procedure, etc." (GF, 2017). This perspective may seem to invite criticism (or skepticism) of nurses and doctors, but it also establishes parents as long-term caretakers.

While websites, social media platforms, and forums can encourage parents and caretakers to engage in dialogue while in the NICU, such online engagement requires constant vigilance and participation, something not possible for all NICU families, for a host of reasons that come up in every stage in the life cycle of early motherhood, such as structural oppression and injustice, economic inequality, and geographical distance from medical resources. As Elisa recollected, "When I read online support groups many of the other moms were basically living at the hospital and for me that would have made me miserable." The driving and parking costs were a burden, especially since Elisa returned to work early to save some maternity leave for her daughter's homecoming (a class-specific option she acknowledged some other parents do not have) (Miller Quinlan, 2017).

Again, Internet and social media resources can be helpful or stressful, contingent on the unique experiences and social capital of each family and even of individuals. Given the particular challenges of NICU care, including cost (which can require an early return to work), access to the facility (distance from home, transportation difficulties, paying for parking, insurance coverage issues), difficulty in family relationships (e.g., partners, siblings, extended family members), and uncertainty or worry about the transition home, Internet authors, journalists, and even individual social media users are now sounding the alarm about the link between premature birth and parental posttraumatic stress disorder (PTSD). For Catriona Ogilvy (2017), once she took her baby home the "support network of the hospital" disappeared "overnight" (n.p.; see also Tarkan, 2009). That loss of support prompted feelings of isolation, stress, and PTSD symptoms such as flashbacks and hypervigilance, which complicate the process of bonding with a newborn in the NICU and at home. Michalik (2017) experienced some of these symptoms at home:

> I was unable to recognize my own anxiety at the time, and [my spouse] was dealing with his own stress (over finances and helping with nighttime feedings). The doctor-recommended seasonal isolation kept us from socializing unless [my spouse] or I went out separately, so it was difficult to escape our little bubble. . . . Life was overwhelming because of multiple factors, and my anxiety kept me from appreciating my time with Lidia. And, as the cycle goes, I felt guilty for having feelings other than sheer elation over Lidia's homecoming.

Elisa delivered early because of severe preeclampsia, which complicated her early experience with the NICU:

> It's an overwhelming experience on every level, especially when you are try-ing to adjust to being a new parent, make complex medical decisions for your child, and process a ton of medical information when you can barely func-tion. The magnesium IV given to prevent seizures (a medication used for pre-eclampsia) has strong side effects which in my case was blurred vision and severe nausea. You are supposed to remain on magnesium for the first 24 hours after birth, which is also the time you are supposed to be bonding with your new child. (Miller Quinlan, 2017)

As we posit throughout this book, the historical consolidation and ascendency of credentialed expertise in America between the late nineteenth century and the mid-twentieth contributed to the bifurcation of technical and lay expertise. Other scholars maintain this same conclusion. Yet the Couney myth complicates this narrative. First, this same consolidation allowed white males (primarily) to "put on" and benefit from perceived technical expertise, as Couney did in his exhibits. His white coat, paired with his gender and race identity, allowed him to transcend expertise boundaries in ways unavailable to women and/or people of color at that time (see also Janik, 2014; Morantz-Sanchez, 2000; Vandenberg-Daves, 2014). Second, the present-day social media focus on the particularities of Couney obfuscates not only the nature of his expertise but also the nexus of other experts (lay and technical) involved in preventing premature birth and attending to the needs of preemies. This myth also obscures the emotional, phys-ical, and financial crises prompted by premature birth, particularly for mothers such as Madeleine Michalik and Elisa Miller Quinlan. Finally, the notion of a primarily oppositional relationship between technical and lay experts does not play out in Couney's story, where some technical experts embraced him prac-ticing medicine in a "lay" space; nor does it play out in the present, when neo-natal physicians and nurses, preemie parents, and other support professionals work jointly to support premature babies. Today this partnership begins in the NICU, not a sideshow.

CHAPTER 6

NOT JUST BABY BLUES

HISTORICAL REALITIES AND SOCIAL MEDIA ACCOUNTS OF POSTPARTUM CARE TODAY

In 1895, a doctor in Boston making his postpartum rounds for outpatients recorded an unusual sight: a baby swaddled and asleep on the mother's bed by a box filled with sawdust and one very young puppy; a second puppy was suckling at the woman's breast. The doctor's report continued: "In the course of this convalescence, this patient was presented, by some friend, with two puppy dogs; [they] were used to suckle the woman's breasts as she had 'too much milk.' I suggested the danger to her; and recommended sending the dogs back, telling her I could remedy the excess of milk. She readily complied with my request and took [magnesium sulfate] instead" (Boston Lying-In, 1832–1981). In the long-form entry in the Boston Lying-In Hospital outpatient volumes labeled "Clinical Memoranda," the doctor noted that upon hearing of the labor, a neighbor had immediately gone into the community to procure the youngest puppies she could find and delivered them within 24 hours of the home birth. There is no evidence that this was a typical practice among the immigrant communities in 1895, as this is the only record of the practice in hundreds of records (see also Morantz-Sanchez, 2000). Still, for this neighbor the procurement of young pups was not a response to postpartum milk production issues; it was a response to news of labor, implying that for her the practice was a routine component of postpartum recovery.

Early in our research we wondered about the use of Twitter as a place where stories of infanticide or postpartum suicide influence depictions of postpartum depression (PPD) and postpartum psychosis. We also wondered how technical experts and lay users discussed traditional treatment for these maladies such as pharmaceuticals and/or alternative therapies such as meditation. Then, in the archives at Francis A. Countway Medical Library in Boston, we realized we had failed to consider the fundamental question of the postpartum stage in the life cycle of early motherhood: namely, do mothers with access to the health care system in the United States receive adequate care and support, particularly in the first six weeks after childbirth?[1] After examining hospital records between

1885 and 1901 in the Northeast, we concluded that women from the newest immigrant groups, those without education and with insecure or no income, were surprisingly likely to have access to consistent, supportive postpartum care, particularly within those first few weeks. Of course the care they received varied and was only as effective as the medical science of the day could accommodate. Still, it is striking that today many U.S. women, across the class and race spectrum, don't receive any routine postpartum care (PPC) before the six-week mark, and many are unsatisfied with this lack of technical or lay (medical) support. In the late nineteenth and early twentieth centuries, a very small minority of women delivered in hospitals, whereas nearly 99% of women do today. Currently, patients can receive PPC and support—if they can pay for it, demand it, work around the system, or experience a severe or near-death health crisis—but they have to seek it after they leave the hospital. This may help explain the shocking maternal outcomes in the United States, which spends an enormous amount per patient and has the highest maternal death rate in the entire industrialized world (Martin & Montagne, 2017b). In 2015, over 1,000 women in the United States died because of childbirth, a number much greater than in New Zealand (7 postpartum), Australia (19 postpartum), and Canada (26 postpartum) (Global, 2016, p. 1784). The gap is significant and growing (CDC, 2017; Global, 2016; Martin & Montagne, 2017b).

The World Health Organization (WHO, 2013) described the first six weeks postpartum as the most critical and most neglected phase in the lives of mothers and babies, given the high number of deaths that occur during this period. Some scholars and lay practitioners note the importance of the postpartum period up to 6 to 12 months after birth, given ongoing adjustments in maternal health and mental well-being (Akpinar, Ipekci, Gulen, & Ikizceli, 2015; Fahey & Shenassa, 2013; Negron, Martin, Almog, Balbierz, & Howell, 2013). The days and weeks (especially the first six weeks) following childbirth are still a critical time in the lives of mothers and newborn babies, as most maternal and infant deaths occur then (Burns, 2017; WHO, 2013). According to WHO (2013), "This is the most neglected period for the provision of quality of care. Lack of appropriate care during this period could result in significant ill health and even death" for both mothers and babies (p. 6). Yet, "rates of provision of skilled care are lower after childbirth when compared to rates before and during childbirth" (WHO, 2013, p. 1). Additionally, WHO (2013) stated, "The critical maternal health outcome considered [in this report] was maternal morbidity (including haemorrhage, infections, anaemia and depression)" (p. 7) and proposed home visits as a way to maintain the postpartum health of the mother-child dyad and prevent health crises.

In this chapter, we explore the impact of technical and lay expertise on patients seeking PPC in the first six weeks postpartum, at the turn of the twentieth century and today. As we have seen, a binary understanding of expertise fails to represent the care systems during this stage, both then and now. In the archival records we investigated, technical experts included both male and female physicians and nurses, who operated within and outside of the clinical setting (e.g., in the hospital and the home). In outpatient records, midwives and doctors in other systems are mentioned, though it is unclear how physicians categorized these practitioners. As we discussed in chapter 4, the definition of "lay expert" in the birthing room was in flux at the turn of the twentieth century and remained so for decades, as obstetricians began to take on more births and pregnant patients considered new hospital maternity wards for birth. Still, in the Boston Lying-In outpatient records, we found that neighbors, women, midwives, husbands, and even "spiritual advisers" were called upon for everything from emotional support to bathing and dressing the new baby and holding the fundus in place after birth (Boston Lying-In, 1832–1981).[2]

At present, the vast majority of U.S. births occur in the hospital, with obstetricians and nurses and, increasingly, midwives or nurse-midwives (CDC, 2014; Craven, 2010; Morbidity, 1999; see also Wolf, 2009). Yet in the postpartum period today, particularly during the first six weeks, nearly the entirety of care happens via lay experts. Friends and family often come to visit and/or help out, deliver meals, and perform other tasks. Postpartum doulas work within a rapidly expanding market in the absence of other standardized medical PPC, offering feeding support, newborn care and sibling care, overnight help, and referrals to other resources (American Pregnancy Association, 2017a; Campbell, Scott, Klaus, & Falk, 2007; Lynn, 2012; Meyer, Arnold, & Pascali-Bonaro, 2001; Pevzner, 2015). Postpartum patients seek social supports from friends and family but may also call on or visit lactation consultants (LCs), seek out other postpartum support groups, or join postpartum fitness groups (Birthfit, 2017; Druxman & Carl, 2006; Evans, Donelle, & Hume-Loveland, 2012; Negron, Martin, Almog, Balbierz, & Howell, 2013). All of these support systems could be classified as lay, though they involve experts with varying levels of medical knowledge and practical experience. Many of today's lay practitioners, particularly LCs and postpartum doulas, perform the work physicians handled in the late nineteenth and early twentieth centuries (see also Lynn, 2012). Today's postpartum lay experts are a result of shifting definitions of technical and lay expertise and emerged to fill a void in PPC for American women, which blurs the line between technical and lay experts in our medical system.

To compare the PPC available over a century ago with that today, we begin with a discussion of inpatient and outpatient PPC in two hospital systems in Boston between 1885 and 1901. We discuss the work of medical practitioners, the length and nature of care, the role of family and community members, and the idea of a "normal" postpartum recovery experience at the time. In the casebooks we read, the postpartum care records were part and parcel of birth records, normalizing the recovery period (which could extend for weeks or months) as part of having a baby. Again, medical records did not break out the postpartum period from the birth—they simply continued until mother and child were well enough to leave, which took days, weeks, or months. We examine the early postpartum period, which scholars and practitioners today define as the time immediately after birth and lasting for about six weeks (Kansky & Isaacs, 2016).

Next, focusing on the contemporary era, we discuss some of the research on PPC in the United States and explore the PPC data we collected through informal interviews and Radian6 (R6) (Barkin, Bloch, Hawkins, & Thomas, 2014; Fahey, & Shenassa, 2013; Suplee, Gardner, & Borucki, 2014). Currently, the U.S. medical system allows for a gap in care between birth and six weeks postpartum, and as a result social (and medical) expectations are focused on "bouncing back" and monitoring the health of the newborn. As such, we address the body erasure inherent in PPC and discuss the ways social media addresses or does not address the social, emotional, and physical needs of postpartum patients during the first six weeks.

A Rapid and Uneventful Convalescence: The First Six Weeks Postpartum, 1885–1901

To understand the postpartum period in the late nineteenth century and early twentieth, we focused on two sets of records: the Boston Lying-In Hospital (hereafter referred to as Boston) records for outpatient maternity cases (home births and PPC with physicians) between 1895 and 1901 and the New England Hospital for Women and Children (hereafter referred to as New England) maternity records between 1885 and 1900. New England's maternity records documented inpatient cases, while Boston's outlined outpatient PPC, even though Boston also offered inpatient maternity care. Ultimately, the patient records themselves described routine PPC, including changes to care over time (for example, magnesium sulfate replacing licorice powder as a stool softener). They also depict expectations for both technical experts (physicians) and lay experts (postpartum women and their support systems) regarding normal recovery and PPC care and support. These resources provided valuable information as they are nearly complete for more than 20 years—a rarity among nineteenth- and early twentieth-century hospital systems (see also Johnson & Quinlan, 2017).

Historian Regina Morantz-Sanchez's (2000) examination of similar and overlapping institutional records and annual reports provided a general framework through which to understand the medical and social goals of each institution.[3] Morantz-Sanchez (2000) aptly described nineteenth-century hospitals as "institutions of the urban poor," though she insisted they were not homogeneous in their approach. Some acted as a last resort for the ill and dying, while other "voluntary" hospitals utilized a sliding pay scale or nominal or no fees to the working poor (p. 226). Both Boston and New England can be characterized as voluntary institutions, yet they attracted differing clientele (Boston Lying-In, 1832–1981; Morantz-Sanchez, 2000; New England Hospital, 1885–1900).[4]

Morantz-Sanchez (2000), who based her research on inpatient records only, characterized these hospital systems according to their pay scale and perceptions of patients. New England hospital practitioners and administrators focused heavily on the moral and spiritual influence of the female-run hospital space. They considered the moral standing of patients, first by charging extremely modest fees—but expecting patients to pay as a form of empowerment—and then by refusing unwed mothers after their first child (Morantz-Sanchez, 2000). New England was one of the first hospitals for women and children launched and staffed by female physicians. From the hospital's opening in 1862 until the early 1890s, when competition and resistance to modernization and new systems marred the institution's sterling reputation, New England was the leading training center for female physicians studying maternal health. The hospital used an incubator in 1900. At that time incubators were often ineffective in saving premature babies, as we noted in chapter 5. But the fact that New England had one speaks to its interest in state-of-the-art infant care technology, even as hospital leaders resisted change in other areas (see also Morantz-Sanchez, 2000).

Conversely, the Boston Lying-In Hospital was a teaching hospital for Harvard Medical School (Morantz-Sanchez, 2000), so it is likely that many of the practitioners recording their outpatient work were medical students or residents completing an obstetrics rotation. In the outpatient records we viewed, all practitioners seemed to be men. Doctors arrived with necessary equipment, tools, and medicines, and if they ran out of supplies, they sent a messenger to the hospital to request more. Postpartum visits often included supportive care, medicines, and herbal supplements provided by the visiting practitioner as well. Morantz-Sanchez (2000) noted both Boston and New England refused to care for unwed mothers birthing their second child. In the Boston outpatient records, unwed mothers are listed, though the signifier "primipara" (meaning first birth) was not always noted, meaning unwed Boston outpatients may have accessed care for subsequent births. Morantz-Sanchez cited 23% of inpatients paid fees at Boston, while we saw no evidence of charges or an exchange of goods for services in outpatient cases.

Given that we examined Boston outpatient and New England inpatient records to gain a wider representation PPC, we came to different conclusions about the nature of PPC. In contrast to Morantz-Sanchez, we found Boston's records more complete since we focused on outpatient records, albeit from a practitioner perspective. Boston's outpatient records included Clinical Memoranda as well as a Case Record, which listed vital signs, medicines, and procedures during birth and throughout the postpartum period. The Clinical Memoranda often included directions for other doctors (e.g., a detailed description of steps for stopping hemorrhage), blunt (and occasionally demeaning) assessments of patients, moments of vulnerability (e.g., trepidation and hunger), and times of levity, including the line "with nothing but a placenta to my credit," a recurrent joke by one practitioner that designated his oversight of a successful birth (Boston Lying-In, 1832–1981). Other entries outlined training practices: a medical student attended by teaching physician Dr. Newell recorded, "Before making the vaginal examination I received instruction on the aseptic technique" (Boston Lying-In, 1832–1981). Finally, there are red and blue markings throughout, suggesting these records were reread and evaluated. New England inpatient records were detailed, professional, even pristine, but generally lacked detailed description, unless a unique or critical case presented (e.g., a congenital hand deformity in mother and child) (New England Hospital, 1885–1900).

Morantz-Sanchez (2000) characterized the maternity care (including postpartum care) at New England as lasting "from four days to three months," while inpatients in Boston Lying-In checked out at around 14 days (p. 227). Given that we viewed both inpatient (New England) and outpatient (Boston) records, our observations differed from those of Morantz-Sanchez slightly. We agree the length of stay for patients at New England was generally much longer, with more direct care, and as Morantz-Sanchez noted, some Boston patients may even have been "virtually ignored after delivery," staying only 14 days on average, a full week less than those at New England. For example, in 1885 one patient checked in on January 7 and did not check out until January 29; she sat up on January 22 (New England Hospital, 1885–1900). Fifteen years later, patients stayed for a similar period—20 or more days being routine (New England Hospital, 1885–1900). New England patients received checks from doctors and/or nurses two to three times per day, and extensive observations of the baby are apparent in trifold records. Here, as with Boston outpatients, mother and child were treated as a patient dyad, with individualized but parallel records. While Morantz-Sanchez (2000) identified lackluster postpartum support for Boston inpatients, we observed personalized, engaged care for outpatients (Boston Lying-In, 1832–1981). Practitioners normally visited daily for PPC and two or even three times per day if there was evidence of fever, infection, or other issues (e.g., edema) (Boston Lying-In, 1832–1981). The PPC period varied depending on the nature of the birth and the individual recovery process. Between 1896 and 1901, outpatients received care for 9, 10, 11, 12, 13, 16, 18, 20, and 21 days (for which the practitioner's notes said, "convalescence was exceedingly slow"); for one patient a doctor made three visits in just one day (Boston Lying-In, 1832–1981). The average length for outpatient cases we viewed fell between 10 and 16 days, which is significantly shorter than that for New England, but the records indicated more consistent and involved care for Boston outpatients than Morantz-Sanchez found for inpatients.

We attribute the variance in length of in- and outpatient care to three factors: First, patients may have recovered more quickly at home, with the support of friends and family and the comfort of familiar surroundings. Breslaw (2012) claimed that in the mid-nineteenth century, "one went to a hospital to die, not be cured" (p. 181) (see also Morantz-Sanchez, 2000). While conditions had changed by the early twentieth century, it is likely many patients still preferred to recuperate at home. Second, outside of the hospital setting, doctors had less control over patient activity level, something that frustrated Boston doctors. One recorded that a patient "got up today, against orders," and another patient "got up on the 6th day & this caused her temperature to rise" (Boston Lying-In, 1832–1981). Their irritation is understandable given the risk of death from puerperal fever at the time (Morantz-Sanchez, 2000).[5] Doctors and nursing staff at New England had more control over patient behavior since they could monitor patients at all times. Third, although postpartum injuries don't appear worse in the Boston records and antiseptic measures and treatments are commonplace between 1895 and 1900, the female physicians at New England recorded internal exams, including details on previous birth injuries to cervix and perineum, and far more patients seemed to have cervical tearing or laceration listed. In one case, wherein the mother did not sit up until the 20th day, the case notes said, "Cervical erosion treated with $AgNo_3$ [silver nitrate]" (New England Hospital, 1885–1900). It is unclear whether increased cervical treatment was a result of birth methods or prior maternal health or whether there was more extensive internal monitoring at New England than Boston. While it is possible that patients admitted to New England were in poorer health than those who gave birth at home, we can't demonstrate a marked differential between in- and outpatient health outcomes.

Also different from Morantz-Sanchez (2000), we observed that medicinal support, especially pain relief, was standard for both New England inpatients and Boston outpatients. In the cases we viewed, Boston outpatients appeared to live in tenements (e.g., ten family members living in two rooms), and doctors noted lack of food, conditions of poverty, lack of sanitation, and, in a handful cases, flea bites and other evidence of "vermin" biting babies. The level of detail in these observations suggests that even poor outpatients received ample attention and care (e.g., medicine, antiseptic measures, supportive care) commensurate with New England inpatients, though for shorter periods (Boston Lying-In, 1832–1981). Furthermore, in the Boston outpatient records, we noted the obvious role played by family members and neighbors, who were recorded in the room during or after birth, assisting the doctors with the baby after birth, bringing food and tea, and holding the fundus in place (Boston Lying-In, 1832–1981). At times doctors even expressed consternation over the meddling of neighbor women in the room (Boston Lying-In, 1832–1981). Still, both lay and technical experts were available to postpartum patients, and as we discuss later, lay experts advocated for health care on behalf of new mothers, and doctors responded.

The overarching similarities we discovered between these sets of records include a minimum of around ten days with daily PPC, with medicinal support focused on pain relief, antiseptic protection, and comfortable and consistent bowel movements. Doctors in both systems closely examined the position of the uterus, the state of the perineum, and any stitching throughout the recovery period, using similar supplies such as glycerin tampons and pads treated with aseptic solutions. Boston outpatient physicians often prepared pads for their patients and left a supply behind. Patients with both Boston and New England had daily contact with a physician before being discharged from care, and if they complained of pain, discomfort, or other potential health problems, they received an examination. Patients in both systems depended on technical experts for the care of their newborns, which included cord clamping, washing, eye care, weighing and temperature tracking, and overall health assessment. Patients in both systems received referrals to further care, even after weeks of daily PPC. At New England, a patient in 1900 stayed for nearly a month before referral to a "local dispensary" (New England Hospital, 1885–1900). A Boston outpatient was advised "to go to the hospital within about 3wks to have perinaeum [*sic*] operated upon," and in 1901 another Boston patient with milk supply issues received a referral to a clinic (Boston Lying-In, 1832–1981).

The most striking aspect of these casebooks is the extensive and individualized care patients received. Routine challenges included constipation, after pains, nipple soreness, issues with nursing, complications with stitches; babies faced "sore eyes" (treated with silver nitrate), had issues with feeding and weight gain, and suffered cleanliness issues with the umbilical stump. Medicines distributed with the most frequency were ergot and opium for placenta delivery and after pains; Epsom salts (taken internally and used externally) for issues with blood pressure, water retention, and perineal healing; warm baths, licorice, rhubarb pills, and eventually magnesium sulfate for bowel movements; and flaxseed poultices, ice, and hot compresses for complaints such as abdominal swelling and abscess (Boston Lying-In, 1832–1981; New England Hospital, 1885–1900). Doctors often provided compound cathartic pills (C.C. pills) for constipation (Boston Lying-In, 1832–1981; Hare, Caspari, Rusby, Geisler, Kremers, & Base, 1907; New England Hospital, 1885–1900). Outpatient cases that involved all these supports were uniformly described as "uneventful and rapid" or "getting along first rate" (Boston Lying-In, 1832–1981). In 1896, Boston physician Dr. Robert Porter managed an outpatient maternity case and visited daily for 12 days. His care included the following: "Check[ed] pulse and temperature, tightened binder, changed pads, left corrosive pads in a corrosive towel [with further directions for use], had nipples washed with castile soap & water . . . [and] <u>clean</u> towel after each nursing. Inquired how long, how often baby was fed gave instruction about it. I examined, breasts, sleep, pains, headache, tenderness about abdomen" (Boston Lying-In, 1832–1981). At the end of this case, the doctor characterized it as "normal." Another Boston doctor noted, "nipples sensitive, nipple shield . . . C.C. pill" and concluded, "convalescence was without event" (Boston Lying-In, 1832–1981).

The risk of death was ever present, even in this period when aseptic measures were becoming more common, so physicians likely perceived aches and pains, bleeding, and abdominal tenderness—without fever—as a regular part of recuperation and signs of recovery. In the early twentieth century, 40% of maternal deaths resulted from sepsis, meaning that practitioners had to focus on life-saving aseptic procedures and rely on daily tracking to alter maternal outcomes (Morbidity, 1999).

In both hospital systems, practitioners provided daily care for the immediate postpartum period, focused on cervical, perineal, and nipple and breast care. They administered medicines and abdominal or breast binding to lessen routine pain and discomfort and assisted with bathing, personal sanitation, and the cleanliness of the bed where mother and baby recuperated together. Physical support, care, and monitoring were not only reasonable but extensive. PPC in the immediate postpartum period defined uneventful, healthy, and rapid postpartum recovery. Importantly, practitioners realized childbirth and the postpartum period had potential health complications for bodies, in part because so many women died at the time. The expectation among practitioners within both systems for regular recuperation could not be more different from PPC expectations today.

We are not arguing for the reconstruction of late nineteenth- and early twentieth-century PPC systems, even if that was possible in U.S. society today. Paternalism certainly played a role in the Boston Lying-In outpatient program, as male practitioners did not hesitate to use force when women failed to comply during birth: "By using a good deal of force and persuasion her husband and I got her on the bed" and "together we [two male doctors] held her down" (Boston Lying-In, 1832–1981). Similar to the present, practitioners maintained strong opinions about diet: "Found a mother in bed eating a piece of bread fried in lard. Scolded her and threw the bread out the window. Baby doing well" (Boston Lying-In, 1832–1981). This type of condescension occurs today (Hodges, 2009), but it is not purposefully routine or deemed healthy communication with patients (Epstein, 2006; Hall, Roter, & Katz, 1988). Furthermore, PPC was likely predicated, in part, on the assumed weakness inherent to females (Morantz-Sanchez, 2000; Smith-Rosenberg, 1985). In these records, weeks of daily care characterized rapid and normal recovery, and language disparaging women, in particular, did not appear, though claims about class and ethnicity did (e.g., "and many other ailments common to the Jews") (Boston Lying-In, 1832–1981). Medically speaking, too, many methods and treatments prominent in historical health care need to remain where they are—in the archive (e.g., dosing newborns with brandy when they seemed weak).

Still, these casebooks revealed doctors with a keen interest in their patient's well-being. In June 1896, one doctor documented, "As she was very poor, I gave her a diet order and a little money on several occasions" (Boston Lying-In,

1832–1981). Doctors with both Boston and New England acknowledged patient wishes on infant feeding and supported women who could not or chose not to breastfeed, though these women composed a small minority of patients. In 1896, a physician recorded, "The woman told me that she was not going to nurse the child . . . the child was fed first on diluted fresh milk . . . the child and mother were both well when I discharged them" (Boston Lying-In, 1832–1981). On one occasion, family (lay expert) advocacy prompted a resident to prescribe a placebo: "On the 14th day [postpartum] they [her family] sent to the hospital saying the woman was sick. As I was absent, Dr. Weil went down and they declared to him that she was 'swelling up.' They knew a woman who had 'swelled up on the 9th day and died' and now 'she was swelling.' He could see nothing wrong but to comfort them gave her some licorice powder which evidently produced the desired results for we heard nothing more about swelling."

Swelling in the postpartum period can result from postpartum edema (from excess fluid in bodily tissues), which today warrants further medical investigation. In rare cases, edema can point to conditions like peripartum cardiomyopathy, a potentially life-threating cardiac condition, which emerges up to five months postpartum (Akpinar, Ipekci, Gulen, & Ikizceli, 2015). In each of these examples, even those concerning physical force and food control, women had reliable access to medical care. In the swelling incident, the patient's family advocated for further care just nine days postpartum and the doctor took their concerns seriously, despite finding no medical issue. Routinely, Boston outpatients in the early twentieth century likely benefited from home visits in the first weeks, wherein practitioners checked for infections, checked for signs of and treated hemorrhage, and monitored overall health (Boston Lying-In, 1832–1981). We see, then, that the expectations among both lay (e.g., family members) and technical experts included regular care, adequate diet, and monitoring for potential health complications in the early postpartum period of weeks or months.

Strokes and Stitches: What We Wish We Knew

Given that individuals who give birth in the United States today do not see practitioners between the first few days after giving birth and the six-week postpartum appointment (unless there is a critical health issue), it is urgent to consider that the lack of rest and recovery negatively impacts maternal health, physically and mentally (see also Borreli, 2013; Dagher, McGovern, & Dowd, 2014). For instance, Dagher, McGovern, and Dowd (2014) reported that in the first year postpartum, more extended maternity leave and more recovery time are associated with a decline in depressive symptoms. According to the researchers, this demonstrated that a longer leave allows mothers appropriate time to rest and recover (Dagher, McGovern, & Dowd, 2014). Findings also indicate that current leave time (i.e., recovery time) provided by the Family Medical Leave

Act is insufficient (see also Borreli, 2013). Moreover, social isolation, lack of contact with medical providers, and a compartmentalized approach to care, which considers mother and baby separately, shape today's PPC, also increasing the risk of depression and anxiety.

NPR and online investigative news agency ProPublica are currently collecting individual accounts of U.S. postpartum health crises online, to support research on the causes of postpartum maternal health crises and death (Gallardo, Martin, & Montagne, 2017a). In Texas, nearly 60% of maternal deaths occur in the first six weeks or shortly thereafter; many of these deaths happen not during or immediately after childbirth but in the period of medical neglect in the weeks following delivery (Martin, 2016). The investigation also uncovered that "more American women are dying of pregnancy-related complications than any other developed country," and the number continues to rise, despite the fact that some of these deaths are preventable (Martin & Montagne, 2017a; see also CDC Foundation, 2017). Overall, the maternal death rate in the United States has not declined since 1982 (Morbidity, 1999).

To be clear, U.S. maternal death rates are still far better than those in some low-income countries, including Haiti, Afghanistan, Congo, and a host of others. However, these numbers can be misleading. First, the United States has a much higher rate than every other industrialized country at this time. For comparison, we have a death rate six times the rate in Ireland and nearly seven times that in Finland (Global, 2016; see also Martin & Montague, 2017b). While we have better outcomes than the poorest countries on the planet, we don't do better than many countries that spend far less per patient on medical costs and have fewer medical staff and supplies at their disposal. For example, in 2015, compared with the United States' more than 1,000 lost mothers, Chile lost 48, Venezuela 381, Paraguay 141, Iran 281, and Iraq 729 (Global, 2016).[6] To begin to understand this discrepancy among countries and between the past and present in the United States, we investigated postpartum care today.

As such, we engaged in informal interviews with 17 friends, family members, colleagues, and acquaintances, in addition to investigating social media accounts (described in the next section). To the best of our knowledge, these individuals all had some form of health insurance; most were educated, and the majority were white, heterosexual and married, and lived in urban or suburban areas. We noticed that postpartum individuals were unprepared and couldn't ascertain the difference between "normal" postpartum recovery and health crises in the first six weeks after birth. Meredith said, "I had very little guidance on taking care of myself postpartum . . . I didn't get much information about what was appropriate for activity level in the days/weeks following." Kandace (2017) remembered, "While visiting my OBGYN they informed me that the hospital should have given me a spray bottle to help with urinating, numbing spray for the area, and instructions for a sitz bath. I received none of that information before I was discharged." This reflects the reality that as late as 2012, newly trained doctors in maternal-fetal medicine "didn't have to spend time learning to care for birthing mothers" (Martin & Montagne, 2017a, n.p.).

Postpartum patients report that because of the intense focus on the health of the baby (during childbirth and in postpartum period), their own health needs (physical, emotional, and mental) were not addressed (Martin & Montagne, 2017a), reflecting the splitting of the "mother-child dyad" in health care models today. For instance, Kandace (2017) remembered that she contracted MRSA at the hospital and struggled to access follow-up treatment: "We were sent home from the hospital on Friday afternoon and had no other access to care over the weekend. My OBGYN and pediatrician were both closed. . . . At 1.5 weeks post-partum I saw my OBGYN. . . . I was experiencing excruciating pain when urinating and when having bowel movements. . . . It was another 8 months to a year before I was ordered a colonoscopy to discover the tear in my anus that had occurred during delivery." When mothers express concern about their own health or recovery process, they might be dismissed or even ignored by technical experts.

Deadly or critical postpartum health experiences for mothers vary and include infections like MRSA, edema, blood pressure issues, hemorrhaging, and others (Martin & Montagne, 2017a). NPR journalists Gallardo, Martin, and Montagne (2017) recounted the postpartum care experience of patient Marie McCausland, who suffered from severe preeclampsia (very high blood pressure) just four days after giving birth. She described her childbirth discharge materials as vague, confusing, and "really quite useless" for ascertaining whether or not her symptoms were critical (Gallardo, Martin, & Montagne, 2017, n.p.). McCausland visited two hospitals before her concerns were addressed and she finally received treatment. At the first hospital, she received feedback that her chest pain and obvious edema were "normal postpartum symptoms" (Gallardo, Martin, & Montagne, 2017, n.p.). Interviewee Meredith (2017) was not even examined in the hospital and had to contact her doctor for hospital discharge: "I wasn't seen by a doctor until 40 hours after labor, and I had to call my doctor's office to send somebody to sign paperwork the following day so that I could check out of the hospital. . . . When I got home from the hospital, I had zero faith that I was healing ok since I'd never really been looked at, so I called my practice and said I was worried about infection (a lie) and went in. That was about a week [postpartum]." In this instance, Meredith advocated for herself by getting herself out of the hospital, only to lie so she could get the care she should have received immediately postpartum. Unlike the working-class women in Boston at the turn of the twentieth century, Meredith did not receive any afterbirth care and could not depend on any regular check-in or a home visit from a medical practitioner. The most disturbing and common themes found in these recollections are that the new mothers lacked critical information *and* their symptoms were dismissed. Given the risk of health crises in the postpartum period, dismissal can be deadly.

Individuals also discussed the added pressure to put their own needs aside to care for their newborn in the first weeks and months postpartum. We had several conversations since the birth of our daughters about how we wished someone warned us about how difficult the first six weeks would be, even as we experienced the excitement around having a baby with friends and family. Dana (2017) echoed our sentiments: "I wish someone had shared with me how hard it would be (in a loving/caring way) . . . I really wasn't prepared, and I would have liked to be!" The lack of attention to the health and well-being of the gestating parent was almost universal among those we interviewed. Most even acknowledged their baby's health was paramount. Dana (2017) reported her postpartum experience as a litany of doctor's visits and check-ins but only for her healthy son. Dana also scheduled an appointment with an LC twice during the first six weeks. We probed, "But in those first six weeks no one seemed that concerned about your health?" She responded, "It certainly didn't seem like a priority. My son was the main concern (and for me also! Even if I had had problems, I probably would have put them on hold or downplayed them). . . . The providers I saw kept telling me to 'hang in' and 'things would get better,' . . . but it really wasn't helpful . . . I think the main concern is for the baby . . . but how can a baby be taken care of if the caregiver is not also being taken care of?" As Karen fervently proclaimed, "[It was] completely on me to seek out any additional help that wasn't . . . built right in to the standard plan of care."

Maggie, Bethany, and interviewee Lorelai recalled the difficulty of scheduling appointments for ourselves and baby, with different doctors and sometimes across medical systems (see also Martin & Montague, 2017a). On the day of a pediatric appointment, caregivers have to navigate bundling up babies, leaving the house, and driving across town. Pediatric visits are frequent (48 hours postbirth, 1 week, etc.) during the first six weeks—a time when individuals are still in active recovery, perhaps dealing with stitches or C-section wounds, prolonged bleeding, or the more critical health concerns addressed above. Karen (2017) also mentioned the difficulty of leaving the house: "I was also too scared to leave the house, so I was not as proactive there as I could have been." Lorelai (2017) confided, "With both births, I sought out support from lactation consultants and had multiple appointments with them prior to the 6-week mark. I needed a ton of breastfeeding support and am glad I went for help but wish there had been an easier way to get that care (other than carrying a newborn to and from the office for appointments)." Maggie, who has a family history of PPD, experienced breastfeeding anxiety (as did her husband) since no one helped them process the trauma of her daughter's breathing cessation from an improper breastfeeding position just an hour after birth. An LC coming to the house and showing her how to breastfeed on her couch or bed rather than on a hospital lactation ottoman/

glider that she did not own would have been extremely helpful. Six months later, she finally found the courage to teach herself how to nurse laying down—the LCs hadn't demonstrated it. Maggie was fortunate that her insurance covered several visits to a LC, but she would have needed to pay for a visiting LC.

Others recalled frustration over the design of health care today in that OBGYNs and family practitioners, pediatricians, and doulas/midwives/LCs specialize in either the baby or the mother and don't treat them as a unit. For Boston outpatients and New England inpatients, doctors could attend to both mother and baby; as we discussed in chapter 5 and will discuss in chapter 7, pediatrics emerged in the early to mid-twentieth century in response to infant mortality rates, but it seems that the separation could be negatively impacting maternal health needs today.

In a "What to Expect" chatroom on postnatal support from family and friends, we learned that many husbands/partners were able to take two weeks or less (if any) leave from work, in part because of leave policies, but also because of pressure not to take allowable time off. In a country without universal paid family leave, leaves tend to be short. And a lack of paternal or partner leave removes the one in-home support system available to most postpartum individuals, especially when friends and family aren't available. STEPHABEE50 (2017) posted, "With my first I had basically no postpartum support. I delivered on a Friday and by Monday my husband went back to work and I was alone at home with baby. I had one friend bring a meal. The lack of support wasn't healthy for me and I think contributed to my developing PPD." One friend bringing a meal (while needed and appreciated) certainly can't meet the full scale of postpartum support needed and desired. When compared to archival historical records, these women are merely expressing normal postpartum desires, and experiencing physical and emotional challenges categorized as "normal" over a century ago. The increased isolation of American parents and caretakers today reflects added emotional and logistical issues, which can compound anxiety and stress. In contradistinction, Boston outpatient case records showed neighbors stopping by and staying until doctors returned.

Some contemporary mothers did report feeling supported and cared for during the postpartum period. Every individual with a positive experience reported that parents or other family members came to help and most mentioned partners with at least one week off. Finally, self-reported supported individuals mentioned paid supports more than half of the time (e.g., LCs, doulas). Sandra (2017) referred to her midwives as "saving her life" when she hit "rock bottom" and received treatment for PPD during the practice's routine two-week and six-week postpartum appointments, both focused on her health and well-being. Sandra concluded, "I couldn't have asked for better, more compassionate care," noting the importance of the two-week visit for early intervention. Her in-laws also provided childcare after both births. Blogger Hilary (2017), who founded

"The New Mystique," described as "a community exploring the intersection of motherhood and work," had two C-sections; she relied on her husband, mother, and mother-in-law in the weeks following the birth. In an interview, she described their support as "invaluable in keeping my toddler engaged so I could rest and spend some time with my newborn. My [mother-in-law] has helped do light cleaning of my house and do our laundry since my first daughter was born. My husband helped primarily with errands, prescription pick-ups, preparing meals, etc." (Hilary, 2017). This brings up an issue many postpartum individuals face: managing the young children they already have while attending to a newborn and struggling with their own health challenges. Due to her C-sections, Hilary also saw her doctor at two weeks and six weeks postpartum for "wound care, stitches removal and general checkup." She also cited extensive lactation support in the hospital, though that support "disappeared after we were released to go home" (Hilary, 2017). Positive experiences today are similar to those we observed in archival records, with adequate support (from friends and family) time to rest and heal, and help with other responsibilities from friends, family, and neighbors.

Others who reported a positive experience cited help specifically from postpartum doulas. Meyer, Arnold, and Pascali-Bonaro (2001) argued that postpartum doula support provides much-needed assistance, which can reduce feelings of anxiety and isolation. Belly Bloom Birth Services advertises "immediate" postpartum and "extended postpartum" services, providing first feeding support, baby wearing (in a baby carrier, wrap, etc.), and infant massage (jennabrowski, 2017, n.p.) Some doula services focus on household help and assist with bottle feeding as well, supporting parents with diverse needs and practices (Doulas of Charlotte, 2017; see also Lynn, 2012). As Jenna Dabrowski (2017) inquired in a blog post titled "Yes you NEED your postpartum period. You are not a Water Buffalo," "Are the needs of a new mother not worthy of acknowledgement?" (jennabrowski, 2017, n.p.). Jaime (2017), who paid for one-on-one attention from a doula, described her PPC very positively: "I sincerely felt all my needs were met . . . a lot of this came from having regular contact with our doula in the weeks following our baby's birth. Her presence was reassuring and we used her as a night nurse six times over the course of the first 8 weeks." Jaime's experience also reflected the archival record we examined in that a practitioner visited for day shifts, monitored both her and her baby's health and recovery, and offered feeding supports and troubleshooting. The doula provided reassurance and encouragement—critical emotional supports other interviewees desired and lacked.

At the same time, some were exasperated by the price of PPC, wishing they had local friends and family nearby to avoid paying for vital support. Unfortunately, the supportive services offered by postpartum doulas, while funded by health systems in other countries (e.g., France), are not fully covered by insurance companies in the United States (Pearson, 2017; Shapiro, 2008). Maggie lamented, "I wish doula or midwife care was covered, not just an extra expense!" Doulas deserve compensation for their excellent and necessary work (and require it in a capitalist economy). Yet in our health system, these lay experts work chiefly outside of the health system (Chee, 2013). If you want doula help, you need to find it yourself and most likely pay out of pocket for it, which is difficult if not impossible for anyone outside of the upper-middle or upper classes given the cost per hour (Dana, 2017; Glauser, Konkin, & Dhalla, 2015). In the late nineteenth and early twentieth centuries the vast majority of women gave birth at home, but as our research revealed, home births in Boston included a regular point of contact with qualified medical professionals. Today, the vast majority of births take place in the hospital, but maternal care ends shortly after the birth. Unlike the patients we observed in casebooks, today postpartum individuals are (medically) on their own—unless they are newborn babies.

Social Media in the Care Gap: Lay Experts Policing the Postpartum Period

Communication scholar Tasha Dubrwiny (2012), in her media analysis of blogs on PPD and expectations of motherhood, discussed the social construction of motherhood as an integral part of how we imagine postpartum behavior. First, she noted that "good motherhood" is constructed as white, educated, heterosexual, and essentially privileged (Dubrwiny, 2012), as we continue to discover in every stage of the life cycle of early motherhood. Our study takes Dubrwiny's research a step further, analyzing social media platforms. The interactive space of social media also constructs "good motherhood" in the postpartum context. But it does more than that. We discovered that individuals turn to social media for support in the absence of formal medical care or insufficient familial or community support during the first six weeks.

To construct a picture of perceptions of PPC on social media platforms, we analyzed social media discourses by using R6 to analyze English-language, U.S.-based social media postings over a 90-day period (October–December 2017). We conducted R6 searches using the terms "postpartum care" and "support" and "postpartum depression," then analyzed approximately 1,154 pages of social media postings, with over 9,000 posts, tweets, and retweets. We coded more than 200 pages, including 2,056 comments/posts on social media platforms (e.g., FB, Twitter, Pinterest, Instagram [IG]). We kept track of retweets and reposts on these pages before we reached saturation.[7] In our R6 analyses, commenters drew attention to the reality that PPD and postpartum psychosis (while tangible, serious problems) are not the only issues that mothers face during this period. Posts most often included comments about PPD or anxiety but also revealed significant struggles with lack of available PPC and support during the first six weeks. Many posters reported feelings of isolation, despair, and/or anxiety and depression as they longed for care and support they did not receive.

In the absence of the face-to-face, broad-ranging support many postpartum individuals desired, new mothers used social media as a place to ask questions about personal health concerns, such as breastfeeding issues, exhaustion, and healing difficulties. Lorelai (2017) shared, "I also felt little . . . support for related medical issues that came up (hemorrhoids, etc.) and often found myself reaching out to friends/online support communities to find out if my experiences were common." Responses to individual questions varied. FB and BabyCenter chat group/app conversations often prompted debates and disagreements, while Twitter and IG seemed to offer space for venting about lack of support but weren't conducive for extensive dialogue. In a BabyCenter post Aurora679 (2017) identified a lack of support, yet worried her struggles were selfish: "Mommies, I need to vent. I'm a little over 3 wks pp. . . . My mom is a really nice person, but I just can't understand why she wants to leave so soon. . . . This is depressing me even more. I just feel so alone. . . . Am I being selfish?" Some responses to Aurora679 suggest that social media can be a space of policing maternal desires for support, underscoring a tough-it-out ideal of postpartum motherhood. For example, one respondent claimed that Aurora679 should be grateful to receive any help at all.[8] "It's not really your mom's responsibility to help you out with baby. It was your decision to have a baby, not hers. . . . Appreciate the help you were able to get" (Aurora679, 2017). Preggosteph chimed in, "I think you are the one being selfish" (Aurora679, 2017). And 03+05+07 Mommy added, "With my first I had my mom come for one day to show me the ropes and that was only for a few hours. DH (dear husband) went back to work immediately. I had a 3rd degree laceration and was only 21. I managed just fine! You will be fine!" (Aurora679, 2017). These responses reveal that many individuals lack sufficient PPC. Perhaps as a result of that lack and their own struggle through the period, some internalize the message that needing, wanting, or asking for assistance isn't socially acceptable. As a result, online users sometimes police one another through one-upping (Haferkamp, Eimler, Papadakis, & Kruck, 2012) and shaming, moving responsibility for postpartum outcomes onto the individual and neglecting questions about a systemic lack of support. Haferkamp, Eimler, Papadakis, and Kruck (2012) surmised that women share personal information in social networking environments, while men tend to compete through one-upping practices. In our research on the postpartum period we saw women engage in both practices simultaneously—one-upping through the communication of personal information. A few respondents were supportive of Aurora679's (2017) concerns. Mermaidalways said, "Good luck and remember your [sic] not alone" (Aurora679, 2017). Still, throughout this conversation no one questioned, "Why are we struggling? Why did we need more help than we received?" After reviewing Boston and New England postpartum records, we were struck by the reality that many today have internalized isolation and lack of consistent medical, familial, or other PPC supports as normative. In the age of social media, lay experts turn to these platforms for support and to ascertain the severity of their medical symptoms and other concerns early twentieth-century postpartum patients could discuss with practitioners in person and at no cost.

Others also turned to social media to combat isolation; but in some cases this led to increased feelings of isolation. Karen (2017) divulged, "I did reach out on social media. . . . I searched blogs and websites desperate for reassurance. Most of the time, I would end up feeling more anxious than when I started! Any helpful suggestions or stories online would just lead to rabbit holes of all the other horrible possibilities and personal stories that were truly terrifying." Mothers sometimes exited social media after platform use added to feelings of isolation and/or anxiety. Even some who work in the social media world lessened their use in the postpartum period. For example, blogger Hilary initially processed her unplanned C-sections and connected with other mothers through her posts. But she eventually withdrew: "I did use social media a ton to ask questions in the beginning. Facebook groups primarily. . . . I have since pulled back from using social media for this purpose. I found that people's opinions . . . would often send me into a further spiral of fear and indecision, and the FB groups tended to get pretty judgmental and dogmatic about 'their approach'" (Hilary, 2017). As a seasoned contributor to online discourses around motherhood, Hilary perceived social media platforms as a source of stress where every commenter offered an expert opinion and the certainty (and judgment) of others unsettled her during a challenging time. Similar to our findings regarding other stages in the life cycle of early motherhood, we found that during the early postpartum period social media can increase anxiety and self-surveillance and confuse or complicate the boundaries of lay and technical expertise. On the other hand, they can also provide community, relieve fears (e.g., "Is this normal?"), and provide resources at unusual times when most practitioners are not available (e.g., middle-of-the-night feedings).

We came across some mothers in our R6 results who used social media as a way to advocate and bring awareness to PPD. For example, Adriana Neff (2017) reposted an IG post on Twitter: "Did you know that 1:7 women experience Postpartum Depression? I sure didn't. And because I thought I was alone, I suppressed the urge to speak up. Postpartum Depression survivors [can support] other moms through mentorship." There are research-based advocacy groups composed of lay experts (who had PPD) and technical experts (e.g., psychologists) who provide supportive treatment and mentorship, such as through the American Pregnancy Association (2017b) and International Childbirth Education Association (ICEA, 2017). Both organizations were named in tweets advocating awareness and support for women experiencing PPD: "Are you experiencing the baby blues or postpartum depression? Discover the importance of support during this time" (American Pregnancy Association, 2017b) and "Sleep and Support Essential in Treating Postpartum Depression" (ICEA, 2017). These posts link to articles with more information on these topics. The *Huffington Post* reported on a BabyCenter survey in which 90% of respondents knew about PPD but 40% who may have struggled with symptoms did not seek care because of fear of social censure and because of the belief that they could (or should) tough it out (Pearson, 2014; Rope, n.d.).

On August 8, 2017, *Mothering Magazine* posted on FB, "Postpartum depression (PPD) often hides behind a seemingly picture-perfect family." Digging into this post and its responses, we saw how lay experts asserted technical expertise, claiming to have "the cure" for PPD. As Brenda, in response to an article posted on *Mothering Magazine* (2017), proclaimed, "Take your darn progesterone cream you will be fine." After pushback, she continued to defend her position: "My directives are towards caregivers . . . give your patients progesterone" (*Mothering Magazine*, 2017). As a lay expert (and mother seven times over), Brenda felt comfortable giving health advice to other people online, including providing "directives" to practitioners. Unfortunately, she reduced all postpartum issues (physical, mental, social) to a progesterone imbalance, which cannot fix postpartum eclampsia or prevent a stroke. Even in the context of seeking support or expertise on social media platforms, misinformation and/or oversimplification are risks, particularly when categories of expertise are blurred (e.g., sharing personal anecdotes alongside suggestions for hormonal therapy).

While individual solutions to postpartum struggles vary, so does the role social media platforms play for individuals. Interviewees and social media posts reflected the reality that postpartum patients are responsible for monitoring and guiding their own medical recovery, a similar individualized burden of responsibility we address in chapter 3 about pregnancy risks. What is clear is that many individuals in the first six weeks postpartum struggle with unmet needs and health challenges and turn to social media, where lay expertise (helpful or not) offers the possibility of filling this support gap.

QUESTIONS WE STILL CAN'T ANSWER

The terror [associated] with motherhood, particularly [the] postpartum stage, is directly connected to the isolation and dearth of meaningful support. (Rowan Reyes, 2017, personal communication)

In the past and in the present, postpartum practices in other countries protect a period of time during the first six weeks as a unique medical stage in the life of birthing bodies that requires quiet, rest, and supportive care (Gigante-Brown, 2015; Kendall-Tacket, 2017; Tuhus-Dubrow, 2011). In China, the postpartum period is 30 days; 100 days in Korea; 21 days in Japan; 30 to 44 days in Malaysia;

40 to 60 days in India; up to 40 days in various African nations. Across Latin America, the practice of *la cuarentena* or quarantine lasts up to 40 days (Gigante-Brown, 2015; see also Kendall-Tackett, 2017; Stern & Kruckman, 1983; Tuhus-Dubrow, 2011). Yet postpartum patients in the United States will find their six weeks largely devoid of special care and diets and without increased health care or additional physical, social, and emotional supports, unless their families/communities engage in alternative cultural practices or plan for and sometimes pay for PPC (Kendall-Tackett, 2017; Stern & Kruckman, 1983; Tuhus-Dubrow, 2011). Health psychologist Kathleen Kendall-Tackett (2017) argued that postpartum, cis females are "typically . . . discharged from the hospital within 24 to 48 hours after a vaginal birth or 2 to 4 days after a cesarean section. . . . There is a tacit—and sometimes explicit—understanding that she is not to 'bother' her medical caregivers unless there is a medical reason, and she must wait to talk to her physician until her six-week postpartum checkup" (n.p.). Anthropologists Gwen Stern and Laurence Kruckman (1983) also noticed that the management and conceptualization of the postpartum period in the United States "virtually excludes any notion of a post-partum period after hospitalization" (p. 1028). In short, the postpartum patient ceases to exist shortly after the birth. In contrast, the baby gains an expanded definition as a patient and experiences involved and consistent care from a range of available experts during the same period.

While reframing women as competent and influential agents in and after their birth process was a necessary and powerful corrective to nineteenth-century medical understandings of "weak" or "frail" female bodies, this construction risks situating the postpartum period as a time when females who "conquered" birth don't need further care. After all, if women are seen as biologically determined to give birth, it would be expected that they would heal well afterward, perhaps with little intervention (see also Craven, 2010; Gaskin, 2002). Theoretically, PPC should be an extension of an empowered pregnancy and birth experience, where women have access to a wide range of health care resources and support systems. However, we maintain that both contemporary medical approaches and, to some extent, feminist empowerment rhetoric (e.g., "'your body is made to do this' narratives") result in mothers internalizing the message that women should just endure, while minor (and even mortal) difficulties are par for the course. At doctor visits, at the ER, in chatrooms, and on FB, both technical and lay experts left women thinking they must be strong enough to push through on their own. We are still waiting for our revolution in PPC.

Recently, practitioners such as obstetrician Dr. Alison Stuebe have drawn attention to what they call the "fourth trimester," or the 12 weeks following birth (4th Trimester Project, 2017; Strauss, 2016). In an online article for *Slate*, Stuebe described available PPC: "Once the candy is out of the wrapper, the wrapper is cast aside" (Strauss, 2016, n.p.). Media studies scholar Lesley Husbands (2008) has examined popular media representations of the postpartum period and concluded that these images construct a postpartum period in which the body is orderly, clean, and sanitized and quickly returns to the acceptable (meaning white, thin, abled, cis) body. The media display few leaky bodies, few infected stitches, no edema, and no intense emotions here; the mediated postpartum body in recovery is sanitized, anesthetized, and, by extension, erased. Again, this particular representation of the postpartum period reflects the patriarchal, individualist culture in the United States, where postpartum bodies must have a quick recovery, achieve parenting excellence, and return to "normal," without remaining physical or emotional evidence of a pregnancy or birth (see also Hausman, 2007). This bodily erasure also narrows postpartum representation to cis women and their babies and fails to consider surrogates, biological parents who have an adoption plan, individuals who identify as transgender and/or nonbinary, individuals who lose their babies at birth, and adoptive mothers with newborns. Kendall-Tackett (2017) posited, "American mothers often find that people are more concerned about them before birth" (n.p.). If women in recovery don't receive attention, if "good mothers" experience bodily erasure, then these other groups don't exist.

Doula Salle Webber (1992) described PPC care work as checking the health and examining breasts, relieving muscle discomfort (e.g., lower back), monitoring the baby's level of hydration and sleeping behavior, ensuring the mother stays hydrated, changing sheets, performing light housework, talking through health concerns and questions, and ultimately helping produce a clean and calm environment for mother and baby. Though Webber is considered a "lay expert" in today's medical system, she performs work similar to what Boston doctors offered their outpatients. Their records chronicled changing sheets, preparing tea and checking on food sources, monitoring the baby's health, cleaning the birthing room, and directing family or community members to care for the baby while the mother was treated, cleaned, and made comfortable. Then, in recurrent daily visits, doctors monitored breasts and nipples, stitches, and abdominal health and observed discharge, temperature, and pulse while watching for serious complications. In short, they provided the care that scholars, activists, and many technical (medical) experts have called for in the last 25 years and continue to call for today (4th Trimester Project, 2017; Gigante-Brown, 2015; Kendall-Tackett, 2017; Martin & Montague, 2017a; Stern & Kruckman, 1983; Strauss, 2016; Tuhus-Dubrow, 2011).

In the absence of normalized, accessible medical treatment expertise, it is understandable that individuals would experience confusion about their health and how to seek adequate PPC in the weeks and months after birth. Whether or not postpartum individuals would feel comfortable with doula care, as it stands now, there is no option to receive PPC support outside of one's network without paying out of pocket. The assumption is that PPC takes place in the 48 hours after birth, though in reality the health risks extend for months afterward. Post-partum doula care is often outside of the budget of even many middle-class families, and income-insecure families without reliable transportation may struggle to schedule and then attend appointments with LCs or pediatricians, let alone addressing the bodily needs of the caregiver.

A shift in cultural and even medical understandings of the postpartum period and the necessity of PPC must occur before efforts to expand PPC are success-ful (see also Kendall-Tackett, 2017). The first shift would be contending with the reality that the United States has the highest rate of maternal death in the entire industrialized world, a rate that has been climbing since 2000 and is still increas-ing (Global, 2016; Martin & Montagne, 2017a, 2017b). Grassroots efforts to chal-lenge U.S. postpartum norms are gathering energy (Kendall-Tackett, 2017). The ProPublica/NPR investigation suggests a shift in media perceptions of PPC risks and the necessity of care, but this is only a beginning. As conceptualized and advocated in the larger feminist (birth) movement, PPC exists on the contin-uum of "natural birth" as a necessary extension of experiences of pregnancy and childbirth, and a time when medical care and social and emotional support are vital to the physical and mental health of the mother (Lynn, 2012; Strauss, 2016). Poet and feminist activist Adrienne Rich (1976) highlighted the work of schol-ars reframing the postpartum period (as well as pregnancy and birth) in an effort to transform these stages from periods of body erasure to an empowered embodi-ment with adequate social support (see also Arms, 1975).

Unseen by technical experts, postpartum patients don't always understand their embodied experience (e.g., Are these after pains normal? Is this swelling/bleeding/itching normal? Should I feel this anxious?), and lay experts on social media platforms sometimes offered a welcome influx of information. Individuals who did not feel supported socially or medically often lacked access to techni-cal experts. But in seeking to access expertise online, some faced social censure for expressing their anxiety, isolation, and despair, though the expertise of respondents remained unclear. Once commenters reframed physical, emotional, and social needs as "selfishness," the narrative effectively erased the postpartum adult person, policing leaky, recovering bodies daring to step outside cultural norms and good mother narratives.

Thematic throughout our work, particularly in the context of social media, is the reality that the binary of lay and technical expertise doesn't accurately describe any stage of the life cycle of early motherhood. We discovered this in the landscape of PPC as well. One mother had to lie to access care, while others just assumed their needs didn't matter. Still others expressed that they felt sup-ported, but they paid for care or had ready access to family members. Almost universally, individuals reached out to social media networks for medical exper-tise, advice, and support when they believed there was a problem with them-selves or their baby, even if they later found this choice problematic. Without proximity to a wide range of supportive resources due to accessibility (geo-graphical or economical), communities without the assurance of reliable PPC from technical experts may also struggle to find knowledgeable, supportive lay experts, even with access to social media.

Running throughout the social media posts and individual recollections was the specter of postpartum anxiety, PPD, and postpartum psychosis, expressed as the fear that postpartum difficulties would devolve into mental illness or that continuing difficulty and the desire for support itself would intimate a potential mental health problem. Over 30 years ago, Stern and Kruckman (1983) acknowl-edged that "between 60–80%" of U.S. mothers report having experienced the "baby blues," but argued that the continuum of baby blues to PPD most directly reflects a particular social failing in U.S. society: namely, the inability and/or unwillingness to support postpartum caregivers, focusing instead on the baby, to the detriment of both. To combat baby blues, Stern and Kruckman recom-mended (1) demarcating a distinct postpartum period (as other cultures do), (2) socially and medically structuring this period around protective measures and rituals aimed at the new mother, (3) allowing social seclusion, (4) mandating rest, (5) assisting mothers in tasks with help from technical and/or lay experts, and (6) socially recognizing and awarding status to the new mother.

Finally, Stern and Kruckman (1983) linked postpartum isolation, anxiety, and even some depression to lack of PPC in the United States, noting that in cultures with distinct PPC rituals, PPD is rarely if ever mentioned. That is not to say post-partum mental health isn't a valid and pressing issue or that individuals strug-gling with PPD and postpartum psychosis do not deserve formal and informal supports, including pharmaceuticals. We don't know which of these cases emerged as a result of lack of PPC and support. Would instituting Stern and Kruckman's (1983) six components of PPC prevent PPD and postpartum psy-chosis? In 2013, Peltason identified the ongoing gap between awareness of PPD and the "normal" postpartum experience. She noted that individuals are urged to remain vigilant regarding their mental health in the postpartum period—a focus revealed in our R6 findings as well. Peltason (2013) continued, "The prob-lem with that question as our primary approach to the struggles of new moth-erhood is that it suggests that the post-partum experience itself is just fine, unless of course you have a legitimate clinical illness that distorts your perception of it. And the post-partum experience is not just fine. It is immensely, bizarrely complicated" (n.p.).

As we explore throughout the book, difficulty in obtaining PPC is com-pounded by access to care, poverty, and even health before pregnancy, rooted in U.S. structural inequality. Such unequal access to quality resources impacts individuals throughout the life cycle of early motherhood (Martin & Montague, 2017a, 2017c). Difficulty receiving PPC is particularly alarming considering the overall high risk of death in the six-week postpartum period in the United States, which is even higher for African American women, rural women, and individuals facing income insecurity. This reality continues to resurface on social media platforms such as FB (Howard, 2017; Martin & Montague, 2017c). In late 2017, world-renowned athlete and tennis star Serena Williams had to beg for care just days after giving birth to her daughter (Lockhart, 2018). After fighting for the interventions and treatment she needed for a clotting condition, she ruptured her cesarean scar coughing and required surgery, an internal filter to prevent blood clots, and six weeks of bed rest at home (Lockhart, 2018). Even wealth and fame do not guarantee adequate treatment or attention in the postpartum period, particularly for African American women.

By examining historical casebooks and social media discourses around PPC, we conclude that a revolutionary shift would involve offering *any* routine, reliable, supportive care to postpartum bodies in the United States during the first six weeks post-birth. Considering Stern and Kruckman's (1983) six components of adequate PPC and the role of both lay experts and social media in filling in the care gap in our current medical system, two things are clear. First, the United States has made little progress in our understanding of the postpartum period and in providing necessary or even essential postpartum support for birthing bodies. The current maternal death rate in the United States demands a response, even though it is vastly improved from the early twentieth century as a result of medical advancements, medicines, and monitoring systems. Indeed, medically speaking at least, we seem to have forgotten what we once knew.

Second, as we discover throughout this book, social media play a role in providing expertise, offering a resource for individuals in crisis when traditional forms of knowledge are not readily available. However, social media platforms are not only a place of solace—regarding postpartum struggles, these platforms can also increase confusion, anxiety, and social isolation. But in our current health care context, what works? The daily check-ins, the attention to patients' own assessments of well-being and pain level, and the importance of maternal health are elements we can take from this earlier era and better integrate today. In today's social media context, there are also benefits to consider, such as the immediacy of information and the availability of social supports, though both the information and support may not be the perfect fit for each user. Regardless of what methods we return to, continue to use, or start to use, we must take seriously that once a baby is born, birthing bodies exist and all are worthy of physical, emotional, and social support.

PART IV

INFANT LOSS AND
EARLY CHILDHOOD

CHAPTER 7

MEMENTO MORI IN THE VICTORIAN ERA AND ON SOCIAL MEDIA

THE "RIGHT" (WAY) TO GRIEVE

Is it not melancholy to see how the family die off? They have lost five out of seven children. Three in six months. Mama writes that uncle John and aunt M. bear their loss wonderfully well.

—Floride Clemson (Sublette, 1993, p. 146)

On December 20, 1858, three-year-old Cornelia Clemson died of scarlet fever (Sublette, 1993). Nina, as her family called her, was well loved. On numerous occasions, her mother Anna Calhoun Clemson feared she was "spoilt" and suggested that "when she gets older, all the little spoiling can be corrected" (Sublette, 1993, p. 623). Anna Clemson peppers her letters to her elder daughter Floride from 1856 to 1858 with Nina anecdotes, describing the child's personality, teething struggles, intelligence, growing vocabulary, favorite toys, and illnesses (Sublette, 1993). In toddlerhood, Nina's worst habit was "screeching, which she [did] to show pleasure, or anger at the top of her voice" (Sublette, 1993, p. 631). Anna was often effusive: "Nina sends many kisses. She is hearty & quite rosy & gay as a lark—& too smart" (Sublette, 1993, p. 630).[1] In these letters, it is apparent that Nina was a valuable member of the family. Anna discussed Nina in nearly every letter to Floride between Nina's birth in 1855 and her death in 1858. Given the constancy of Anna's discussion of Nina, the abrupt absence of all mention of the child after her death creates a noticeable and uncomfortable silence at the end of each letter, in which Anna mentions Nina's nurse Babette, but no longer ends with greetings from and anecdotes of the family baby (see also McGee, 1989).

Published material from the family letters does not allude directly to Nina's passing, but the family archive provides further information about the grief process as well as attempts to memorialize Nina's passing with new photographic technology. A letter from Anna's mother, Floride Calhoun, just a week after Nina's passing, elucidates this trying time for the family:

> Just this moment received both of your letters . . . the illness and death of our darling little Cornelia, which is indeed a severe shock to me. . . . I feel keenly for you all. . . . I feel for my dear Anna, fearing it may cause her severe indisposition, but her as much as possible to *restrain her feelings* and live for her remaining children, who now require the watchful care of a mother and *resign* her dear child, to God, and view her, a little angel in Heaven. (Letter from Floride Calhoun to the Clemsons, 1858, emphasis added)

In an album of Anna Clemson's unpublished materials, she wrote,

> Oh Nina oh my angel where are you? Why are you taken? When shall I see you again? Never—never . . . when a mother loses her child it is lost forever . . . what should we do without the memory of the loved & lost . . . when alone the closed doors of my heart open & the dwellers in those silent chambers come out & surround me once more. Then my Nina plays around me or climbs my knees & puts her arms around me with loving words . . . but a footstep approaches . . . the heart closes, & life is once more sad and gloomy. (Album leaf on Cornelia, n.d.)

This entry, perhaps viewed only by Anna, suggests a deep grief and longing, indulged only in private spaces.

This personal grieving is reflective of the expectations around loss in Victorian culture—a mastery of public emotions alongside deeply felt sentiments (Hoffert, 1989; Iepson, 2013; North American Women's Letters and Diaries, n.d.; Sublette, 1993; Thomas G. Clemson Papers, 1786–2000). Though Anna's mother urges her not to dwell on her feelings and stay busy, she openly grieves Nina's loss in a letter to her namesake (granddaughter) Floride: "I cannot yet realize that I shall never again see her, dear, darling little Angel" (Letter from Floride Calhoun to Floride Clemson, 1858).

Nina was not the first child Anna Clemson lost. Her firstborn child died at three weeks old, and Anna wrote to her close friend and relative Maria Calhoun of her grief and attempts to master her emotions:

> My illness was very severe & my recovery retarded by the death of my poor little baby—Oh! Maria I am more reconciled to the blow but indeed it was hard to bear at first . . . but I promised myself not to write on the subject for words can now be of no avail. Do not think I permit my feelings to overcome me. . . . Remember I must but I will intrude my feelings on the notice of no one & my sole effort has been to control myself. (Sublette, 1993, p. 219)

The sentiment expressed in Anna's letter, a yearning for control of grief, prompted some historians to argue that parents in the eighteenth and early nineteenth centuries (and before) maintained varying levels of emotional distance from infants and young children, given the high risk of death before five (Ariès, 1981; Calvert, 1992; Pollock, 1983).[2] Zelizer (1994) posited that the long-term process of defining and redefining childhood—definitions impacted by race, class, and gender stereotypes—and the rise of nineteenth-century sentimentality regarding children coalesced to create the "priceless" child of the twentieth century.[3] Nuanced scholarly research addresses the sociocultural constructions of childhood and grief around infant and child loss (Ariès, 1962; Calvert, 1992; Hoffert, 1989; Linkman, 2011; Mintz, 2004; Pollock, 1983).

Today, parents grieve both publicly and privately; some post images of their beloved deceased children on social media platforms. In this chapter, we investigate Victorian grief and memento mori practices and ask, what are the "rules" of grieving such immense loss in today's social mediated world? As with so many aspects of social media behavior, social expectations remain in flux, while grieving families continue to look for resources (lay and technical) to meet their needs, just as families did in the nineteenth century.

In this chapter, we define "technical experts" as technicians aiding parents in recording their grief—photographers, funeral workers, and the technical manuals that guide them, as well as nurses, doctors, or other health workers present at the time of death. In the mid- to late nineteenth century, technical experts included doctors and photographers, though family and community members often acted as technical experts as well (particularly before the rise of mortuary practice) in terms of preparation for burial, "laying out" the body, and organizing the funeral. In the nineteenth century some funerary participants were lay experts present at the time of death including caretakers, friends, and even wet nurses. Today, lay experts include family, friends, and public commenters on social media (e.g., commenters on photographs on the Thanatos Archive, commenters on Facebook [FB] and Instagram [IG]). As ever, the boundaries between technical and lay expertise are fluid and hard to define. For example, in the 1980s, technical medical experts (nurses and doctors) engaged in lay photography (handheld cameras) to help parents document loss.

To ground our understanding of the resurgence of posthumous newborn and infant photography, we examine the Victorian practice of memento mori specifically for infant and early childhood loss, consider the role of technical and lay observers, and then interrogate the ways "seeing" can be misconstrued as "expertise" on social media today. How is grief around child loss policed on social media by both technical and lay experts? We compare the attitudes around child loss and public viewing in the mid-nineteenth century and the present and ask, is there a "right way" to grieve infant loss? We argue that there must be space available to parents for both public and private grief—including private memento mori images kept in the home or today on password-protected blogs and/or on social media and thus publicly available.

To assist us in understanding historical grief patterns and practices, we examined the Clemson Family Papers as well as newly digitized online archives such as the North American Women's Letters and Diaries collection, which includes over 150,000 pages of transcribed text. After examining hundreds of pages in this collection, it is undeniable that parents felt their children's loss in the mid-nineteenth and early twentieth centuries on a deeply emotional level, from the more well-known losses, such as that of Harriet Beecher Stowe's son Charley, of which she penned on July 26, 1848, "This heart-break, this anguish, has been everywhere, and when it will end God alone knows," to lesser-known women who grieved their loss(es) just as keenly (Stowe, 1848, p. 406). In March 1847, Abigail Gibbons wrote, "Sweet angel! hearts idol! our love for thee knew no bounds.... Oh, what a mournful blank in the home circle! deeper and darker desolateness, the more the heart-breaking reality is felt by us!" (p. 395). Hoffert (1989) uncovered the personal impact of infant loss in letters and diaries as well and noted grief-based stress "was perceived to pose a real threat to a mourner's physical and mental health" (p. 176) in the nineteenth century.

In a diary entry from January 1851 that reads as if someone penned it yesterday, Maria Dayton began, "I have come over to mother's to spend the day because it is too desolate at home. Last year at this time Theodore was ten days old" (Dayton, 1851, p. 220). She continued, "I feel that he might have been spared to me.... What can I do, for I can not forgive Dr. G—, I have told him so" (Dayton, 1851, p. 220). Gibbons's belief that her doctor medically mistreated her son intensified her grief. Gibbons's difficulty with the role of technical expertise in the demise of her son also underscores the ambivalence the American public had toward medical practitioners in the mid-nineteenth century, a time before both pediatrics and knowledge of sanitation (Janik, 2014; Vandenburg-Daves, 2014).

In July 1854, Varina Davis scripted, "I have made several efforts to write to you since our loss, but could not. My child suffered like a hero. A cry never escaped his lips until his death, but he would say, 'Mamma, I tired, I wana walk, I wan bed'" (Davis, 1854, p. 580). More than half a century later, on December 2, 1912, Elinore Stewart wrote, "Do you remember, I wrote you of a little baby boy dying? That was my own little Jamie, our first little son. For a long time my heart was crushed. He was such a sweet, beautiful boy. I wanted him so much" (Steward, 1912, p. 281). Nowhere in these diary entries and letters do we see coldness or indifference; instead, the sentiments around pain and loss appear timeless.

These private communications are separate from the public mourning rituals popular in Victorian American culture (Hoffert, 1989; Laderman, 1996; Linkman, 2011). Understandably, some practices differ from the grief rituals engaged in by parents after the loss of a child today. However, the recent resurgence of infant loss photography and the (Internet-based) fascination with both Victorian loss photography often referred to as memento mori (Burns, 1990, 2011; Burns & Burns, 2002; Van Der Zee, Dodson, & Billops, 1978) and Victorian mourning culture as a whole parallel public reactions to present-day loss photography groups like Now I Lay Me Down to Sleep (NILMDTS, 2016). The interest in posthumous photography of infants and young children, past and present, reflects the ongoing struggle over how to deal with the loss of a beloved child.

Contemporary interest in infant loss contributed to a contest of meaning over Victorian grief and by extension over appropriate expressions of grief over infant loss today. This contemporary interest is possible to measure on the Internet and on social media platforms. The Thanatos Archive, an online collection of Victorian memento mori, has a dubious reputation and charges a membership fee for varying level of access to images. Some of these images may be counterfeit versions of originals photographed or scanned from other archives and printed collections; users engage with these images as legitimate archival images (Burns, 2017). Regardless of this online archive's reputation, site members have left hundreds of comments, revealing public perceptions of memento mori as well as assumptions around technical (scholarly) expertise on death and grief rituals as expressed in contemporary social media. In comment chains under pictures of deceased infants, members claim that academics are unwilling to recognize the stark grief of parents who lost children in the Victorian era (Thanatos Archive, 2017).[4] We find the popular, lay notion in this social media discourse of the "cold" expert analysis inaccurate and overly simplistic. From firsthand accounts, we can see that Victorian parents experienced the same devastation from the loss of a child as people do today. Available scholarship reflects an awareness of the depths of parental grief in various periods in history and the ways grief is shaped by cultural constructions of childhood and the "worth" of children from various racial, ethnic, and class backgrounds and across genders (Ariès, 1981; Calvert, 1992; Hoffert, 1989; Iepson, 2013; Laderman, 1996; Mintz, 2004; Zelizer, 1994).

Interestingly, the dissemination of posthumous digital photographs of infants on social media platforms initially prompted censorship and a media firestorm around picture policies on FB and IG. This short-lived scandal illustrates the taboo nature of death in American culture today as well as the willingness of lay experts on social media to police the way(s) that parents grieve and memorialize their lost children. Interestingly in Victorian culture, "mastery of emotions" and public self-control were preferred behaviors, though individuals had an outlet for grief in a wide variety of public grief rituals (e.g., memento mori, mourning jewelry and art). Today fewer acceptable outlets are available to grievers, yet we still expect individuals to discipline their grief so as to not make others uncomfortable. We find reactions to modern-day memento mori on social media consistent with expectations around keeping grief a private affair. Furthermore, the similarities between nineteenth-century memento mori images and the professional photography produced today are striking and suggest a timeless desire to hold on to those we have lost.

NINETEENTH-CENTURY MEMENTO MORI: LOSS AND PARENTAL GRIEF

Long before photography, cultures sought ways to represent their dead and the process of dying (Linkman, 2011). Photographing the dead, specifically children, was widely practiced from the arrival of photography (1850s) until the early twentieth century (Burns & Burns, 2002; Hilliker, 2006; Hoffert, 1989). With the rise of funeral homes and services in the late nineteenth century, death became more institutionalized and postmortem photography began to disappear in mainstream American culture, particularly after World War I. However, in some immigrant groups and among the significant middle- and upper-class African American population in Harlem, New York, the practice continued (Burns & Burns, 2002; Hilliker, 2006; Linkman, 2011; Van Der Zee, Dodson, & Billops, 1978).

As Julia Sublette (1993), the editor of Anna Calhoun Clemson's published letters, stated, nineteenth-century diaries and letters highlight "the constant reminder of the ever-present threat of illness and death" (p. 49). The inability of nineteenth-century medicine and medical technique to prevent, cure, or even adequately diagnose illnesses from bronchitis to cancer is well documented (Breslaw, 2012; Hoffert, 1989; Iepson, 2013; Janik, 2014; Starr, 1982; Ulrich, 1990; Vandenberg-Daves, 2014; Weiner & Hough, 2014). Nationally collected data show that as late as 1900 in some U.S. cities, up to one-third of infants died before their first birthday (Morbidity and Mortality Weekly Report, 1999; see also Meckel, 1990). As a result, "The familiarity with death . . . led individuals to seek consolation and succor from a support network accustomed to the emotional rupture caused by death" (Laderman, 1996, p. 22).

A fascination with the departed, notably the corpse (Laderman, 1996; Linkman, 2011), allowed for the development of a unique mourning culture in Victorian America: cultural practices included complicated dressing rules, the depiction of coded church bells suggesting the age and gender of the deceased, funeral processions, flowery elegies printed with coffin imagery, and symbols such as hourglasses, urns, cherubs, and willows on tombstones and in art. The grieving sought both imagery and artifacts, which included mourning jewelry (and often displayed locks of hair from the deceased), as well as hair from the deceased woven in intricate designs including flowers and other scenes (Iepson, 2013; Laderman, 1996; see also Ariès, 1981). Beginning in the 1840s, artifacts could comprise photographic images, including daguerreotypes, and eventually cabinet cards, tintypes, and finally paper-based photography (Iepson, 2013; Osterman & Romer, 2007; Romer & International Center of Photography, 2005). The posthumous daguerreotypes of infants and young children served as a vital physical bridge between grieving parents and buried children; parents could physically open a velvet-lined case and touch the child's image, as they would a coffin and the physical body (Hoffert, 1989; Iepson, 2013; Laderman, 1996).

In the Clemson family, there is ample evidence of Victorian grief culture in family letters and records. Floride Calhoun wrote to her granddaughter Floride Clemson eight days after Nina's passing, "I have just sent the ambrotype likeness of our dear little Cornelia, as you requested . . . and hope you will receive it safely. I put it in an old case to keep it more secure" (Letter from Floride Calhoun to Floride Clemson, 1858). Floride Clemson left a written record of her entire collection of jewelry, including numerous pieces made with family hair (earrings, bracelets, breast pin, and a cross of gold with her grandfather's hair "cut off in the coffin"), a number of miniature postmortem likenesses (portraits), a locket "daguerreotype likeness" of an uncle, and "Nina's coral bracelets," which were given to children as protection against sickness (Iepson, 2013; Record of jewelry collection, n.d.). There is no record of the ambrotype of Nina referenced by her grandmother, but it may have been in Anna Clemson's possession.

Initially, the daguerreotype boasted the widest popularity among Americans, and the production of these images and their frames and cases became a lucrative business in major cities (Osterman & Romer, 2007; Romer & International Center of Photography, 2005). As Osterman and Romer (2007) argued, American daguerreotypists were particular experts in this portraiture, which featured small, silver plate production and could not be copied. Ambrotypes (a more inexpensive image printed on a glass plate and not a silver one), like the one referenced by Floride Calhoun, overtook daguerreotypes in the late 1850s and early 1860s. Ambrotypes presented a cheaper, faster method—one that middle- and lower-middle-class families could access (Langberg, 2011). By the 1890s, photographs were available in a wide range of sizes in a variety of print styles and media, from paper to pure platinum (Osterman & Romer, 2007). Photography underwent a further "democratization" through the production of inexpensive, user-friendly cameras such as the Kodak Brownie in the first quarter of the twentieth century (Ennis, 2011).

Given the full range of typography of images and price points from the 1870s into the early twentieth century, postmortem photography became a "popular specialty item" (Laderman, 1996, p. 7 8). Memento mori images interested middle- and upper-class Protestant families, rural families (Burns, 1990, 2011; Burns & Burns, 2002, 2015; Laderman, 1996), and families of color particularly in urban areas in the early twentieth century (Holloway, 2002; Rietmann et al., 2017; Van Der Zee, Dodson, & Billops, 1978). As Holloway (2002) noted, "Perhaps as a testament to the familiarity of the experience, African Americans upheld the tradition of formal portraiture of the dead . . . [that] Euro-Americans did not" into the first two decades of the twentieth century (p. 27; see also Ruby, 1995).

As posthumous photography increased in popularity, it became an important tool for memorializing and grieving deceased infants and children. "Images of children assuaged the viewer's grief by suggesting a graceful, delicate, and peaceful death" (Iepson, 2013, p. 94; see also Hoffert, 1989). As Linkman (2011) noted, while infants and young children compose a marked majority of post-mortem photographs, memento mori were "born of love not indifference" (p. 19; see also Jalland, 1996). For impoverished families, the cost of a burial plot could be prohibitive, and their children were buried in mass paupers' graves as a result. As such, a daguerreotype, ambrotype, or some other form of postmortem photographic record acted as a memorial space to grieve in the absence of a burial site to visit (Linkman, 2011).

The twenty-first-century displays of nineteenth-century memento mori photography, such as the Internet collection the Burns Archive (2017), curated collections published in several volumes (Burns, 1990, 2011; Burns & Burns, 2002; Roberts, Johnson, & Dunn, 1986; Romer & International Center of Photography, 2005; Van Der Zee, Dodson, & Billops, 1978) and displayed in traveling museum exhibits (Romer & International Center of Photography, 2005), complicates the notion that parents sought posthumous photography because they lacked any other photographic representation of the child. Finally, the largest surviving collection of daguerreotypes, taken by American masters Southworth and Hawes in the second half of the nineteenth century, includes many dozens of images of living infants and young children, captured with or without family members (Romer & International Center of Photography, 2005). This extensive collection of images suggests that white Bostonian families of more than one economic class had their children professionally photographed while alive (Romer & International Center of Photography, 2005).[5] Photography celebrated living children as well.

Iepson's (2013) work on the death of infants and children in nineteenth-century American culture addressed the ways that memento mori, particularly the posthumous photography of children, helped create an idealized child and reflected the particular religious and sentimental culture of nineteenth-century Americans, which prized the angelic nature of children and childhood and the spiritual purity of women and the young. Postmortem images from the nineteenth and early twentieth centuries are divided into three main categories: sleeping angel images, family portraits, and illusory portraits (Iepson, 2013; Linkman, 2011). After studying the work of Iepson (2013), Linkman (2011), Burns (1990, 2002, 2011), and Van Der Zee, Dodson, and Billops (1978) and viewing and coding hundreds of images available in books and digital archives, we agree with the typographic categories espoused by Iepson (2013) and Linkman (2011). As we coded individual images, patterns emerged, regarding image type, surroundings, props, and lighting, that reflect previous findings and reveal linkages to modern, digitized memento mori.[6]

Sleeping angel images obscured death by suggesting the subject was merely in a state of sweet repose. By positioning the infant or young child as if the child

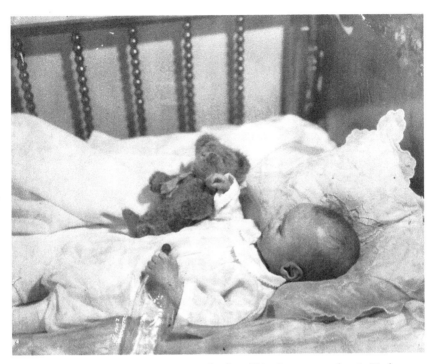

Figure 6. Comfort in passing, 1931. Note the date. This picture was taken in Harlem, reflecting the memento mori practices in that community well into the twentieth century. This image uses the "sleeping angel" motif with favorite objects placed in the tableau. Photographer: James Van Der Zee. Copyright: Donna Mussenden Van Der Zee.

was asleep, parents and other relatives had a relic that illustrated peace and relief, instead of the potential suffering endured before death. By meditating on this image, the viewer could become more at ease with the physical separation and focus instead on peace and new beginnings (Linkman, 2011). Black-and-white prints, soft lighting, babies or children tranquil and at peace on beds, cots, or couches, on clean linens, sometimes with toys, bottles, or other beloved objects nearby, suggest to the viewer the subject has fallen asleep mid-play. The only feature that might interrupt the ruse is a small bouquet of flowers, which sometimes appears in a young child's hands. There is a significant minority of "sleeping angel" pictures featuring newborn or infant multiples between 1850 and 1900, which documents the inherent danger of pregnancy and birth with multiples in a time before widespread sanitation practices, antibiotics, incubation, or neonatal medicine (see Figure 6).

While the majority of memento mori featuring young children and infants relied on the "sleeping angel" motif, family portraits are also common (see Figure 7). These pictures might include living siblings pictured next to or touching deceased babies and children and in some cases large, extended families gathered

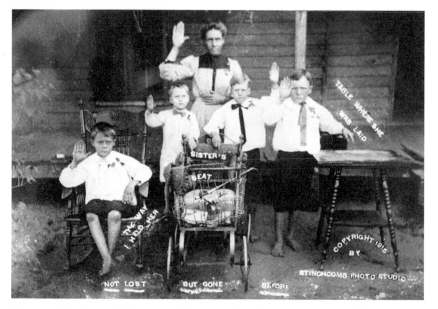

Figure 7. Sister's seat. Early twentieth century. Stanley B. Burns, MD and the Burns Archive.

around a deceased child (Burns, 2011; Burns & Burns, 2002). In other instances, two individuals, presumably the mother and father, are pictured with their child, either held across their lap (Burns, 1990; Burns & Burns, 2002; Johnson & Johnson, 1985; Van Der Zee, Dodson, & Billops, 1978) or, later in the nineteenth century, lying between them in a coffin (Burns, 1990, 2011).

Perhaps most fascinating (and complex) for a modern-day viewer is the death as illusion motif. The viewer may wonder, is the subject alive or deceased? In an analysis of illusory posthumous pictures of babies, Iepson (2013) scrutinized the use of facial tinting on the image (e.g., pink cheeks and lips) and props like pillows, toys (e.g., grasping drumsticks with a drum on the lap), and books. Iepson insightfully targeted the "tells" in these pictures, which include material creased from the weight of a lifeless body, a stiff posture, open eyes with glassy stare, and stiffness apparent in fingers, hands, and legs (see Figure 8). These pictures, while unusual in the present, served to catch a moment, "frozen in time and place, but with a physical presence that denies true loss or departure" (p. 93). Still, the signs of death in this form of pictorial memento mori may force the viewer beyond the acceptance of illusion to confront the reality of loss.

While Victorian mourning culture and mourning artifacts (e.g., rings featuring woven hair) capture public attention on social media outlets today (Dickens, 2011; Lovejoy, 2017), the resurgence of posthumous photography and artifacts memorializing newborns, infants, and young children is striking.

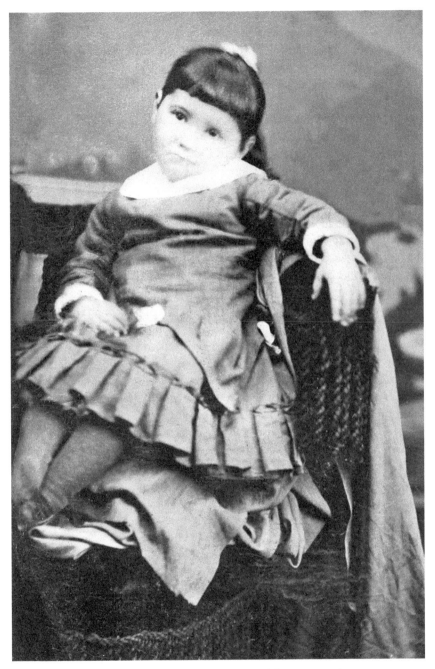

Figure 8. Death as illusion. Stanley B. Burns, MD and the Burns Archive.

Posthumous photography of children reemerged in the 1980s through what Ennis (2011) calls "vernacular photography," or photographs taken by "medical staff untrained in photography," what we conceptualize as lay photographers. Ennis (2011) argued that it followed a particular visual aesthetic (p. 136). In the 1980s, color prints showed a bathed and dressed baby with parents and other members of the family and/or with toys, and detailed shots of hands and feet became common (Ennis, 2011). Ennis (2011) noted that these pictures likely acted as photographic mementos within larger collections that included "hand and footprints, an identity bracelet, perhaps a lock of hair and a toy" (p. 136).

The particular style of 1980s posthumous photography is distinct from Victorian memento mori in that pictures were almost exclusively taken by lay experts. The 1980s photographs were similar to memento mori in that photographs became handheld objects, at least for a time, before the development of digital photography and smartphones. In the Internet age, lay experts include the parents and other grieving friends or family members, willing hospital staff, and other bystanders. Digital cameras record pictures that may never be printed but instead populate computer and tablet backgrounds or simply exist in file folders in "the cloud." Early cell phones captured grainy photographs that could be shared via text, while today's smartphones can capture higher resolution photographs that individuals can edit and enhance through a wide range of free apps; final images may or may not be shared with friends and family members or end up posted on private websites or on FB, IG, or other social media platforms or even be used in projects that create other memento-based artifacts such as pillows or scrapbooks. Hence, the rise of "vernacular death photography" (lay) is a response to "the medical and technological event dying has become, another way of taking control of one's own circumstances. . . . Photography provides a means of reclaiming the deceased from their position as a patient, rehumanising them" (Ennis, 2011, p. 138). This "reclaiming the deceased" occurs in a unique way online since pictures, tweets, and FB posts remain "in memoriam" as long as the Internet exists and in many cases, even after they are deleted (Fertik, 2015). Hence, new technologies may expand the forms of public grief available to parents after the loss of babies and young children.

GRIEF IN THE INTERNET AGE: NOW I LAY ME DOWN TO SLEEP AND SOCIAL MEDIA CENSORSHIP

U.S. infant mortality rates between the mid-nineteenth century and the late twentieth declined more than 90% (Flaherty, 2000; Hoyert, Kochanek, & Murphy, 1999), although African American infants continued to have a much higher rate of mortality despite these improvements (Holloway, 2002; Morbidity and Mortality Weekly Report, 1999). The CDC (2014) reported that the U.S. infant mortality rate in 2014 was 5.82 deaths per 1,000 live births, which Ingraham

(2014) referred to as a "national embarrassment" in comparison to rates in other industrialized nations (n.p.). Still, most American families today have not experienced the death of an infant. As a result, individuals view postmortem photographs differently today, particularly those that capture infant and child loss (Sauber, 2014; Wise, 2013). Historians of photography and social scientists are interested in shifting patterns of mourning and various aspects of death culture as infant loss became less common. They investigate rituals, artifacts, and culturally acceptable expression of grief (Burns, 1990, 2011; Burns & Burns, 2002; Gibson, 2008; Hallam & Hockey, 2001; Linkman, 2006, 2011; Ruby, 1995; Sontag, 1973).[7] These historians note that by the mid-twentieth century, the practice of memento mori photography declined, including among immigrant groups and African Americans communities (Ariès, 1981; Jalland, 1999; Kürti, 2012; Lutz, 2011). A resurgence of the practice began in the 1980s, when lay experts (parents) advocated for access to their children after loss and objects that served as mementos. This revival could reflect the reclamation of death from technicality as well as reclaiming private grief rituals in the public space of the hospital.

Until the 1970s, medical staff often prevented parents from viewing or holding their stillborn babies and encouraged families to forget their loss (Blood & Cacciatore, 2014a; Erlandsson, Warland, Cacciatore, & Rådestad, 2013; May, 2008), similar to the ways hospitals sought to control birth in the mid-nineteenth century (chapter 4). However, research started to identify the negative psychological outcomes attributed to this denial (Lewis & Page, 1978; Malacrida, 1999). Lay activists (parents and their supporters) advocated for birthing places to adopt compassionate baby and child loss protocols (Gold, Dalton, & Schwenk, 2007; Malacrida, 1999), such as honoring the baby's existence and supporting parents to express grief (Blood & Cacciatore, 2014; Capitulo, 2005). Today, social psychology research illuminates the value of postmortem photography as a way for parents to begin sense making and attempt to cope with the death of a child (Blood & Cacciatore, 2014b; Capitulo, 2005; Layne, 2000; Malacrida, 1999).

However, there are still some in mainstream U.S. culture and within the health care field that find memento mori photographs unusual, jarring, or even "creepy" (Cacciatore & Flint, 2012; Hilliker, 2006; Quinlan, 2011; Riggs, 2008). Currently, implementation of posthumous photography remains inconsistent as some families may decline to have images taken for a host of cultural reasons. At the same time, some hospitals hire professional photographers (technical experts) whereas others assign nurses or doctors to take the images (lay experts in photography; Jones, 2002; McCartney, 2007). Other parents may decide to take their own images on smartphones or personal cameras. Johnson and Johnson's (1985) *A Most Important Picture* became a key training manual for technical experts (professional photographers) and lay photographers (family members, friends, and doctors) taking images of stillborn infants. And today, the organization Now I Lay Me Down to Sleep (NILMDTS) utilizes password-protected instruction manuals and recently launched webinars to train photographers in technical and practical details for working with images, families, and hospital staff (Harris, 2017).

Currently, Americans display a strong cultural tendency to avoid direct contact with the dead and with death, in contradistinction to the Victorian cultural practices discussed above (Linkman, 2011). However, as we have shown, one consistency between the past (nineteenth century) and the present is the experience of grief after the loss of a child. In 2005, Cheryl Haggard, who lost her son Maddux six days after his birth, cofounded NILMDTS (2017) with photographer Sandy Puc'. Located in Colorado, this 501(c)(3) nonprofit organization connects mourning families with professional photographers and trained volunteers who provide gratis heirloom remembrance portraits to families. This organization offers both the print and twenty-first-century digitized photographic artifact of loss, the present-day version of memento mori. Currently, NILMDTS relies on nearly 1,700 active volunteers worldwide, including photographers, digital retouch artists, care package assemblers, and more (NILMDTS, 2017). NILMDTS digital retouch artist Bruce Muncy crops images to highlight the baby's unique features: "When I zoom in on the fingertips and toes and little ears, there's fingerprints, they are actually beautifully and wholly formed. So that's to me the incredible thing, how much a miracle each one of those lives are, and for me to be able to record that, and to give parents something to remember that little life by, I think that's all I need to do" (Dashiell, 2012, n.p.). NILMDTS creates private mementos of great significance for grieving families. But public displays of dead infants can be controversial, involving parents in contention about appropriate ways to grieve. In 2012, Tennessee-based mother Heather Walker said she was barred from posting images of her son, Grayson James, on FB because they displayed anencephalic facial and skull deformities. The pictures were reported and deleted, and she was denied access to FB as a result. The photographs included images of her son after his birth, with and without a cap. She said, "They [FB] allow people to post almost nude pictures of themselves, profanity, and so many other things but I'm not allowed to share a picture of God's beautiful creation" (Neal, 2012, n.p.). Neal (2012) stated, "Facebook's community standards state that the company can remove content that contains graphic violence, threats, self-harm, bullying and harassment, hate speech or nudity and pornography" (n.p.). Some people came to Walker's defense, while others critiqued the public display of these images. In 2013 Facebook posted an apology: "Upon investigation, we concluded the photo does not violate our guidelines and was removed in error. . . . Occasionally, we make a mistake and remove a piece of content we shouldn't have. We extend our deepest condolences to the family and we sincerely apologize for any inconvenience" (Andrusko, 2013). Although published articles discussing the FB ban reported that the photographer worked with NILMDTS (Dillion, 2014; "Faith" 2012; Morgenstern,

2012; Quigley, 2012), an interview with chief executive officer Gina Harris revealed that this was not an official NILMDTS session (Harris, 2017). The images shown had the photographer's logo and were in color. The standard gift from NILMDTS is a set of heirloom-quality remembrance portraits, gently retouched in black-and-white or sepia; it never includes watermarked photographer logos (Harris, 2017). Regardless of the source of the image, the larger question remains— who is allowed to critique online loss?

We argue that American society may not yet be equipped to engage with raw images of loss, particularly given that some of these images reveal babies born with disabilities that were (and are) often hidden from mainstream society. Scholars of the history of disability report that in the early nineteenth century "moral blame for most childhood disabilities" was assigned to parents and especially to mothers who lacked economic status (Ferguson, 2002). More and more children were institutionalized (e.g., asylums, reform schools) to separate parents and children with disabilities (Demos, 1979; Farber, 1986; Katz, 1983). We did not compare the number of contemporary images of infants and children with disabilities in postmortem photography on social media versus in Victorian-era archives and printed collections. But we did observe that through the lens of ableism, there appears to be some technical-lay tension related to the depiction of children with disabilities or chronically ill bodies. For example, many of the images from the Victorian era include visual markers such as visible dehydration (from diarrheal illness) and some with cut or shaved hair (from scarlet fever). However, as lay experts ourselves, it is difficult for us to label disabilities in historical images (e.g., ambrotypes), though we did view enlarged heads that suggested macrocephaly. Still, in almost every case, we had to guess, infer, or assume. Today, more images of children/infants with disabilities appear in postmortem photography, but this could reflect advances in modern medicine prolonging pregnancies and the lives of infants and children with complex disabilities or prematurity. Contemporary photographers use similar techniques to "soften" the appearance of deceased infants and toddlers, but some of the lay experts we interviewed expressed mixed feelings about making images of their children acceptable to viewers (i.e., hiding or softening illness and disability). The lack of technical expertise in the form of formal diagnosis complicates our ability to understand how Victorian families and communities dealt with the loss of babies/toddlers who did not appear "perfect/normal" or able-bodied.

The reasons for infant and child loss today differ due to medical advancements, so posthumous photographs happen just before or after the baby or child passes. Organizations like NILMDTS (2017) offer these images free of charge. However, during the Victorian era, families commissioned a photographer. Unlike in the Victorian age, postmortem images today are often captured in the hospital. Still, in contemporary photographs medical technology is removed; digital pictures often match the aesthetic of Victorian memento mori photography, perhaps making the images more palatable to viewers (Harris, 2017). Also similar to the Victorian age, modern-day digital pictures may depict babies who appear to be sleeping, and the innocence and purity of the child are underlined by soft and ambient lighting, cropping, positioning, and very light editing. According to Gina Harris (2017), images are gently retouched to smooth out skin that may be bruised or torn. Images are never retouched to change any unique features of a baby (such as a cleft lip or an extra finger on a hand) but are retouched like professional portraits of living subjects. In the Victorian era, images were also edited; the use of soft, ambient lighting did the work of a modern retouching. Are ambient lighting and retouching ways to "soften" the loss, allowing the viewer a moment of denial or making grief less stark?

In our analysis, the images that receive the least amount of policing are the ones most similar to those produced during the Victorian era (e.g., black-and-white or soft color touches, ambient lighting, "sleeping angel" positions). Gina Harris (2017) reported that NILMDTS had not had any of their images banned. Organization representatives believe that no social media platform or entity should ban any images, whether or not they were produced by NILMDTS and no matter what style or aesthetic the photographs display. Parents should be able to post pictures of their babies on social media platforms (Harris, 2017).

Today, parents report these images as one of the only (and most treasured) keepsakes they have to commemorate a child's life or death and a permanent marker of life (NILMDTS, 2017) (see Figure 9). Still, there is insufficient research on parental preferences for postmortem photography (Harvey, Snowdon, & Elbourne, 2008). As a parent in Blood and Cacciatore's (2014a) study lamented, "I would have liked someone to offer me the choice of spending time taking photos with my deceased child," reflecting the wish of many parents that they had more photographs or keepsakes to aid in the grieving process (p. 5).

When a family living in the Seattle area unexpectedly lost their daughter Amaiya after her birth, Amaiya's parents went through the process of taking photographs with a local NILMDTS photographer. In shock after their loss, the couple's doula and midwife suggested the photographs (Anonymous personal communication, 2017). In a local hospital room otherwise used for medical procedures, the parents were allowed to stay with their daughter as long as they wanted. Though some of her own vitals were slightly unstable, Amaiya's mother and father declined further monitoring and assessments and chose to leave the hospital in the middle of the night. She said they needed to let go of Amaiya's physical body to begin the process of saying goodbye to her. Today, their NILMDTS pictures, which the mother initially hesitated about having taken, are treasured mementos of their time with Amaiya and of her life (Anonymous personal communication, 2017).

Erin Willer, a communication studies scholar at University of Denver who experienced the loss of her son Milo (survived by twin Matilda), remembers feel-

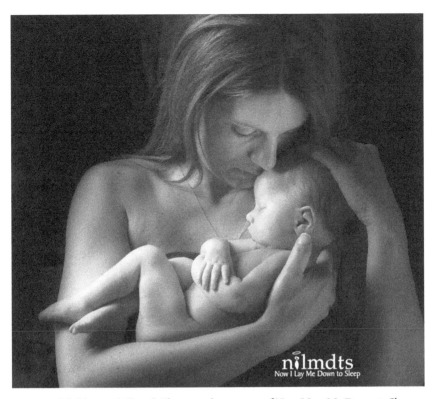

Figure 9. Maddux and Cheryl. Photograph courtesy of Now I Lay Me Down to Sleep, taken by Sandy Puc', photographer, of Cheryl Haggard, NILMDTS cofounder, with her son, Maddux Achilles Haggard.

ing proud to post the beautiful black-and-white postmortem photographs of her son Milo (Willer, 2017). Yet the full-color pictures best reflected her lived experience and her time with Milo; she recalled that she finds healing in those color images. However, Erin understands that color images are shown less often and viewed as "too harsh" for the rest of the world (Willer, 2017). She also noted that seeing memento mori of babies without abnormalities or who looked like sleeping, live babies ("sleeping angels") prompted complicated feelings of envy (Willer, 2017). Perhaps viewers struggled with images of her son who was born with a cleft pallet because he did not look "perfect" in the ways other infants do.

Grieving parents are vulnerable to online policing by lay community members who are uncomfortable engaging death and dying on social media platforms, even when pictures are discreet (illusory) or show infants or babies as "sleeping angels." Despite cultural discomfort with and avoidance of death, the dead, and the dying, grieving parents desire (and deserve) a way to mark the loss of beloved children. Even after FB's censorship of NILMDTS images ended, parents report ongoing tension around the decision to share the story of their

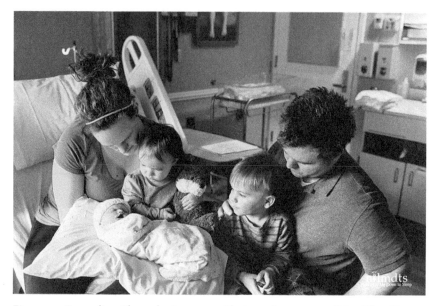

Figure 10. Evangeline Alexandra Lawrence. Photograph courtesy of Now I Lay Me Down to Sleep. Photographer: Sarah Sweetman.

children's birth, on social media or in face-to-face conversations (Willer, 2017). Willer remembered posting about the loss of her son Milo on FB. She observed that people often commented or "liked" postings about her living daughter Matilda more than her son who died; perhaps some FB contacts were uncomfortable or uncertain about what to say when she posted about her loss? Willer noted that in 2013 when her twins were born, FB allowed individuals only to "like" images, but now that there are more options (through emoticons), people have more ways to acknowledge posts about grief and loss. She wondered, how can parents with babies with disabilities or preterm babies with physical differences share their images—their grief—in public? (See Figure 10.)

In the wake of these tensions and complications, lay experts—many of whom have experienced various forms of baby loss, including miscarriage and stillbirth—continue to fashion mourning tokens and items for remembrance. In this way, lay individuals turn their "expertise," often fashioned from loss, into a resource for others. For example, the agency A Heart to Hold (AHTH) (2017a), a 501(c)(3) nonprofit, had a mission "to offer comfort to families who have experienced pregnancy or infant loss with the gift of a weighted handmade heart" (AHTH, 2017b). After the loss of Abi and Dave Crouch's son, a friend sent them a heart-shaped pillow that was the same weight as their son Corbin (Pearson, 2014; Ternus-Bellamy, 2014). They both cherished this pillow and eventually established a nonprofit to create weighted pillows and ship them free of charge to others who experienced pregnancy and infant loss. The pillows allow grieving parents an opportunity to hold and touch an item patterned after the child they lost. When Willer received a heart pillow that weighed 2 pounds 14 ounces (the same birth weight as Milo), it put "a weight to the memory of him—an embodied memory" (Willer, 2017). The demand for these pillows was so great that after a little media coverage they had orders for 600 heart pillows almost overnight. By 2014, after producing over 3,500 pillows, the organization was no longer active but provided directions on its website for individuals to create their own or make one for a grieving parent.

Erin Willer's journey with grief extended beyond social media, where she continued to post family pictures that included representations for Milo at holidays (e.g., a pumpkin for Milo next to Matilda and son Fyo at Halloween). Her journey of loss intersected with her work in 2010, when she worked with the local community to create the Scraps of the Heart Project (SOTHP). The website states that the group is "a collective of parents, health care providers, artists, students and researchers working together to empower families and educate communities about baby loss through story and creative arts" (SOTHP, 2017). This is an example of scholarly (technical) expertise coming together with lay expertise (e.g., artists, students, parents) to positively impact the community. In March 2017, SOTHP had an exhibit at the University of Denver showcasing their artwork. On the SOTHP website, individuals can learn about their workshops and research projects and purchase grieving cards and a children's book. At this stage in the work, Erin realizes that art is a way to connect with her son Milo, to show the world he is real and has an identity as a son and brother.

There is also a growing demand among the bereaved parents for an outlet online—particularly in social media contexts. For example, CarlyMarie (2017), a mother who lost her son Christian, has developed Capture Your Grief, a campaign where individuals can post images representing grief. There are FB groups and blogs dedicated to providing opportunities for individuals to share their stories (Healing Hearts Baby Loss Comfort, 2017; Ross-White, 2013). In Internet spaces, parents and particularly mothers make their loss and grieving process public—by displaying artifacts, joining support groups on FB, following blogs, and even posting videos of grief rituals, such as balloon releases. What we see from these online rituals and objects is another return to the past. Like Victorian mourning jewelry and art and the small, handheld daguerreotype, which opened to reveal a stunning "sleeping angel" surrounded by gold scrolling and rich velvet, the weighted pillows, scrapbooks, blog-based grief journeys (CarlyMarie, 2017), miscarriage jewelry (La Bella Dame, 2017), and digital photographs of today perform similar work. These memorial objects, rituals, and posthumous photographs not only provide a physical link to a lost child but also keep the child's name and identity from disappearing; they mark a life lived, however short.

As Amaiya's mother explained to us, the photographs she placed in a physical album and shared with friends and family through a password-protected website played an important role in her grieving process, which is ongoing: "For me . . . underneath it all . . . I wanted to celebrate our daughter and I wanted everyone else to celebrate with us, but knowing that only two others that we know met her, I knew that it wouldn't be real for other people. She was never real for anyone else" (Anonymous personal communication, 2017). As Amaiya's mother found, the act of creating both digital and physical mementos became a way of "reclaiming the deceased" by marking her daughter's place in the world. In the midst of staggering loss, parents rely on both technical and lay experts to support babies and children through birth, treatment, and end-of-life care, and then technical medical experts, technical photography experts, or lay experts to take photographs and fashion other memorial objects with which to memorialize their children.

Memento Mori: Access and Representation in the Nineteenth–Twenty-First Centuries

Despite the strictures of Victorian culture regarding behavior based on race, class, and gender, there was acceptance of public displays of grief through rituals for remembering the dead, including infants and young children. However, Victorian culture also required some self-policing through "restraining" emotions. Today, lay experts on social media have the power to police and constrain parents as they seek to memorialize their children through digital photography, communal grief projects (e.g., online Capture Your Grief project), and other social-media-based markers that parallel celebrations of birth and baby milestones for parents with living children. The lack of obvious historical context for grief rituals and memento mori for infants and young children specifically could factor into public fascination with Victorian memento mori as a provocative, "foreign" practice, while the work of NILMDTS and other groups is helping create broader cultural acceptance for public, social-media-based grief and memorializing (Burns & Burns, 2015).[8]

In both the past and the present, mourners deal with constraints around memento mori traditions. Currently, families may lack access to the Internet/ social media or lack knowledge of agencies like NILMDTS. If hospitals provide access to NILMDTS, the family may not own the digital technologies necessary to interact with the photographs. Previously, hurdles included access to photographers and studios, funds for artifacts like mourning jewelry, and access to burial sites. "Sister's Seat" (see Figure 7) is a photograph showing a family gathered around the chair of a child who died months previously; the family still desired a kind of postmortem photograph but had to wait for an itinerant photographer to arrive (Burns, 1990, no. 102). This illustrates the access issues that plagued rural families, including those with means. In the second half of the nineteenth century, the Civil War, Reconstruction, and Jim Crow laws became barriers for African Americans seeking to memorialize lost children. More-over, African American families also faced an infant mortality rate double that of white families, and this enraging disparity continued through the entirety of the twentieth century, decade by decade, in both rural and urban communities (Holloway, 2002; Morbidity, 1999).

The impact of structural inequality and violence experienced by African Americans during this period (and over more than four centuries) reminds us that "Victorian" is a descriptor with conceptual limitations in terms of class and race or ethnicity. Despite the universality of grief and loss, surviving material in the archive may provide only limited information on the experiences beyond white, middle- and upper-class individuals, who had the physical security and means to create, care for, and pass on physical tokens of mourning culture. To explore the experiences of African American communities, the work of Hollo-way (2002), Smith (2010), and others (Rietmann et al., 2017) is instructive, as are the posthumous photographs of revered African American photographers Van Der Zee, Dodson, and Billops (1978) and Richard Samuel Roberts (Roberts, John-son, & Dunn, 1986). Smith (2010) noted that as early as 1772 in New York City, the funerals of enslaved individuals could be held only during the day, with no more than ten attendees, for fear that gatherings could lead to uprisings. In Virginia in 1800, a group planned a rebellion at the funeral of an enslaved infant (Smith, 2010). Afterward, a white owner or clergy member had to be present at all funerals (Smith, 2010). In 1926, Charles C. Diggs secured land outside of Detroit for a black cemetery. When the local white population protested, he buried a stillborn infant on the property "to be sure the land could not be reclaimed for other purposes" (Smith, 2010, p. 65). Thus, the African American history of public grief and loss, which places mourning rituals under white sur-veillance, is a stark departure from Victorian traditions of home gatherings and communities walking the dead through the town to their final resting place, further still from the Southworth and Hawes daguerreotypes of beloved infants and children kept from burial long enough to be held tenderly, one last time. In this sense, James Van Der Zee's posthumous photographs of infants and children are not only memento mori; they are evidence of advancing social and politi-cal freedoms.[9]

Van Der Zee, Dodson, and Billops's (1978) photographs situated African American families and deceased children in seemingly intimate spaces, though they were often taken at funeral homes (Rietmann et al., 2017). Van Der Zee's memento mori work from the early twentieth century wasn't published until the 1970s, but it offers a snapshot into the practice during the Harlem Renaissance and afterward. Babies are placed in "sleeping angel" positions, pictured with toys. Kept privately, publicly displayed in the home, or sent to relatives, these images, their uses, and their locations are similar to earlier Victorian grief rituals, even if the cultural context and contours of grief were unique (Rietmann et al., 2017).

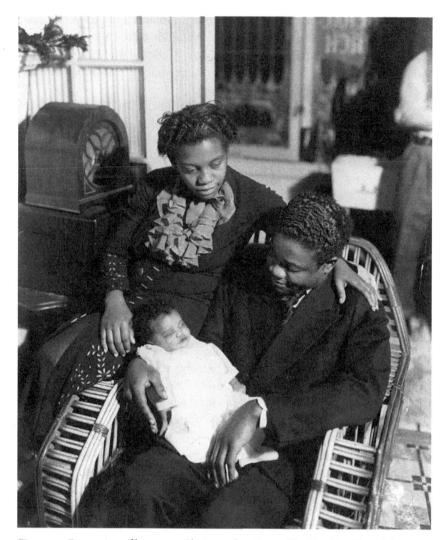

Figure 11. Expression of love, 1945. Photographer: James Van Der Zee. Copyright: Donna Mussenden Van Der Zee.

These photographs reveal the ways in which urban families in Harlem sought and achieved middle-class lifestyles, even in "their tenuous social position, in the face of death" (Rietmann et al., 2017, p. 7) (see Figure 11).

Observing African American memento mori of children in the twentieth century with the knowledge of grossly unequal infant mortality rates and the very real dangers of racial violence elucidates the complexities of grief for African American parents who lost a baby or young child. As Rietmann et al. (2017) remind us, W. E. B. Du Bois lost his firstborn, a son, and at the burial found his pain tinged with relief, knowing his child would not live to face racial discrimination, exclusion, or violence (see Du Bois, 1903). Again, while grief over child loss seems constant across sociocultural groups and across time, for African Americans the landscape of loss, the meaning behind memento mori, and the nature of public grief reflect a unique and painful history. Ruminating on the particular history of black lives in America, Holloway (2002) approached the body of her deceased son thusly: "Without recalling then that the first thing I had done those many years ago with my new four-year-old son was to braid his hair, I found myself doing a last thing like the first. I asked for scissors and then cut locks of his hair to give us something, some little, small touchable thing left of our child to come home with" (pp. 11–12). Holloway's loving act reflected a common urge for memento mori that extends back hundreds of years and reflects the rituals of many communities, despite divergent histories and narratives. Here, the locks of hair are an artifact of loss and longing again strikingly similar to those of nineteenth-century Victorian mourning culture.

While these similarities do not address the disparities in experience, they underscore the importance of making adequate, uncensored space for individuals to grieve the loss of any child, for any reason. Similar to the Victorian period, there are public and private forms of grief. While memento mori kept in drawers and parlors aided in private grief, sharing these same artifacts on social media interrupts the public/private divide. After interviewing mothers who posted images of their children and yearned for an uncensored, public space to express their grief, perhaps the lay community can honor these experts by considering how to bear witness to their grief on social media and more broadly within our culture as a whole, rather than disciplining or curtailing this process by making our comfort paramount.

CHAPTER 8

"BETTER BABIES"

EARLY TWENTIETH-CENTURY SCIENTIFIC BABYHOOD AND CONSTRUCTIONS OF TWENTY-FIRST-CENTURY INFANCY ON INSTAGRAM

On October 14, 2017, the Washington Parish Free Fair (WPFF) Better Baby Contest commenced in Louisiana (WPFF Better Baby Contest, 2017). Parents or guardians were encouraged to bring birth certificates and proof of residency to the Fairgrounds Exhibitors' Office. Reflecting historical anxiety about better babies contests being misconstrued as beauty contests, organizers warned competitors on their Facebook (FB) page, "NO PAGEANT DRESSES OR SUIT AND TIE" (Better Baby Registration, 2016; WPFF Better Baby Contest, 2013; see also Biddison, 1913; de Garmo, 1900–1985). Between 1908 and the late 1930s, contest advertisements reminded entrants that the true purpose of these events was "to serve parents and children" by finding and correcting defects, not ranking the softest curls and deepest dimples (de Garmo Papers, 1900–1985). Still, the impulse to present beautiful babies carried the day for 2017's WPFF Better Baby Contest winners, who wore dresses and headbands festooned with large flowers in various colors or vests and ties (WPFF Better Baby Contest, 2017).

The WPFF began in 1911, but it is unclear how many years Better Baby Contests were a feature at this fair. In *Louisiana Life Magazine*, reporter Melissa Bienvenu (2009) referred to the contests as "a long running staple" and fondly reminisced about her own towheaded, blue-eyed second son taking home the blue ribbon (n.p.). The largest Better Baby Contest at the Louisiana State Fair occurred in 1921, when 615 babies entered the contest from towns across the state (de Garmo Papers, 1900–1985).

The long-running tradition of better babies contests began in Shreveport, Louisiana, in 1908, which could help explain their ongoing popularity in Louisiana today (de Garmo Papers, 1900–1985).[1] These contests emerged nationwide at local and state fairs and in print magazines and newspapers as well. Wildly popular, baby contests initially served as a way for parents to receive feedback on their parenting and, later, pediatric health information. There is some evidence that twentieth-century better babies competitions actually lowered local infant mortality rates (Stern & Markel, 2002). Still, such events were not without controversy; critics of early baby beauty contests decried the public spectacle of private family life (Pearson, 2008). Historical research also shows how better babies contests perpetuated early twentieth-century eugenics ideals of white supremacy and ableism and contributed to the focus on early childhood milestones. The first three decades of the twentieth century developed and deliberately displayed emerging "norms," a codification of eugenic perfection that would reflect the intersection of appearance, health, and character. Of course, "fascination with our own and others' babies is not a new phenomenon" (Dorey, 1999, p. 79). At the turn of the century, as now, parents worried about their baby's health and well-being. Early twentieth-century better babies contests focused on "breeding" defects out of "the race," while today parents use apps and social media to measure and monitor their child's milestone achievement.

In the early twentieth century, medical researchers proposed theoretical developmental milestones or child development stages that "normal" or "typically" developing children progress through. We now know that there is wide variation in children's development caused by genetic, cognitive, physical, family, cultural, nutritional, educational, and environmental factors (Wachs, 2000) and each child develops uniquely. Nevertheless, these modern developmental norms formed baseline expectations for infants based on a given week or month through the first year of life and beyond (e.g., physical, motor, cognitive, language, social, and emotional; CDC, 2017a, 2017b). Today's developmental guidelines emerged (in part) from Dr. Arnold Gesell's work in the early twentieth century, which overlapped the popularity of better babies contests (Gesell, 1925, 1928). An assistant professor at Yale University, pediatrician, and psychologist, Gesell first published on monthly milestones for infants in 1925 and utilized charts to track developmental expectations; early better babies material contained similar charts (de Garmo Papers, 1900–1985; Dorey, 1999; Lovett, 2007; Richardson, 1913b; Schaffer, 2011; Stern, 2007). Similar to better babies judging materials, Gesell's (1925) standards were exhaustive, including "some fifty behavior items—four for each month of the first year of life" (p. 208). Yet Gesell and colleagues (1943) cautioned practitioners, warning that norms "are readily misused if too much absolutist status is ascribed to them," and predicted anxieties about development guidelines (Gesell, 1930, p. 141).

Recent research confirms that newborns have more abilities than Gesell realized (Crain, 2011), and baseline standards are far more flexible than originally believed (Day, 2010, 2014). Therefore, norms are useful only in helping experts such as pediatricians to find deviations in child development and report significant divergences (Gesell, Ilg, Learned, & Ames, 1943; Hulbert, 2004; see also Day,

2010). Still, despite the caution and skepticism that Gesell and his collaborators themselves encouraged regarding their work (1943), pediatricians, psychologists, educators, and infant specialists still use Gesell's norms to determine what babies "should" be able to do at various ages (Crain, 2011; Gesell Institute, 2017). Development guidelines and better babies contests often ignore other factors (e.g., environmental, cultural) and overestimate the importance and possibility of uniformity (Hupp & Jewell, 2015; Rathus, 2004), which can cause stress for parents monitoring developmental delays.

The preoccupations of an era shaped by a merging of scientific motherhood and eugenics find a fascinating echo in today's social media environment. After a discussion of the history and impact of late nineteenth- and early twentieth-century baby contests (both beauty contests and better babies contests), we consider how Instagram (IG) in particular might reconstruct better babies contests in the present, with lay experts arbitrating the well-being and milestone achievement of infants and young children. In the early twentieth century, open platforms like IG didn't exist and whiteness ruled the day, while middle- and upper-class norms defined child rearing. There were newspapers and magazines (e.g., the *Crisis*) with a dedicated nonwhite readership, but they didn't have the reach of the *New York Times* or *Good Housekeeping*. Currently, social media platforms allow users, posters, and commenters of all races to contribute to a digital narrative on milestones and "better babies," but the demographic nature of this narrative and the impact of these posts are difficult to represent given the volume of posts and responses.

In this chapter, we define both historical and contemporary lay experts as individuals participating in, planning, or discussing "better babies contests" in the media (e.g., parents, volunteer organizers, journalists) and their contemporary iterations on IG (and other platforms like FB). We define historical technical experts as medical professionals involved in scoring better babies entrants and choosing contest winners (e.g., pediatricians, dentists, nurses, ophthalmologists). Technical experts today monitor milestones at pediatric appointments and provide expertise through award-winning smartphone apps like the Wonder Weeks. This app is based on the popular book by professor of developmental psychology Dr. Frans X. Plooij and coauthor Hetty van de Rijt; it tracks developmental milestones and norms (Plooij, 2017; Wonder Weeks, 2017).

To better understand how social media users perform parenting babies and young children on social media, and IG particularly, we examine how IG promotes milestone culture, increases policing by lay experts, and enhances self-surveillance around babies and young children's health and development (see also Johnson, 2014). For example, does your child eat enough or too much? Should your baby be rolling over, grasping, standing, talking? Smartphone apps may eventually allow parents to compare their children's medical data against others', a digitalized version of the query "Is my child normal?," with data to biomedically define what "normal" milestone achievement looks like (Johnson, 2014, p. 342). We argue that IG allows for this already, sans actual data, which again empowers judgment without context. While IG is not conducting a formal better babies contest, we argue that IG itself is a better babies contest, one that never ends, and one that no one wins.

Currently, parents are expected to be "expert patients" (lay experts) on behalf of their children. Gender scholar Sophia Johnson (2014) noted that mothers most often perform the role of expert patient on behalf of their offspring, and these perspectives emerge online, particularly on social media platforms, where users enact and reenact lay expertise, with and without evidentiary support. *New York Times* reporter Bruce Feiler (2017) noted that "millennial parents," who give birth to five out of every six babies each year, "spent their formative years steeped in personal technology" (n.p.).[2] As a result, many social media users feel comfortable directing their expertise at one another, armed with a wealth of (potentially) inaccurate information, making health judgments about babies and young children. On IG, feedback is posted beneath pictures curated and edited for public consumption (Callahan, 2015; Howorth, 2017). Meanwhile, it is difficult to situate commenters on social media today. What are their educational or expertise backgrounds? Are these technical experts posting through personal or professional accounts? It is not always clear.

To conclude this chapter, we concentrate on the impact of better babies' scorecards and charts on pediatric norms, then and now. We explore the impact of both nineteenth-century baby beauty contests and the "pediatric tyranny" of early twentieth-century better babies contests in online parenting today. Specifically, IG allows for and encourages this performativity through platform-specific curation, filtering, and picture editing, along with strategic hashtag use to gather platform followers (Cadalo, Flavián, & Ibáñez-Sánchez, 2017; Calkin, 2015). This performative reality can create a crisis experience for parents in which they continually doubt their decisions and abilities while comparing themselves to a constructed norm. At the same time, as we suggest throughout this book, social media and smartphone apps both enlarge and constrain communicative and learning possibilities for mothers and other caretakers.

BABY CONTESTS: FROM BEAUTY TO SCIENCE AND BACK AGAIN

The Learning Channel's (TLC) controversial reality TV show *Toddlers and Tiaras* first aired in 2009. It features babies, toddlers, and young children competing in beauty and talent pageants for money and prizes (Ames & Burcon, 2016; Dejmanee, 2015; Tamer, 2011). Edited deceptively, reality television is meant to portray real-life events and interactions in a compelling way, with an emphasis on the most provocative and salacious elements of these competitions (e.g., a child in a padded bra and undergarments mimicking Dolly Parton; Adams, 2012). Backlash to the show eventually prompted a three-year production hiatus (TLCgo, 2017). This backlash is not new, and neither is the American tradition of publicly displaying cute babies for prizes. The first public contests for babies occurred in 1854, in Springfield, Ohio, 155 years before *Toddlers and Tiaras* (Dorey, 1999; Pearson, 2008). Similar to *Toddlers and Tiaras*, these contests focused on beauty and appearance, whereas better babies events focused on health and milestone achievement. Some of the specifics are different. First, *Toddlers and Tiaras* is an edited television show with a social media presence (e.g., FB account). Second, the styles of clothing, music, and prizes and the application of spray tans obviously do not reflect Victorian trends and fashions. Still, some specific methods and models remain unchanged, such as events at county fairs, involvement of newspapers and magazines, and competition for cash or other coveted prizes.

In the early twentieth century these contests overtly eschewed beauty and denied the supremacy of "glossy golden curls," even as they underscored the dominant cultural preference for white and able-bodied babies. Judging materials ensured a focus on health markers and milestones: muscle development, age-appropriate intelligence, racial superiority, physical ability, and adequate nutrition (Dorey, 1999, p. 77). By the twenty-first century, the social media platform IG offers an amalgamation of these contests by creating an image-forward space where parents can depict their babies and young children at their "best," meeting milestones, and curating their cutest moments for friends, family, and followers. Although the vast majority of users avoid claims of racial superiority, very few (if any) IG posters engage with the ways normative language may or may not be ableist or privilege white bodies and middle- and upper-class cultural norms. The use of pictures to illustrate the health and beauty of children is nothing new either, and pictures of "winning" babies in both kinds of contests, reproduced in local and national newspapers and magazines, helped create expectations for normal and healthy children throughout the late nineteenth and early twentieth centuries, just as social media do today. In what follows, we examine baby beauty pageants, the emergence and popularity of better babies contests, the public response to these contests, and their impact on pediatric norms today.

(BABY) BEAUTY FOR PUBLIC CONSUMPTION

That first American baby beauty contest (often called baby shows in the nineteenth century) aimed to draw visitors to the Clark County Fair in Springfield, Ohio, with famous judges, including newspaper magnate Horace Greeley and famed abolitionist and women's rights activist Lucretia Mott (Pearson, 2008).

News of the fair spread quickly in newspapers throughout the country, and similar events immediately occurred in small rural towns and bustling metropolitan centers. By the end of the nineteenth century, these beauty contests were commonplace (Dorey, 1999; Pearson, 2008). Atlantic City, New Jersey, held a baby show on the boardwalk, and one of Thomas Edison's first films showed the "baby parade" that officially ended the contest (Library of Congress, 2017). Not one to miss out on an economic opportunity, P. T. Barnum (of circus fame) immediately added baby shows to his entertainment roster at the American Museum of New York City (Pearson, 2008). While Barnum turned a profit, women's clubs and community organizations held baby beauty contests to raise money and complete community projects (Pearson, 2008). Almost as soon as the events began, newspapers and magazines held their own print versions of baby beauty contents and mothers sent the best pictures of their children and subscribers voted for their favorites (Pearson, 2008).

From the outset, baby beauty contests drew praise and censure but remained wildly popular and well attended and attracted ample media coverage. In 1891, Los Angeles held a contest with 150 entries, and even small towns reported dozens of participants (Pearson, 2008). To maintain objectivity, judges were sometimes chosen for their lack of connection to babies: bachelors and childless married women were preferred choices (Pearson, 2008). Hence, lay experts played an important role in assessing the prettiest babies. Most baby beauty contests separated participants by age, gender, and, in some cases, race, with novelty categories and prizes as well (e.g., fattest, smallest, reddest hair; Dorey, 1999; Pearson, 2008).

Critics questioned the public display of babies like cattle, cabbages, or other objects traditionally judged at state and county fairs. In the very early years of these contests, some abolitionists wondered if they would normalize slave auctions (Pearson, 2008). Some decried making profit from displaying mothers and babies, and P. T. Barnum received criticism for displaying babies like other human oddities or museum curios (Pearson, 2008). Still others found maternity venerable in the home but grotesque in public, and the suggestion that some attended the contests to look at the figures of beautiful women (as these were presumably the sort that had lovely babies) resurfaced often. While platforms, stages, and raised daises physically separated entrants and their parents, the contests introduced a display of adult bodies and the mother-child dyad that many nineteenth-century Americans found provocative or distasteful. However, by the end of the nineteenth century, the popularity of baby beauty contests continued, while concerns over the contests and critiques around the contests' focus and impact largely disappeared (Pearson, 2008). In the twentieth century, an interest in "social hygiene" and other eugenic principles, alongside detailed judging materials based on infant development imbued the new better babies contests with a scientific air.

A Contest of Scientific Motherhood: Better Babies

Are you the proud father and mother of a Prize Winning Baby? Then, let me
warn you that you have responsibilities of crushing weight. . . . It is your duty . . .
to surround your own child with such intelligent and loving care, that it may
develop into the highest physical, mental and moral type of humanity. (de Garmo
Papers, 1900–1985)[3]

Perhaps owing to an increasing interest in scientific parenting (Ehrenreich &
English, 2005), better babies contests found immediate success and popularity
with the wider public, even more than baby beauty contests did. At state and
county fairs, both baby beauty and better babies contests received top billing and
ample press coverage for decades, though at first articles on the better babies contests conflated them with baby beauty contests (Dorey, 1999). Organizers tried
passionately to separate the competitions; some discouraged using the events as
fund-raisers to maintain distance from baby beauty contests and underscore
their scientific nature (Dorey, 1999). In 1908, contest founder Mrs. Frank de
Garmo, a lay expert, retired teacher, and dedicated volunteer, organized the first
"better baby contest" in Louisiana, prompting nationwide events popular for the
next three decades (de Garmo Papers, 1900–1985; Stern & Markel, 2002).
Described by Selden (2005) as a "peripatetic organizer," de Garmo clearly took
pride in her work on better babies contests and identified as their true origina-
tor (p. 207; see also de Garmo Papers, 1900–1985).

By 1911, *Women's Home Companion* (*WHC*) organized the Better Babies
Bureau, producing streamlined materials (e.g., signs, charts, measurement tools)
and certificates of participation. In Indiana, Dr. Schweitzer advertised better
babies contests on the radio in the mid-1920s and used her own scoring rubrics
(Dorey, 1999; Lovett, 2007; Richardson, 1913b; Stern, 2007). In Mecklenburg
County, North Carolina, the *Charlotte Observer* trumpeted that "steady nerves,
good digestion—these and not pink cheeks, soft hair and dimples, make a better baby and a prize winner" ("Should enter," 1914, p. 6). These public health
events leaned on technical experts (e.g., doctors, nurses, public health officials)
and judged health and hygiene, which did not necessarily have any connection
to lustrous hair, cute smiles, or perfect outfits (Dorey, 1999; Richardson, 1913b).

Like baby beauty contests, better babies competitions drew large crowds, and
organizers were so inundated with entrants that they often had to turn away
potential participants. At the Oklahoma State Fair, 488 participants showed up
to enter when organizers expected 50 (Dorey, 1999, p. 88). In Indiana during the
1928 fair season, 67,000 people visited the better babies complex (Stern & Merkel,
2002). The free examination by a physician was an enormous draw in rural areas,
where the expense of a comprehensive health assessment was cost-prohibitive
for many families (Dorey, 1999). The size of these crowds also illustrated the

advantages and disadvantages of bodies on display. Since better babies contests ensured good fair attendance or ticket sales, the examination portion of the event required a separate, sanitary space with examining tables and room for medical staff (Dorey, 1999; Stern & Markel, 2002).

As with the preemie displays at fairs in Coney Island discussed in chapter 5, live demonstrations came with challenges. While allowing public observers increased access to the events, both babies and physicians who were unaccustomed to being on display found it difficult to concentrate (Dorey, 1999). In Michigan and Kentucky, better babies contest buildings separated contest entrants and examiners from gawkers by long windows or "transparent walls" (Dorey, 1999, p. 89). Some felt a viewing public sullied the event, just as critics of baby beauty contests questioned the ethics of judging infants like prize-winning goats or jams (Pearson, 2008). Literacy was a real hurdle for those trying to educate the public about infant health. To promote visual education, public health officials successfully advocated for the construction of permanent, elaborate, and sometimes lavish buildings on public fairgrounds (Dorey, 1999; Stern & Markel, 2002).

For better babies contests, permanent buildings allowed more entrants because they offered dependable examination space, public viewing spaces, protection from the elements, and educational exhibits for those waiting or viewing the event. The extensive examination at the center of the better babies contest set it quite apart from baby beauty contests. Nurses were often on staff to assist physicians and to provide professional childcare in adjacent childcare centers. Set up for tired babies and active toddlers, free childcare also provided mothers with time to view the fairgrounds unhampered and perhaps make purchases (Dorey, 1999). Resting spaces in permanent buildings and a trained nursing staff were a necessity due to the extensive, even exhaustive scoring systems used by many better babies contest organizers. Every physical facet was examined and scored. Some contests had both ocular and dentition measurements, gathered a full family health history, and conducted tests for soundness of intelligence and mental health (de Garmo Papers, 1900–1985; Lovett, 2007; Pernick, 2002; Stern, 2007; Stern & Markel, 2002). Similar to baby beauty contests, entrants were categorized by age, but also by rural or urban addresses (Stern, 2007).

In Indianapolis, mothers and babies entered the building, handed over their enrollment card for check-in, and visited a booth where a volunteer recorded a full health history. Afterward, a psychologist conducted age-specific tests. To deemphasize appearance and symbols of status or class standing, volunteers dressed babies alike (see Figure 12).

Each infant or young child began with 1,000 points and then received deductions by category (Stern, 2007). For example, scanty hair, scaly skin, receding chin, enlarged adenoids (thought to create a "stupid countenance"), nail defects,

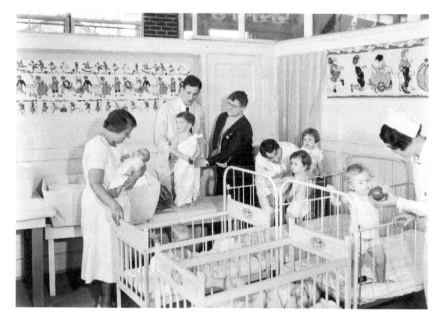

Figure 12. Day nursery in the Better Baby Contest Building at the 1931 Indiana State Fair. Indiana Historical Society P0490.

and any deviations from height and weight norms prompted deductions. So too did being ill-tempered during examination (Dorey, 1999, p. 136; de Garmo Papers, 1900–1985; Stern, 2007). Stern (2007) noted that in Indiana these standards, generally met by white, middle-class entrants, merely served to reinforce long-standing race and class prejudices and "accentuated the disquieting fact that only plump white babies could achieve perfection" (p. 27). Better babies contest judging materials also recorded heredity and milestone achievement, then recommended specific nutritional and sanitation practices to strengthen and improve future generations of Americans (Pernick, 2002).

There is ample evidence that better babies contests celebrated eugenics, and groups around the country integrated eugenics theory as part of contest design (Pernick, 2002). As Stern (2007) maintained, eugenicists included "biologists, physicians, industrialists, psychologists, socialists, feminists, and traditionalists" (p. 5). Eugenics supporters eagerly anticipated the lessening of social maladies (e.g., crime and drunkenness) through scientific solutions involving engineered "breeding" of the American population (Stern, 2007). Immigration and eugenic marital laws were already in place in the 1920s, and states such as California, North Carolina, and Indiana ran active, state-sanctioned sterilization programs (Hamer, Quinlan, & Grano, 2014; Stern, 2007).

Charles Davenport ran the Eugenics Record Office, responsible for much of the early public campaign on eugenics in the United States (Stern, 2007). He urged better babies organizers in Iowa to award a full 50% of the score based solely on hereditary history (Lovett, 2007). A handful of pictures survive, which illustrate better babies contests held in eugenics buildings at fairs or adjacent to them, as well as photographs of eugenics learning exhibits (interactive displays designed to increase support for eugenic principles and policies) integrated with the prejudging waiting area (Dorey, 1999; Lovett, 2007). Most contests collected a "hereditary history" prior to the physical examination and in some locations scored this history apart from physical examinations (Biddison, 1913; de Garmo Papers, 1900–1985; Lovett, 2007). Whiteness and health both reflected eugenic ideas of racial hierarchy, quite popular at that time. In the early twentieth century, experts linked family traits of alcoholism, laziness, promiscuity (in women), and "idiocy" (a scientific term, used interchangeably in the nineteenth century with "feeblemindedness") to an unhealthy heritage or hereditary history, in ways that reinforced predominant class and race prejudices. Some historians asserted the centrality of these contests to the American eugenics movement through the 1930s, particularly with regard to what is termed "positive eugenics" (Dorr & Logan, 2011; Kline, 2011; Lovett, 2007; Pernick, 2002; Stern & Markel, 2002). Coined by Sir Francis Galton in 1883, "eugenics" refers to the scientific improvement of the humans through targeted breeding methods, based on methods used with plants and other animals (Dorr & Logan, 2011). "Negative eugenic" policies such as immigration and marriage restriction (e.g., the Chinese Exclusion Acts and anti-miscegenation laws) were in place well before the turn of the twentieth century. However, "positive eugenic" policies sought "fit" marriages (e.g., between two healthy, mentally and intellectually "sound" individuals) and supported scientific parenting to ensure infants and children gained the lifelong advantages of a healthy beginning (Dorey, 1999; Dorr & Logan, 2011; Pernick, 2002). As historian Alexandra Minna Stern (2007) argued, educational exhibits set up for parents at these contests discouraged the reproduction of impoverished immigrants and nonwhite individuals, promoting a negative eugenic practice (see also Pernick, 2002).

Contest exhibits taught visiting parents that "examinations and medical treatment could prevent a defective childhood," "defective" being a eugenics buzzword (Dorey, 1999, p. 136). In the de Garmo Papers (1900–1985), Mrs. de Garmo's handwritten notes proclaimed that better babies contests "awoke the world to the value of eugenic child raising and ways of living" (n.p.). In Iowa, organizers Mary T. Watts and U.S. Children's Bureau director Julia Lathrop planned "Eugenic Expositions" with their contest (Lovett, 2007, p. 136). Dr. Ada Schweitzer in Indiana informed audiences that the better babies contest would help improve the human race (Stern, 2007). *WHC* published an article that claimed, "Better babies mean fewer hospitals, fewer asylums, fewer prisons . . . more sunlight and less shadows for your children and mine" (Richardson, 1913a, p. 25; see also de Garmo Papers, 1900–1985).

Pernick (2002) noted that "maternal feminists" embraced better babies contests because they created an avenue to increase infant and child health through "scientific motherhood," which aimed to empower mothers to use all available scientific knowledge to rear the healthiest, most intelligent children possible (Ehrenreich & English, 2005; Pernick, 2002). Lay expert organizers, particularly middle-class, white, female community leaders, embraced and promulgated eugenic theory, through their work as reformers engaged in progressive politics, maternal feminists, supporters of scientific motherhood, or some combination of these (Pernick, 2002; Stern & Markel, 2002). In the early twentieth century, the nuances of a range of influences on babies' development garnered little discussion. Instead, scientific motherhood and eugenic social engineering would produce "better babies." Better babies could meet eugenicists' goals for an improved population.

Mrs. de Garmo, perhaps a maternal feminist herself, originally called her event the "Scientific Baby Contest" and wrote that her work in Louisiana and later in Missouri would improve the health of young children around the country (de Garmo Papers, 1900–1985; Seldon, 2005) (see Figures 13 through 15). Her papers include staged studio pictures of herself, a nurse and/or doctor assessing a child using better babies standards, copies of scorecards and standard tables, and a detailed history of the contest's beginnings in Missouri, all materials supporting her status as a better babies expert (de Garmo Papers, 1900–1985). As the popularity of better babies contests exploded, physicians willingly assisted lay experts in these events nationwide. Lay experts from WHC worked directly with medical practitioners to make scoring cards, charts, and other materials, then distributed these materials to parents (Richardson, 1913b, 1914; see also Brosco, 2001). These systems of ranking and measurement, along with research-based development theory (Gesell, 1925, 1928), became the standards by which technical experts gauge "normalcy" in infants and young children today.

WHC writer and editor Anna Steese Richardson may have identified with de Garmo as an organizer and reformer; she was an outspoken supporter of eugenics and, as a writer with WHC, engaged in protoscience journalism as well (Tomes, 2002). As the in-house director of the WHC's Better Babies Bureau, she penned a 12-part series on "Babyology" to great acclaim among the WHC readership (Dorey, 1999). In her publications, Richardson often returned to the standardizations created and distributed by the Better Babies Bureau, which reinforced the gospel of scientific motherhood, reflected eugenics standards, and set the stage for the work of Gesell and other technical experts in early child development. She connected WHC-backed better babies contests directly with eugenics, "the most misunderstood and abused of social sciences" and noted, "The baby health contest form[s] the connecting link between the scientific minds . . . the marvelous theories of eugenics and the mother minds which will put those theories into everyday practice" (Richardson, 1913a, p. 25; see also de

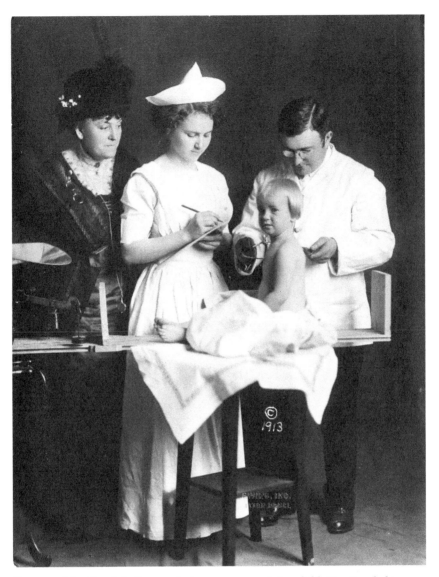

Figure 13. Mrs. Frank de Garmo, doctor, nurse: examining child. Mrs. Frank de Garmo Papers, MS 1879, University of Tennessee, Knoxville Libraries.

Garmo Papers, 1900–1985). In our terms, Richardson understood better babies contests and the work of the Better Babies Bureau and the *WHC* as transactional expertise—eugenicists and physicians imparted knowledge to mothers, who took this technical expertise and infused and combined it with the lay expertise of the "mother mind" to raise a new, "hygienic" generation of Americans.

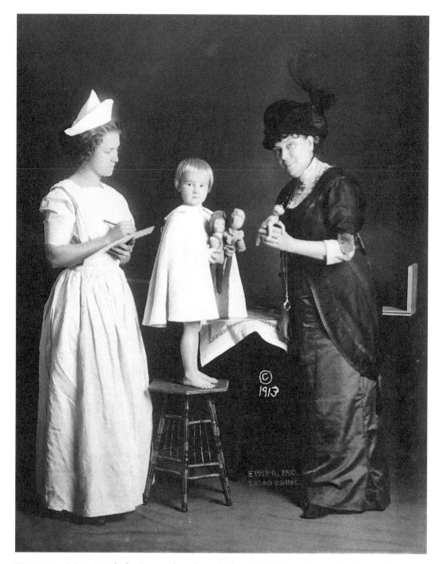

Figure 14. Mrs. Frank de Garmo handing doll to child. Mrs. Frank de Garmo Papers, MS 1879, University of Tennessee, Knoxville Libraries.

When newspapers eventually published better babies news, many publications initially replicated the themes and style of the nineteenth-century baby beauty contest (Dorey, 1999; Pearson, 2008). Maude Murray Miller of Columbus, Ohio, wrote a column in which she regularly chronicled better babies contests in the area; in New York City, the *Evening World* partnered with *WHC* and a baby welfare association to hold a contest and provided ample media coverage (Dorey, 1999). In North Carolina, the *Charlotte Observer* reported on better

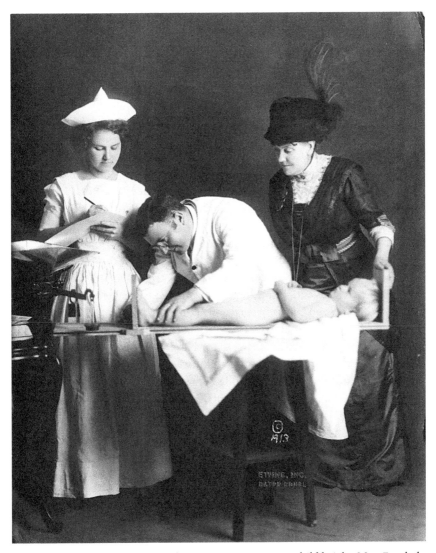

Figure 15. Mrs. Frank de Garmo, doctor, nurse: measuring child height. Mrs. Frank de Garmo Papers, MS 1879, University of Tennessee, Knoxville Libraries.

babies week ("Prizes awarded," 1921), during which doctors spoke to crowds of entrants and onlookers, giving talks such as "Proper Food for the Infant and Child" ("Better babies contest Saturday," 1916, p. 7). Contest organizers and lay experts like Mrs. de Garmo encouraged and sought media attention and coverage for contests, while journalists such as Maude Murray Miller and Anna Steese Richardson (1913b) were lay experts who ensured their publications focused on spreading "the gospel" of better babies (p. 22). This print publicity, coupled with free materials distributed at events, encouraged the dissemination of scientific parenting as well as eugenics ideals.

These contests and standardized measurement materials doubtless had an impact. In Indiana alone in just 12 years, Dr. Schweitzer "had examined 77,583 children, registered 55,171 mothers in instructional classes, show[ed] health films to 606,364 viewers," and distributed more than 1 million pamphlets (Stern, 2007, p. 23). The Better Babies Scorecard (BBS), released by the Better Babies Bureau, attempted to streamline and organize national contests, ensuring that all doctors examined all children using the same (exhaustive) standards. Richardson's (1913, 1914) articles in *WHC* specifically cited the benefits to "little folks between the ages of one and three years" tested against the "Better Babies Standard Scorecard" (p. 90). The *WHC* published a pamphlet about how to hold a better babies contest and claimed that the BBS was used in 150,000 examinations nationally—just during the 1913 fair season (Lovett, 2007; Richardson, 1913b).

WHC's Better Babies Bureau aimed to change women's caregiving practices in the home and, to that end, produced a pamphlet, *Hints to Mothers*, expounding on BBS standards and scientific parenting methods; the Better Babies Bureau gave out over 600,000 copies in 1913 alone (Dorey, 1999, p. 134). Building upon the popularity of these contests, organizations like the Auxiliary of the Babies' National Alumni Association (BNAA; for babies who placed in an event and their parents) sought new members to influence caregiving practices and maintain the standards that led to the child's contest prize (de Garmo Papers, 1900–1985). The BNAA suggested that parents take the scorecard, based on better babies scorecards, into their home, and fill it out "daily weekly or monthly . . . and with unfailing regularity" (de Garmo Papers, 1900–1985). The stated goal of the BNAA was to "establish a new standard for normal children" (de Garmo Papers, 1900–1985). Mrs. de Garmo participated in "Baby Week" as the best way to "spread the better baby gospel" (de Garmo Papers, 1900–1985). Hence, by the end of the 1920s, child rearing and the individual parenting choices previously kept within the home became a matter of public debate—and public record (Dorey, 1999). The contests also helped link normalcy and perfection: able, flawless bodies, measurable (and comparable) social and intellectual ability, and freedom from disease became normalized along with the display of "perfect" specimens of childhood (Dorey, 1999).

Unfortunately, the minutia of these scoring methods and the multiplicity of guidelines likely discouraged some families without sufficient means from attempting the recommendations at all. Moreover, printed materials required literacy, a skill not available in some families most in need of the information. And if a baby or child did not meet or failed to continue to meet contest standards—the "new normal" for children under the auspices of scientific parenting—who failed? Well, likely the parents and more specifically the mother

(Dorey, 1999; Richardson, 1913b, 1914). As with the other crises we've studied in this book (e.g., infertility, pregnancy, premature birth), experts of all kinds offer methods for success, but the responsibility for a positive outcome is never structural; it is individual.

Presently, the milestone guidelines of the Centers for Disease Control and Prevention and the World Health Organization reflect the work of Gesell and other child development researchers from the early twentieth century, as well as better babies charts used by the Better Babies Bureau, Mrs. de Garmo, and others (de Garmo Papers, 1900–1985; Richardson, 1913a, 1913b; Stern, 2002, 2007). Better babies contests momentarily shifted responsibility from technical experts (physicians) to lay experts (parents) and intermediaries like Mrs. de Garmo, suggesting that their ability to follow contest mandates at home would produce healthy children; today, parents are continually directed back to their pediatricians for advice and guidance (Dorey, 1999). The professionalization (required by both technical and lay experts) and the "scientification" (through standardization) of better babies contests influenced the twentieth-century system of pediatric norms, upheld through scorecards, charts, graphs, and measuring tools. For instance, the WHC Better Babies Bureau materials suggested that at two years a child should be able to use a paper and pencil (de Garmo Papers, 1900–1985). Most parents who fill out the "milestones" questionnaires at the pediatrician will remember being queried about their child's ability to hold a pencil and copy a line or scribble at or around two years (CDC, 2017b). Today, on the CDC (2017b) "Milestone Tracker" smartphone app, a two-year-old "should" make or copy "straight lines and circles." CDC and WHO guidelines allow parents to monitor their baby's progress and, in partnership with health care providers, detect delays, like parents at better babies contests in the early twentieth century (CDC, 2017a). The danger in these standardized milestones is their potential to falsely separate "normal" and "abnormal" children without accounting for variations in development.

Now parents have a seemingly endless array of expert sources with the advent of social media platforms such as IG. Like the print media of the 1920s and 1930s, IG's photo-forward design lends itself well to the exhibition and comparison of babies and young children, further entrenching pediatric norms and development milestones and not necessarily reflecting how the norms were intended to be utilized. While earlier newspapers and magazines required reader letters to compile votes and pick a winner, today IG allows for instantaneous likes and comments—a space for immediate feedback on one's child, which can both reassure and increase anxiety around the health and development of infants and young children.

As patients turn to social media and smartphone apps to manage health in the digital realm, both become important elements in the rapidly changing techno-logical environment "around pregnancy and the transition to first-time moth-erhood" (Johnson, 2014, p. 330; see also Feiler, 2017). The impact of both baby beauty and better babies contests, at fairs, in magazines, and in newspapers, resurfaces on social media, where many parents post pictures of their children and where healthcare practitioners can find themselves using social media to defend or define their own expertise (Khouri, McCheyne, & Morrison, 2018; Thon & Jucks, 2016).

In the contemporary moment, we see "best" or "cutest" baby photograph con-tests, often sponsored by magazines or retailers, such as Gerber, or ongoing radio and magazine contests (Dorey, 1999). The focus today is less on eugenic physical features or on teaching a semiliterate population about child health, development, and milestones. Now, on social media, the authors receive requests from friends and family members to "vote" for their children for various online contests. Although we have declined to participate with our children, we wonder how the emergence of informal competition and related constant comparison on social media uncritically reinforces ideals from better babies contests, par-ticularly the focus on meeting milestones. To better understand this continua-tion, we turned to the image-focused platform IG, which imitates photographic contests in older print media (e.g., by collecting "likes" as "votes") and also sets up a public viewing area similar to better babies exhibitions.

Since its launch in 2010, IG has become the second most popular social media platform (Pew Research Center, 2016). Today over 700 million users post more than 95 million photographs daily; users like 4.2 billion posts each day (Aslam, 2017) with more than half of all users logging in daily (Pew Research Center, 2016). In 2014, a report in *Business Insider* alleged individuals spend 21 minutes a day on IG (Shontell, 2014). Pew Research Center (2016) reported that 38% of users on IG identify as women, while 26% identify as men; 70% of users are between 18 and 50, and 68% have some college education or have completed col-lege; 28% of Americans use the app regularly. IG remains a racially diverse online space, and currently use is nearly equally split across income classes (Krogsdad, 2015; Pew Research Center, 2016). Finally, use is demographically diverse in other ways; in the United States, rural and urban users outpace suburban users, though IG account holders are represented across the country (Pew Research Center, 2016).

Part of IG's popularity stems from its unique design. While images on social media are ubiquitous today, they were not in 2010 when IG launched. IG is a smartphone application that allows users to upload their own photographs or videos with descriptions, to follow others' accounts, and to like or comment on public posts. Additionally, most IG users post images with hashtags (e.g., #mommalife), phrases or buzzwords that, once hyperlinked, allow people to connect with others discussing similar cultural topics (Calkin, 2015). By clicking on a hashtag, users see a curated feed composed of images using the same hashtags anywhere in the world and can follow these other users. The editing and filter functions are also quite popular. Users can crop images, apply a series of filters, and adjust brightness, contrast, and many other settings previously available through desktop programs like Adobe Photoshop (Ridgway & Clayton, 2016).

Thus, images, videos, hashtags, and comments allow individuals to intentionally or unintentionally construct their IG identities (Calkin, 2015; Mascheroni, Vincent, & Jimenez, 2015). Johnson (2014) termed the "device-ification of motherhood" the intrusion and integration of social media platforms in our everyday lives through smartphone apps, tablets, and mobile devices: "Apps and social media are not simply sources of information, but also act as performative devices" (Johnson, 2014, p. 333). Here, we extend Johnson's ideas about the use of these devices and the (self-)production of knowledge, particularly mothering practices and/or the mothering of infants and young children.

Other scholars have found that social media create stress and anxiety for new mothers (e.g., Kotenko, 2013; Pelletiere, 2014; Pinterest stress, 2013). For example, in an article about social-media-based stress, one mother said, "My life on Facebook is an airbrushed and Instagrammed image of my real life. . . . Most of the time, I think I'm a decent mom, and I think I'm giving my kids a pretty good life" (Pinterest stress, 2013). A mother of two said this about social media: "For new moms it's a great place to ask for parenting advice, but then on the other side, you get some who are too opinionated and that can get in the way" (Pelletiere, 2014).

Users' motivations for engaging in social media in the first place are complex. They may seek simple entertainment or desire to keep in touch with family and friends by setting up an account or hashtag for their child and posting pictures of a baby for faraway relatives. But most of these seemingly straightforward behaviors and activities involve heavily curated posts and strategic posting and editing behaviors. For example, parents post monthly milestone pictures of beautifully clad, clean babies in comfortable surroundings, with messages outlining all the babies have achieved or learned that month or pictures of feeding, clothing, bathing, and otherwise caring for their children (#parentingwin, #momlife). Rarely will a picture of a baby crying be posted in the context of milestones, unless the poster strategically seeks community support or solidarity (#parentingishard).

As new mothers, we acknowledge that this device-ification has increased the pressure to publicly perform our parenting. We wonder if the design of IG encourages parents who do "parenting right" or "check all the boxes" to post more, which limits and narrows what is considered acceptable parenting—further alienating or disciplining those who do not uphold specific (yet mutable) standards. For instance, Maggie crops out the background of pictures so that people will not judge the cleanliness of her home and does not post images where her daughter is by the water without a lifejacket or in a car seat for fear someone will post a negative comment regarding her child's safety and thus her parenting. Maggie admits to feeling anxious when posting to IG and checks for likes, hearts, and comments. We both reflexively edit and curate our posts to avoid censure, critique, and exposure as "bad mothers," whatever "bad mothering" means to us individually. In a personal interview, Rowan Reyes (2017) admitted their struggle to "resist the urge to compare myself to the stream of polished, flawlessly lit photos of the myriad mom blogs, ads [and] Instagram feeds."

We witness #badmom IG confessions that, on the surface, complicate the expectations for intensive mothering and proper care and feeding of infants and young children. While the hashtag highlights moments when parents are "doing it wrong," the underlying message is that it is difficult to meet the standards. To pursue and achieve the "tyranny of pediatric perfection" results in frustration (Howorth, 2017; Stern, 2002). Drawing attention to messy houses, "bad parenting" or "mom fails" are a particular form of counternarrative in which users reveal their "real life." However, even these "raw" IG depictions are handpicked for sharing by the user, potentially cropped, edited, and filtered. Hence, attempts to step "outside" strategic or unrealistic depictions of life on the platform still require the use of IG and its tools to perpetuate an edited version of reality, even one of failure or struggle. We argue that this is pseudo-empowerment (see also Dubwriny, 2012). While these posts aim to "draw back the curtain" and reveal the lived experience behind a constructed social media identity, users produce these "revealing" or "vulnerable" images for public consumption. On the one hand, failure hashtags and posts can offer a way for mothers/parents/caregivers to relax or acknowledge the unobtainable social construction of the #perfectmom. At the same time, IG perpetuates a culture underscoring the power of self-surveillance as new mothers become hypervigilant about child development milestones (e.g., safety of a baby by position), seeking their "better babies." Furthermore, pictures of "failure" by feeding one's toddler McDonald's reflect a particular class and cultural hierarchy, and many of these mom hashtags deepen the ongoing silence about the role fathers and other caretakers play in shaping infant and childhood health outcomes.

IG and other social media are integral to the mothering/parenting experiences of a new generation (see Figures 16 and 17). As noted by Feiler (2017), #hashtagbaby has become a hallmark of millennial parenting (mid-20s to late 30s), with many millennial parents making up a hashtag for their children before or soon after their arrival (n.p.). The "crushing weight" imposed by scientific standards and pediatric norms, nationalized in part because of better babies contests in the early twentieth century, can now be experienced imminently and

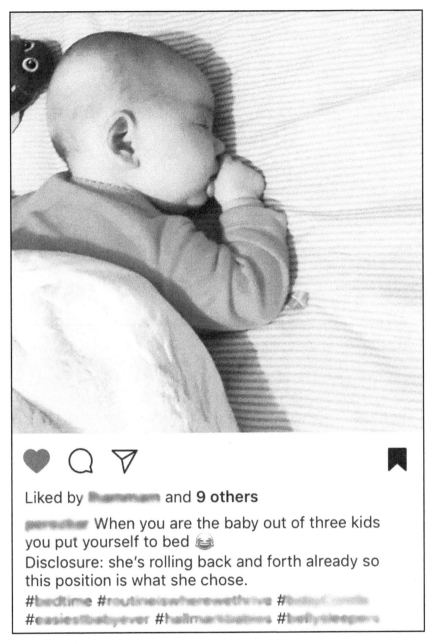

Liked by ██████ and **9 others**

██████ When you are the baby out of three kids you put yourself to bed 😂
Disclosure: she's rolling back and forth already so this position is what she chose.
#bedtime #routineiswherewethrive #█████████
#easiestbabyever #hallmark██████ #babysleeper

Figure 16. Baby Camila on tummy. Instagram.

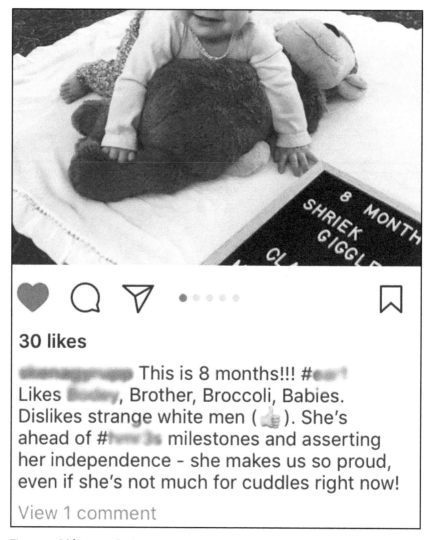

Figure 17. Milestones. Instagram.

constantly because of IG and other social media platforms. And this generation's babies will have records of their curated developmental stories as soon as they are old enough to learn how to search for their own hashtag (see Figures 16 and 17). How could this fail to impact our parenting practices?

As we maintain throughout this book, social media transform expertise, refracting it into numerous murky categories, obscuring the educational and professional backgrounds of users, and dividing posters by the minutiae of parenting choices on questions such as screen time or making versus buying baby food. While parents at better babies contests wondered if their child was performing well according to established norms promulgated by doctors and psychologists, contemporary parents have access to ever-increasing expertise, some of it dubious. Today's definitions of healthy, developmentally on-track babies are being contested and negotiated by a dizzying array of expert commentators with various forms of training, interests, and pursuits.

Today's IG-reinforced fixation on these charts and tables continues to cause anxiety and narrow our sense of the wide range of normal behavior and development possibilities during infancy. As Hadley Leggett (2009) pointed out on wired.com, even though "there's a huge amount of data on the internet about normal developmental milestones," half of normal children fall above or below these averages, and this information is often excluded (n.p.). Perhaps because of mothers'/parents' lived experience of their children's deviations from "norms," many parents discuss the stress these milestones caused them on social media. Others advocate resisting them altogether. Parenting.com writer Margaret Renkl (2010) urged parents to remember that "your child can look very different . . . and still be completely normal" (n.p.). Alessandra Macaluso (n.d.), a blogger for ScaryMommy, said, "Because here's what I think of traditional milestones: Fuck them. Oh, they almost made me crazy in the very beginning." Macaluso (n.d.) continued, "So let's make new milestones. . . . The first time you realize that you are your child's only mother, which means it's OK to smile, nod, and then disregard the 'advice' coming from someone you love when it doesn't feel right to you." Others like jillianleitt (2011) pose questions on discussion boards at sites like Babycenter.com: "So i've read several articles/books that state the sooner a baby hits milestones the more Intelligent the baby is. I also read that if a baby gets a tooth early that baby is more likely to hit other milestones early. Thus getting a tooth early=smarter baby? I personally think it's a crock. . . . Opinions?" Interestingly, jillianleitt questions the logic of milestones even while asking the community for feedback on her resistance. Again, we find that individuals question expertise within Internet and social media spaces, while relying on those same spaces to find expert opinion and/or to confirm their own practices or perspectives.

In earlier generations, parents generally tracked milestones by visiting the pediatrician every few months and recording growth on height and weight charts (if they were willing, or able, through health care access, to participate in those rituals). Now, many new mothers receive weekly emails or have apps on their smartphones that give birthdate-timed developmental updates (Feiler, 2017; Leggett, 2009). There is evidence that smartphone technology and social media are increasing interest in milestones, much the way better babies campaigns did, but with far more data. The tracking of infant and toddler milestones is a profitable marketplace where families can buy apps or other tools to record and monitor data on baby cries, diaper changes, and risk for and developmental delays. Wearable devices keep track of how often you talk to your child and babies' breathing and heartbeat. Toys record how long children play with them. All these data can be used to compare progress to developmental norms (Leggett, 2009).

Celebrities who post pictures of their children on public accounts are sometimes beset by commentary from users with no discernible health expertise who hold forth on the well-being and safety of children based on extremely limited (visual) evidence. For example, in 2016, after reality star Kristin Cavallari posted a picture of her sons in their swim trunks at the beach on IG, she received backlash that her sons were too skinny. One IG user commented on Cavallari's picture, "I understand you live a very strict dietary lifestyle but these children are very obviously nutritionally deficient" (Pyskaty, 2016). There is no evidence this poster saw Cavallari's children face to face; one can't necessarily determine the nutritional health of a child from a picture on IG. Nor is there any evidence this person has technical expertise in nutrition or child development. Still, she felt qualified to claim nutritional deficiency in a public forum, labeling another person's children as malnourished, a categorization that can cause the removal of children from a home. Cavallari bitingly retorted to the "haters:" "Yep, I starve my children. . . . Just blocked the most people I've ever blocked in my entire life. Happy 4th hahaha" (Pyskaty, 2016). Other IG users might lack the confidence to simply block followers, internalizing critical feedback whether or not it is accurate, since some turn immediately to technology with questions about the health and development of infants and young children (see also Feiler, 2017). And if images on IG aim to depict an ideal child, how can parents with babies and children who vary from the desired norm feel confident that their children are healthy and meeting milestones? What if their children will never meet traditional milestones?

Lay Expertise on Social Media: The Contests Everyone Loses

This example is a reminder that, on social media, judging better babies is primarily a lay expert affair, in spite of the continuing structure of data-driven milestones offered by a wide variety of more credentialed experts. When mothers view posts and comments like those under Cavallari's image, the dialogue may act as a disciplining mechanism by framing the health of children visually, where viewing alone creates an expert. At early twentieth-century better babies contests, the space reserved for the viewer remained removed from the infants and young children as well as the technical experts scoring their health. We are not arguing better babies scoring methods or charts were accurate, nor that standards remained free of class and/or racial bias (Stern, 2007). However, the standardized charts and measurement tables created by the Better Babies Bureau of *WHC* as well as Dr. Schweitzer in Indiana were formulated by that era's credential experts and were intended for universal use in states or at the federal level. Our analysis of IG suggests that today's expertise is far more slippery and contested and can add a more volatile sense of a moving target of health, propagated by so many purported experts. While on IG, individual posters pass judgment, offer support, or confirm developmental milestones or the health status of an infant or young child, based on their (lay) expertise viewing an edited photograph. To be fair, while better babies contests were one prominent way people engaged with health commentary about their babies, it undoubtedly occurred in other social contexts as well, such as at church or at a relative's home, and community members likely equated appearance and health in spite of or because of what doctors said. Each era has its day-to-day social context, but social media speed up the exchange, allowing moment-to-moment feedback, from far more commentators and often anonymous ones.

Unexpectedly, although parents have greater access to milestone-based and other development data through smartphone apps, IG nonetheless perpetuates the practices of "beauty baby" contests from the nineteenth century. Lay experts praise delightful, chubby cherubs, pink cheeks, bright eyes, and soft curls as well as the harder to ascertain standards promulgated by better babies contests, such as standardized height and weight ratios. At the same time, IG commenters (like those on Cavallari's post) construct themselves as experts in the vein of pediatricians at better babies contests, creating an amalgam of previous contests. IG measures beauty and health, milestones and cute outfits, nourishment and hairstyles. Once one begins posting pictures of one's baby and uses hashtags to enter the global IG community, the judging begins. Does it end? What is clear is that social media platforms like IG may increase anxiety for mothers in particular, who feel the pressure for perfection and experience feelings of inadequacy, whether the pressure begins internally or comes externally from social media or they work in tandem, increasing perceived external and internal pressure. As Feiler (2017) suggested, millennial parents are "confused about the 'right way' to do things and harshly judged by friends and relatives" (n.p.). And these friends and relatives may be viewing your baby's milestone developments largely through social media applications.

Importantly for IG users, abstaining from social media comes with its own social costs, including "a loss of cultural and social capital" from interacting in high-visibility online spaces, "not receiving invitations to social events or the sense of isolation and disconnection from friends [and] family" (Calkin, 2015, p. 109). Johnson (2014) discussed a digital performance called "puppeteering mother" (p. 337) in which a mother projects her baby instead of herself. This practice allows mothers "to accrue self-worth that might otherwise be difficult to attain" or to achieve through other social forums, such as clubs, moms' groups, or religious organizations (p. 338).

The publicizing of what was once a very personal sphere of intimacy to virtual friends and acquaintances, neighbors, and even family members "suggests a new way of measuring social status" (Johnson, 2014, p. 338). Calkin (2015) discussed the rhetorical functions of the "like" and comment capability on IG, which allows people to give their "stamp of approval" or the heart as a visual declaration of love (see also Fetterman & Robinson, 2013). If someone goes out of her way to click on the comment button, there is an implied investment in a post. Additionally, captions and hashtags allow the poster to define, brand, explain, and comment on posts of all types (Barton, 2015; Calkin, 2015). Our cultural obsession with milestone achievements can act as a form of social currency among peers with children. As Rowan Reyes (2017) shared in an interview, "I . . . found that there was always someone who seemed to be perfecting the art of motherhood [on social media]." As Brown and Webster (2004) argued, social media technologies are "socio-technologies" (p. 334), impacting users on a social level we have yet to adequately measure, at least as it impacts parenting and individual perceptions of infant and child health and wellness.

Johnson (2014) noted that social apps and social media platforms are "important elements in the rapidly changing environment [around] the transition to first-time motherhood," which includes "digital health" (pp. 330–331). As such, "maternal subjects" may use apps and social media to monitor their "children's development and health" (Johnson, 2014, p. 330). We argue that IG allows for comparison and the monitoring of the development and health of other children as well, either confirming or calling into question the health and well-being of your children. In the early twentieth century, parents whose children failed to place at better babies contests contacted doctors in person and through letters, pleading with them to expound on their babies' faults so they might correct these defects in due course (Dorey, 1999; Stern & Markel, 2002). Today, IG can foster a sense of crisis regarding a baby or young child's health, weight, height, milestone achievement, and overall development.

IG can also reinscribe dominant discourses and social hierarchies in ways that are difficult to measure or quantify, just as better babies contests directly or indirectly entrenched the pediatric norms we measure babies and young children against today (Brosco, 2001; Stern, 2002). Is IG "good" for babies and mothers? It is difficult to characterize platforms like IG, where people with various abilities, races, beliefs, and cultural practices ideally have equal access. However, the "follower" function on IG measures popularity, and accounts with more followers are more readily available in searches. Despite user diversity or near universal access, popularity signifies impact. In fact, popular accounts with impact, hosted by individuals termed "influencers" on IG, are more likely to be middle or upper class, white, cis, heterosexual, and able-bodied when their feeds focus on young children and parenting (Becker, 2017). In short, these accounts have commonality with families in the early twentieth century whose babies won better babies contests. Moreover, on IG, popularity can overlap with expertise, as users may look to influencers (e.g., Kristen Cavallari) as models of the ideal experience during the life cycle of early motherhood. These tensions not only reveal the potential for and obstacles to social media platforms as tools for social change but also underscore the difficulties of assessing expertise versus popularity and beautiful curation.

In each chapter we have wrestled with the issue of how each potential crisis in the life cycle of motherhood impacts groups differently, across race, class, gender, and other socially constructed boundaries. If, as Stern (2007) argued, better babies contests reinforced and mirrored the eugenics movement as awardees were almost always white and of Northern European descent (see also Johnson, 2014), what does it mean when we expect edited, digitized curations of the lives of babies and children to reflect our success as parents and, more specifically, as mothers? Grouping all IG users into one community (e.g., parents, mothers) erases the particularities of identity and experience on a platform where "everyone is allegedly permitted to freely exist" (Calkin, 2015, p. 84). Yet IG infamously deletes pictures of women nursing, giving rise to hashtags such as #Freethenipple, in which nursing individuals push back against the idea that nursing pictures are salacious, particularly on a platform that protects the posting of nipples in other contexts (Calkin, 2015; see also Olszanowski, 2014). And barely visible on IG are mothers of disabled children or of babies or young children with developmental delays. Similarly absent are mothers who cannot afford to "eat clean" (e.g., avoiding white sugar and preservatives) or who don't have access to a grocery store with a wide range of healthy foods. The pictures act as the new scorecards while continuing to perpetuate class-based notions of motherhood and ableism and an emphasis on mother over father (or other) caregivers.

We wonder, can IG offer opportunities for counternarrative, and if so, how? How can IG offer images of underrepresented mothers and caretakers as well as underrepresented babies and children? A recent *Time* magazine article questioned the social pressure mothers feel, including on social media, arguing that these pressures create a "kind of over-preciousness about motherhood. It's obsessive, and it's amplified by the Internet and social media" (Howorth, 2017, n.p.). As Howorth (2017) acknowledged, the potential for social media to offer a counternarrative is needed: "Social media can just as easily help celebrate our individual experience and create community through contrast" (n.p.). We hope mothers on IG can find a safe place to celebrate their experiences in supportive environments. Yet because of public posts, in which individuals can accrue a lot of "followers" or tag their posts with multiple hashtags, the very structure of IG could preclude the support desired. It is imperative that we continue to look for, tabulate, and analyze counternarrative structures across social media as a way to widen our expectations for and understandings of the life cycle of motherhood.

Throughout the research for this book, we had conversations with individuals engaged in mothering at the margins, and as we discuss in the conclusion, we believe that future scholarship and future social media platform development must include subjugated voices. Indeed, most crises are defined by and through a certain type of mother—educated, middle class, white, cis gender, and able-bodied. But most of us do not fit into this mold in one or more ways. We want to contest these limited categories, pay heed to the wisdom of the life cycle of early motherhood on the margins, and continue to rail against binary under-standing of expertise as merely "technical" or "lay" in the age of social media. However, unpacking this binary can be difficult, since social media creates space for individuals who frame themselves as experts, but their training, knowledge base, status, and loyalties are hard to decipher. Decentering the widely agreed-upon credentialed experience of the twentieth century allows more voices, but other voices are also capable of reproducing social hierarchies (e.g., race, class, gender), not just institutional ones. The "in-between" or self-proclaimed experts we've observed throughout this book can also produce maternal anxiety by pre-senting expertise that may not be helpful or accurate. Yet by saying "this is my/our experience, and it is different; here is what we do/do not understand yet," individuals can reduce self-surveillance even as they expand the available nar-ratives on parenting, motherhood, reproductive health, and expertise.

CONCLUSION

As we penned this conclusion, Bethany received a bill from her obstetric/midwife practice asking for full payment of her second child's birth before 26 weeks of gestation. The letter suggested that failure to pay could result in the termination of care. Letter in hand, Bethany requested a meeting with the administrator who sent her the letter and asked a series of questions about the letter's language, the process of creating the estimated bill, and the policies and practices expressed in the missive. While taking notes on the physical document, she was informed that she must pay in advance because this was "elective care" and that she was the "only one to ever complain about this letter." Bethany brought up the conversations local mothers were having on Facebook (FB) about this very letter and the difficulties many had understanding the new policy and how it intersected with their insurance policies. She was told these conversations were meaningless, even immaterial to the practice's policies. Even after studying these dynamics, publishing on them, and working on this book, Bethany felt silenced and disempowered by the exchange.

That very week, we tracked two conversations about this same office, with hundreds of comments and directions about how to circumvent the policy, called "global bill pay." Commenters in this private FB group offered detailed information on rejecting the policy, including language to use in conversations with the office manager. Despite the belief of Bethany's office administrator, social media conversations were actively equipping patients to make individual health choices with direct consequences to both office policy and new patient traffic.

Historically, these conversations developed through print media and in organizational structure and the boundaries between technical and lay were more apparent, though still insufficient to describe the exchange of information. Today, on social media platforms and smartphone applications, these distinctions dissolve further, offering more expertise but perhaps fewer answers. To refuse to acknowledge the impact of social media discourse during the life cycle of early motherhood is to willfully misunderstand the way many patients make health choices for themselves and their children during infancy and through the toddler years.

(Dis)empowering Potentialities of the Technical-Lay Binary

New mothers have long sought and received expertise from community members or lay experts, including family, friends, and acquaintances, who provided advice through the lens of their own experience. Sometimes, these lay experts may have had training in technical medical expertise (as family doctors, nurses, and eventually pediatricians) or had training in or knowledge of alternative medical practices. In the United States, medical history is punctuated by both efforts by traditional experts to discount or curtail the activities of practitioners they felt unqualified to practice (e.g., midwives, doulas) as well as waves of populist medical movements, mainstreamed and upheld by the American public (e.g., hydrotherapy, homeopathy) (Breslaw, 2012; Curry, 1999; Grant, 2012; Janik, 2014; Starr, 1982). Female-identified individuals have long participated in protecting the health and wellness of their family and community members, as both lay and traditional experts, even as these definitions have changed; for example, midwives have transformed from community leaders and technical healers to lay practitioners. By the mid-twentieth century, the practitioner-patient relationship (more specifically the doctor-patient relationship) had crystallized into an ideal of the sacred, insulated medical relationship, arranged in a top-down fashion (practitioner *to* patient) and legitimized by technical experts, the shift from home to hospital care, and the corporatization of medicine (Starr, 1982).

For the last three decades, historians and health communication, feminist, and medical humanities scholars working at the intersections of these fields have insisted on the need for a model of practitioner-patient communication that empowers both patient and practitioner and creates a dialogic model of health care, pivoting on clear and open communication and the conclusion that physician-dominated discussion is counterproductive (Ellingson, 2007; Geist-Martin, Bollinger, Wiechert, Plump, & Sharf, 2016; Marsh & Ronner, 1997; Morantz-Sanchez, 2000; Sandelowski, 1984). This research points to the need for caregivers to encourage open communication so as not to overlook important information. Caregivers can also work to ensure the patient does not feel belittled and therefore leave out vital information in fear of critique or censure from the caregiver (Jensen, 2016; Sharf, Geist-Martin, Cosgriff-Hernández, & Moore, 2012). Scholars across these fields continue to wrestle with this delicate communicative balance between patient and practitioner.

Today we understand that the practitioner-patient boundary is highly and even imperceptibly permeable; social media further erode a boundary that was never as clear as many doctors wished, even though technical medical systems have yet to acknowledge or fully engage this impact (Briggs, Burford, De Angeli, & Lynch, 2007). Despite how technical experts, hospital administrators, public health officials, and policy creators may feel about social media platforms and smartphone applications, they can no longer say, "Don't Google it." That ship has sailed, and to continue to deny it is folly. As this book demonstrates, the reach of social media extends much further than Google, WebMD, Fitbit, or blogs; social media platforms allow instant, person-to-person expertise dissemination, particularly in moments of crisis and during hours when technical experts are not easily accessible, unless they too happen to be active on social media. As we've observed, doctors and nurses are active on social media, doling out expertise, but often through private accounts. As we saw in chapter 3, nurses sign on in their personal accounts and then provide their professional affiliation and speak on behalf of their institutions. Though some systems have a policy about personal and/or professional social media activity, many still do not.

From a dramaturgical perspective, sociologist Erving Goffman (1959) made a crucial distinction between "frontstage" (behaviors that are visible to the audience as part of the performance) and "backstage" (behaviors where no audience is present). Health communication scholars have tended to narrow the focus to the frontstage of medical encounters and health care settings (e.g., formal/bounded patient-provider communication) and have often downplayed informal/unbounded interactions that constitute a majority of communication among patients and providers (Sharf, 1993; see also Ellingson, 2007). However, using this framework, Ellingson (2005, 2007) and Atkinson (1995) focused on backstage communication among providers and its impact on patient-provider communication. This monograph extends this research by examining performances in which patients communicate with each other and with providers in the backstage (e.g., private FB groups or Instagram [IG] accounts, patients' letters to each other or their providers) as well as the frontstage, throughout history and on social media (e.g., publicly accessible blogs or letters to the editor in historical newspapers). While writing each chapter, we highlighted implications of these performances for individuals, health care teams, and the overarching U.S. medical establishment.

Implications for Medical Professionals

"Telemedicine" is now generally accepted by physicians as a legitimate way to deliver medical care and/or expertise. However, social media expertise and how it operates, how it is defined, and how it affects patient choice and individual health choices, are less understood. Our research suggests that the impact of social media is ignored by the health care establishment where it intersects with the life cycle of early motherhood. We are not talking about the ample research available on the use of apps or other interfaces to monitor health vitals and/or interact directly with practitioners, including password-protected email and the applications created by and for health care systems. Throughout this text, we have addressed conversations and decisions happening almost entirely outside of these resources, where technical practitioners may enter the dialogue as lay experts without identifying their employment status or educational or professional background; other times, through their personal accounts they construct their technical identities firmly and provide advice as medical experts. As previously stated, the policies about behavior on social media platforms trail engagement considerably.

More engaged communication with patients leads to less burnout of caregivers, but today this will require that caregivers acknowledge and engage with social media use by patients as a source of medical expertise (technical and lay, traditional, nontraditional, alternative, etc.). Throughout the book, we have reminded readers of the established importance of social media platforms and smartphone apps to new parents, and self-identified mothers most specifically (Bartholomew, Schoppe-Sullivan, Glassman, Kamp Dush, & Sullivan, 2012; Edison Research, 2013; Johnson, 2014; Khouri, McCheyne, & Morrison, 2018; Landry, 2014; Madge & O'Connor, 2006; Pew Research Center, 2016).

Patients openly discuss their experience with technical medical practitioners, but they also share information about practitioner career trajectory and suggest other offices and/or practitioners. One FB post included a query about a specific doctor at a specific clinic and respondents weighed in: "For those of you who see [doctor's name] at [name of practice] I just found out as of last Friday, he no longer works there. Does anyone know any details?" (Private Facebook, 2017b). One commenter, referring to another private FB group, replied, "Someone in my neighborhood FB page said he is joining a practice in [name of town]. They didn't say which one though" (Private Facebook, 2017b). Another responder added, "My guess is he realizes how poorly [name of practice] is doing and wanted to get out before his name went own [sic] with them. I know several others have left for this reason as well" (Private Facebook, 2017b). The poster meant to inform the community to make choices about who cared for their young children—perhaps they would switch doctors within the office or move to another practice. Facebook group chats, public and private, can directly impact where patients seek care and their choice of practitioners.

Throughout this book, we have shown that, alongside seeking social support, users seek the advice of medical experts and/or construct their own expert identities, within and outside of the technical/lay expertise binary. The resistance we continue to face from many practitioners (technical, lay, and everything in between) to acknowledge and engage with these social-media-based conversations, particularly through platforms that seemingly have no connection to medical expertise, such as IG, is the newest chapter in the long history of resistance among medical professionals to engage with and embrace communicative change. As we saw in chapter 4, practitioners resisted Twilight Sleep but grudg-ingly responded to public pressure because of printed media, while in chapter 5 we saw that doctors eventually embraced "freak show medicine" for premature babies when the public and most print media supported Martin Couney's efforts.

Some practitioners may see social media as informal communication, while others use the platforms to advertise their practices, such as educating potential patients via eCourses or YouTube videos; we argue that information that impacts individual patient choice is never purely informal, never entirely background communication. Whether or not they are comfortable with or agree with patients using social media platforms for medical expertise and advice, practitioners need to acknowledge the frequency and importance of social media use for individu-als in the life cycle of early motherhood. This is all the more important because the professional, experiential, and educational background of social-media-based expertise is unclear, unstated, or potentially misrepresented.

Implications for Practitioner-Patient (or Patient-Practitioner) Communication

Practitioners, policy makers, scholars, and individual users must recognize that social media platforms are an integral part of health care's backstage and a pri-mary space for improving patient care (Ellingson, 2005, 2007; see Goffman, 1959). The backstage of health care is ever expanding since it can increasingly include interaction with a greater percentage of people from your local area and with individuals across the world whom you would never speak to (or even recognize) off social media. These findings will have implications for how care is provided in the frontstage. First, social media are part of the "health care team" now, which requires an acknowledgment that patients are not passive recipients of knowl-edge. Instead, they actively engage directly with other patients and practitioners (e.g., alternative practitioners and individuals with varying of expertise) on social media and then make health decisions based on these interactions (e.g., choosing practitioners, treatments, alternative or complementary thera-pies, eCourses, etc.) (see Ellingson, 2005; May, 2007; Young & Flower, 2012). Second, if we consider notions of collaborative or transactional communication models, how do we imagine these models interacting with social media in the "backstage" of patient experience? When will the dissemination of medical exper-tise through social media platforms be engaged as a part of medical education or professional development? How can practitioners across all traditions engage with information patients glean from social media, acknowledge the exchange of expertise, and still support patients' efforts to find reliable information? As discussed in chapter 2, historical understandings of reproductive health can resurface through alternative/complementary health models on social media platforms. In the absence of success with traditional medicine, patients often turn to these methods, for example, to examine and/or control emotions or to increase fertility. Meanwhile, health systems continue to consider integrative health treatment modalities, borrowing from multiple medical traditions. Yet the implications of social media platforms as dissemination sources of integrative health information remain understudied.

Implications for Health Policy Makers

Health policy makers must also acknowledge that these conversations and interactions are a part of medical expertise dissemination and public health knowledge—whether or not the material is accurate. Social media discourse as a whole has implications for the creation of health policy, specifically, whether a policy will be a reaction to social media discourse or help shape it, or both. Considering the "global bill pay" example above, if patients are suggesting how to circumvent hospital policy (as we also illustrated in chapter 4), this will eventually erode the success of such policies, which will need to change. Here are some of the suggestions for circumvention offered by the members of this private FB group: "[Insurance] told us . . . technically they cannot bill you for services you haven't received . . . we opted to not pay and asked them to bill us after the delivery" (Private Facebook, 2017a); "I refuse to pay the global bill. Its total horseshit for the parent to float the doctor's office a zero interest loan" (Private Facebook, 2017a). Other commenters asked for suggestions on refusing to pay in advance: "How did you go about not paying it?" (Private Facebook, 2017a). Posters even referenced information they found in other FB conversations: "Someone in another group recounted a story of where she had to pay for a C-section she didn't have" (Private Facebook, 2017a).

Two commenters established their expertise to contextualize a critique or offer expert advice. The first relayed, "I worked as a medical coder and office manager in PA so I knew what I was doing and looking for . . . never saw anything like it here. I didn't even know you could even have multiple deductibles, and I was trained in this!" (Private Facebook, 2017a). The second said, "I work in insurance and from what I understand you can opt out of paying that Global Fee! You might have to push it but refuse to pay it!!!" (Private Facebook, 2017a). How would we categorize the expertise here? The first person is posting as a patient/lay expert about her own birth experience but using her technical expertise to question and critique the policy of this hospital system. The second is using her personal account but providing her professional expertise and advising patients how to ask questions and potentially resist office policy by refusing a new, mandatory payment plan policy. In one sense, this is a continuation of what lay experts did in newspaper and magazines in the early twentieth century, urging patients to resist, ask questions, and/or demand methods of care or policy change (see chapters 2, 3, 4). However, the dialogue above occurs in real time, with individuals confounding the traditional technical-lay binary. The goals are similar but the methods and framework are new.

Policy makers and public health officials have to understand that policy change may result from these social media exchanges, which are not addressed at this time in a meaningful way from the patient or lay perspective or from new categories of expertise that may emerge. Conversations about the impact of social media on health care professionals and public health and health care are available (Dosemagen & Aase, 2016; Mack, 2017; Ventola, 2014). As Mack (2017) reported on *Mobile Health News*, social media are a powerful way to spread information and have "proven to be a valuable tool in healthcare" (n.p.). A cardiologist in North Carolina, Dr. Kevin Campbell, exemplifies a needed awareness of the importance of social media as a place "where our patients, customers, consumers, as well as our colleagues are, and that's where we need to be" (Mack, 2017, n.p.). He cited Twitter and FB as powerful tools but noted the difficulties presented by compliance (Mack, 2017), something that also emerged in our research (e.g., using private accounts but revealing one's professional affiliation in an exchange). Dr. Campbell cautions against engaging in a doctor-patient relationship online, and we observed the difficulties in both understanding and maintaining this boundary. He concluded, "Mobile is where it is at for communication, and it will soon be the same in healthcare" (Mack, 2017). While Dr. Campbell represents a forward-thinking perspective on social media platforms and expertise dissemination, by and large these pieces consider shifts in technology from the view of the provider and few (if any) address the conversations we analyzed—those taking place largely extant to the practitioner-provider relationship.

Implications for Mother-Child Dyad (Broadly Defined), Parents, and Caregivers

We recognize that "mother" remains a complicated term: many caretakers of infants and young children are not mothers like the traditional hetero- and cis normative model. Yet institutions and social structures continue to engage with the mother-child dyad from and through this model (see also Crenshaw, 1991; Weedon, 1996). After completing our research and the first manuscript draft, we realized our own perspectives on communication with our peers in the life cycle of early motherhood shifted. Now we are cognizant of how easily folks dole out directives to mothers and other caregivers as if they were themselves experts, ourselves included. The commentary we studied in turn-of-the-twentieth-century newspapers and magazines as well as what emerged on social media platforms were strikingly similar in that most engaged in the discourse felt they had *the* answer for *all* people (e.g., Twilight Sleep, grief rituals, progesterone for postpartum mental health issues). Yet what worked for you or a close friend may have no use for someone else. The issue is that we (the public) are often not trained to find reliable and credible sources in social media spaces, and this is also a limitation of our research. We couldn't map the complexities of credibility and also create a system for educating individual users on finding credible sources, particularly when individual needs vary so widely during this life cycle. But we all need to increase our health information literacy; this extends to us as well.

Our social media use patterns also altered during this book. On the one hand, we engaged more often and more deeply because we were seeking answers to questions that directly impacted our day-to-day work. Our research also helped us key in on posts more quickly, and friends and family constantly sent us links, tagged us in posts, and even sent us screenshots to see if we were interested in the material. Since we both became pregnant during the writing of this book, the material felt very personal at times, and we both sought refuge from social media platforms when they became a source of stress and anxiety. Bethany coined the term "Reconnaissance Model" for social media use: get in (don't get "sucked" in), get the basic information you need, get out. As we've stated elsewhere, this research prompted ambiguous feelings about the value of social media for mothers/parents/caretakers during the life cycle of early motherhood. These platforms and apps could be a boon—a real source of desperately needed encouragement and reassurance. However, these same spaces can cause anxiety, become disempowering or shaming, or cause feelings of worry (see also Nielsen, 2015). For example, we often monitored discussions in which potentially dangerous health advice was proffered confidently and communicated as expertise, and we weren't equipped to engage in these exchanges without setting ourselves up as health experts. For example, we've seen pictures of rashes in bad lighting and people asking what the rash was; many posters gave confident diagnoses. Ultimately, we wonder if these posts relieve anxiety because of the immediate responses or prevent individuals from getting treatment. Waiting and watching is something many medical practitioners advise, yet how can anyone accurately surmise from a picture on FB if a rash is critical (e.g., an allergic reaction) or worth waiting to see what develops?

Methodological Implications

Because of our commitment to providing a voice to individuals in/at the margins, we believe that our innovative methodology allowed us to tell a complicated story of the medical expertise individuals encounter during the life cycle of early motherhood. For each chapter, we began in the archive to discover how experts approached these crises in an earlier media "epoch." Working with personal papers, letters, and patient records allowed us to consider the similarities and differences between our contemporary experiences and those of whom we studied. After anchoring ourselves in historiographical literature and primary sources, we studied conversations captured on social media through our personal accounts as well as collecting publicly available posts and comments via Radian6. When we wanted more detailed information about individuals' experiences, we reached out to online commenters directly or contacted online groups, friends, colleagues, and acquaintances who wanted to discuss their struggles (e.g., personal communication and interviews from previous research projects). Many interviewees told us they had never been asked about these crises; many wanted to remain anonymous or use a pseudonym because of the stigma around sharing honestly about health crises and responses during the life cycle of motherhood. At the close of this project, we are struck by the ways scholars still need to attend to the discourse of individuals in the life cycle of early motherhood on social media, as they have done with archival records.

As mothers (with toddlers and both pregnant while writing this book), we are part of these conversations and experienced some of these crises ourselves, which allowed us to account for some of our experiences autoethnographically. We openly address our own experiences throughout the book (Ellis, 2004). As friends and coauthors, we shared some of our deepest anxieties, stereotypes, and inadequacies as we composed each chapter, embracing/questioning our different parenting styles and "good/bad mom" moments. In many ways writing this book served as a therapeutic space to explore our own experiences within a mediated environment; we often sent screenshots or text messages of what we were viewing and experiencing, including images from social media platforms that intersected our own experience (or did not). At times, the project created anxiety as we navigated our lives as "academic mamas." For example, Maggie became more aware of her use of social media and removed FB and IG from her phone in the fourth trimester of her second pregnancy, acknowledging the unhealthy ways social media were impacting her.

Both of us were very guarded about our second pregnancies on social media, in part because of our previous research on infertility (we wanted to be sensitive) and our "advanced" (geriatric) maternal ages. After four years of failed infertility treatment and two spontaneous and unexpected pregnancies, Bethany experienced gestational diabetes during both pregnancies, and though she monitored her health and diet closely, she resisted sharing her experience in social media spaces, despite a commitment to feminist activism and advocacy. Moreover, we both approached our second postpartum period much differently from our first and considered when and how we would use (or not) social media during that period. The countless hours spent on social media for "research" purposes provided a lot of space for reflexivity. In short, the embodied experience of reproduction during the project both simplified and complicated our approach, but also allowed us to immerse ourselves in various crisis conversations addressed in the book on social media. We still question the depiction/use of the mother-child dyad on social media—many users post health questions on behalf of themselves or their children, but in a health system that separates the dyad in its care models, individual users seemed to uphold this separation. Here again there is more work to do.

The methodology of this book is part of its broader contribution. We are not aware of other scholarship that brings together historical research and qualitative and rhetorical analysis on the life cycle of early motherhood. For example, collecting data through Radian6 (a relatively new program for historians and health communications scholars) helped us to see the broader conversations for each topic. We were mindful when reporting the stories of women who had experienced crises, knowing that they may remain anonymous (or use pseudonyms) because many of the topics covered in this book are taboo and highly stigmatized. We hope that our methods will serve as a model for future scholars' transition from theory building to praxis. What does it mean to articulate our findings in the context of mothering identities and the formation, training, and management of teams in health care settings, where social media are a silent, backstage "team member" of dubious quality? We remain passionate about the ways that social media can provide space for counternarratives by allowing those oppressed by structural inequality and injustice to share their stories, seek and provide knowledge (from their unique perspectives), and advocate for each other. To be trusted with any part of a narrative that amplifies voices at the margins is an honor; our contributors were both patient and generous. There is still a lot to learn, and we continue to wrestle with our own privilege.

From a crystallization perspective (see Ellingson, 2009), we hope these conversations continue, and we remain committed to translating our research findings into multiple research products. For example, we are in the process of creating a website to provide full bibliographic access to our historical and mediated resources. Thus far we have written blog posts (e.g., ART of Infertility; *Vital: On the Human Side of Health*, sponsored by the National Endowment for the Humanities), given radio talks on NPR, and partnered with local news stations to talk about our research projects. We have mentored and trained graduate students, created an ethnographic documentary on infertility treatment support, and used study findings to generate greeting cards for individuals experiencing infertility (Johnson & Quinlan, 2015, 2017; Johnson, Quinlan, & Evans, 2017; Latos, 2017). There is a great deal more to accomplish here, and we will continue to engage in and off social media, with the public and with our peers.

LIMITATIONS AND FUTURE RESEARCH

We remain passionate about investigating and deconstructing the taken-for-granted power relations in health care as well as the larger sociohistorical context of modern medicine in the United States. At the close of this project, we understand that studying forms of medical expertise on social media alongside the particular patterns of expertise dissemination can transform our understandings of public health policy, binary categories of expertise, patient health literacy, and individual health choices. The archive was a vital resource throughout the book, particularly in chapter 6, where we compared postpartum care to the lack of care regularly available today. Without this perspective, our interviews and observation of social media discourse would have rankled. Juxtaposed to the casebooks we studied, the difficulties postpartum individuals face in the United States today are enraging. Across our research, we found plenty of similarities (e.g., populist movement, self-advocacy, grassroots activists using technical expertise to empower lay actors) alongside some striking differences, such as the immediacy of communication, the observable influence on individual health choices, and the difficulty of categorizing forms of expertise.

Scholars and policy makers need to continue to develop models of care (e.g., transactional communication model) where patients and caregivers engage in collaborative care relationships and caregivers and patients are peers, making mutually satisfying decisions while acknowledging differing perspectives and levels of training. Additionally, there is a pressing need to consider a transactional patient-practitioner relationship and the social media impact on that relationship (e.g., practitioners using FB live to discuss medical advances; doctors and patients communicating about infertility medicines on IG). Scholars need to examine the benefits and drawbacks of the communication already taking place, during and outside of the life cycle of early motherhood. We did not fully contend with the "how" of finding "good" information in these spaces and understand that unique needs require unique and varied solutions and thus expertise.

One of the challenges for addressing these dialogic constructions is that we lack the language necessary to describe the various forms of expertise we observed throughout this project (e.g., technical experts communicating medical advice through private/lay social media accounts). Future scholarship must wrestle with the boundaries around "technical" and "lay" and help examine, excavate, and redefine the forms of expertise social media make possible. Moreover, it must be acknowledged that patients may be "bringing social media" into the "room" as an expert in and of itself, but we did not have space to adequately explore the complications of social media as a space where expertise is disseminated, exchanged, and even transformed. For example, the amount of information that is incorrect, misleading, dangerous, or decontextualized is well established by scholars. Furthermore, experts of all kinds must take seriously the implications of social media in the room, given what we observed regarding the impact of these platforms on individual choices for parents dealing with health crises for young children.

Another looming concern is the recent challenge to net neutrality made official by the Federal Communications Commission on December 14, 2017 (Collins,

2017). If net neutrality is overturned (a decision currently being challenged in our court system; Collins, 2017; Denisenko, 2017; Granados, 2015; Savov, 2017), it may impact access, particularly for apps and platforms that require the use of cellular data (e.g., FB, IG, Twitter). For example, will private FB groups become less populated if there are tiers of access? Will information become more or less reliable if telecommunication companies can control what information is available to the public? If media companies decide which pieces of information reach the public (e.g., articles, news events), how will this throttle the potential for marginal groups to exchange information and expertise? How will it alter how individuals engage and what forms of expertise they have access to? If net neutrality is abolished and the ability to access social media platforms and smartphone applications shifts dramatically, this monograph may become only historiography—a snapshot in time when individuals sought support for crises with infants and young children online, before they moved to other technologies or methods of communication.

Additionally, we are interested in the policy and or/design implications for the people who run/format/invent/organize social media platforms. Having consulted on apps for practitioners, we are aware that design and function play key roles in the dissemination and perception of expertise. It may become complicated for FB or IG (the organizations/companies) to rate individual expertise and nearly impossible to contextualize it in real time for users. Moreover, social media programmers may not have the training/experience or health literacy to assess health information on many of these crisis topics related to the life cycle of early motherhood. Scholars might address some of the consequences for the exchange of expertise, particularly in private and/or protected spaces and on social media platforms as well as the implications for design and function.

Finally, as feminists, we remain committed to those who are not adequately addressed in this book: disabled mothers; mothers who do not identify as female; mothers in prison; surrogates; mothers who have an adoption plan; adoptive or foster mothers; queer mothers, fathers, and parents; and a host of others. As Rev. Elizabeth Hagan (2017), who chose adoption, reminded us, "Mothering has everything to do with how we label each other and ourselves." Communication scholar Laura Ellingson (2017) leans into "aunting," while artist, activist, and trained social worker Rowan Reyes "left the mom groups and unfollowed the mom feeds to quiet the noise," even as they battle the "good mom/terrible mom dichotomy." Reyes (2017) strives to battle an invisible, chronic illness, even as they seek to be a generous, tender parent to a toddler. Communication scholar Julie-Ann Scott reminded us that "caretaking is profoundly emotional, but people think of it as physical," noting that her diagnosis of cerebral palsy makes time management difficult, but it doesn't preclude her ability to be a loving parent. Jessica (2017), a trans woman, said she would "greatly enjoy being called a mom," while scholar and communication studies scholar Chad McBride (2017) wrestles with the idea of "mothers" and the assumption that a "maternal presence" is vital, while parenting a son in a same-sex marriage. He shared,

> [There] are discourses that reinforce the need or the assumption that [children] at least need a mother-figure (and ideally a mother and father). . . . I struggle with this. I know that culturally mothering is equated for the nurturing, caring, etc. And certainly all children need this. However, even in cross-sex parenting relationships, it is not always the female who does this sort of parenting. . . . So neither of us are exclusively the "mother-er." And I would hope that in straight couples this would be the case as well, which makes the notions of mothering a complete misnomer.

If labels around mothering and parenting need modification, so do categories of expertise and our understandings of the impact of social media on individuals making health care choices for themselves and their infants and young children. As these discourses continue to shift and transform alongside and because of technology, our understanding of the life cycle of early motherhood has to transform as well.

In this book, we started the process of understanding the similarities between the historical "boom" of newspapers and magazines (Douglas, 1999) and the current "boom" of social media interaction. We also articulated the stark differences between these technologies, including both the limits (e.g., heightened self-surveillance and anxiety) and the possibilities (e.g., space for counternarrative and marginality) of social media interaction. We have yet to build a language for the patterns and types of expertise we see emerging in smartphone application chats, in private FB groups, on Twitter, in IG comments, and more. And now, at the boundaries of language, with questions yet to ask and answer, let's begin.

METHODOLOGICAL
APPENDIX

Study 1: "Practitioner-Patient Communication:
Individuals' Experiences with Reproductive Endocrinology," Approved
July 15, 2014, IRB #14-06-26

The goal of this project was to study practitioner-patient communication during reproductive endocrinology in infertility (REI) treatment. Participants were 18 years or older, identified as female, and spoke English. Participants self-identified as heterosexual or homosexual, lesbian, or queer. All had a diagnosis of "infertile" or had worked with a reproductive endocrinologist within the previous three years. For this study, (heterosexual) "infertility" was defined as the inability to conceive within 12 months of unprotected sex (Chandra, Copen, & Stephen, 2014).[1]

Participation in the study was entirely voluntary and required the participants to take part in an in-depth qualitative interview focused on their experiences with patient-practitioner communication during REI treatment. We concluded interviewing when we reached saturation, after 28 interviews, when our participants shared incidents covering the same themes and no new or divergent themes emerged (Morse, 1995). Interviews were digitally recorded and transcribed verbatim. Each participant received a $25 retail gift certificate. The final sample was slightly heterogeneous in terms of social characteristics. Table 1 provides a summary of demographic information for the sample.

We interviewed each woman during an in-depth session, focusing on their communicative experiences with medical practitioners during REI treatment. Due to ethical considerations, we were unable to observe interactions between patients and practitioners; instead, interviewing allowed women to make sense

TABLE 1

PARTICIPANT CHARACTERISTICS ($N = 28$)

Characteristic	Data
Age	30 to 50 years ($M = 36$)
Marital status	Partners at time of study ($n = 25$), single ($n = 3$)
Race/ethnicity	Caucasian ($n = 21$), "White" ($n = 1$), African American ($n = 2$), Native American ($n = 1$), no response ($n = 3$)[a]
Religious affiliation	Attempting Buddhism ($n = 1$), Christian ($n = 11$; including Presbyterian, Catholic, lapsed Catholic, Methodist, and Episcopal and Metaphysical Christianity), Jewish ($n = 1$), Spiritualist ($n = 3$), undecided ($n = 1$)
	Those without a reported affiliation include: none ($n = 7$), no response ($n = 4$)
Sexual orientation	Heterosexual/"straight" ($n = 24$), lesbian/ homosexual ($n = 4$)
Occupation	Health-related field ($n = 10$), professor ($n = 5$), worked in the home ($n = 3$), marketing or sales ($n = 2$), lawyer ($n = 1$), human resources ($n = 1$), marketing manager ($n = 1$), academic administration ($n = 1$), small business owner ($n = 1$), acupuncturist office receptionist ($n = 1$), did not name specific occupation ($n = 2$)
Diagnoses	Most frequently reported diagnoses: unexplained infertility ($n = 6$), age-related infertility ($n = 3$), endometriosis ($n = 3$), polycystic ovarian syndrome ($n = 3$)
	Additional diagnoses ($n = 1$ each): autoimmune disease, blood clotting disorder, diminished ovarian reserve, early onset menopause, high LH [luteinizing hormone], high BMI [body mass index], ovarian failure, premature ovarian failure
	No official diagnosis ($n = 2$)
Male factor fertility issue	1–2 [unconfirmed in one case]; 1 had a trans male partner, who required donor sperm
Household income	Range: 40–225,000 ($M = 100,000$)
Geographical location	Midwest: CO ($n = 3$); Northeast: NY ($n = 7$), MA ($n = 1$); West Coast: CA ($n = 1$); Southwest: AZ ($n = 2$); South: NC ($n = 8$), FL ($n = 5$)

Characteristic	Data
Interview location	In person at private acupuncturist's office or private home ($n = 7$), via telephone ($n = 21$)
Length of interview	35–130+ minutes ($M = 90$)

[a] Participants were invited to choose their own label or diagnosis; we did not offer a list of options for this question to allow participants to label themselves.

of their interactions with REI practitioners retrospectively. We asked questions about how they attributed meaning (i.e., thoughts and feelings) to often painful topics for participants, which we could not observe during treatment. At the beginning of each interview, we asked each participant to choose a pseudonym, explained informed consent procedures, and encouraged participants to ask clarification questions about the study.

Our iterative analytic process included making notes about themes, categories, patterns, and conceptual associations as we conducted and transcribed interviews (Strauss & Corbin, 1998). We used a constant comparative method (Fram, 2013) to create categories describing data collected by particular question sections.

During analysis, we read each other's interviews and came together to discuss the major themes emerging from the work. In the second stage, while remaining open to additional themes, the focus of the final reading relied on a deeper analysis of the codebook created in the initial analysis. To maintain the trustworthiness of our data (Lincoln & Guba, 1985) we engaged in member checking to confirm or clarify the researchers' interpretation of the data and sent a draft of our findings to the participants quoted. We also appeared on a local National Public Radio station to discuss our research and sent a link to this broadcast to all participants. The radio link served as a method to complete a member check with those not quoted (Sandelowski, 1993).

For more information on our findings, see these sources:

Johnson, B., Quinlan, M. M., & Myers, J. (2017). Commerce, industry and security: Biomedicalization theory and the use of metaphor to describe practitioner-patient communication within Fertility, Inc. *Women's Reproductive Health, 4*, 89–105. doi:10.1080/23293691.2017.1326250

Johnson, B., Quinlan, M. M., & Marsh, J. S. (2018). Telenursing and nurse-patient communication within Fertility, Inc. *Journal of Holistic Nursing, 36*, 38–53. doi:10.1177/0898010116685468

Study 2: "Greetings in the Gap": Participant-Generated
Support Messages and Emotional Support for Fertility Patients,"
Approved June 20, 2016, IRB #16-05-19

The purpose of this study was to examine patient perceptions of desired emotional support compared to the support received from family, friends, intimate partners, and practitioners. This study used quantitative ratings and qualitative questions to design support materials to distribute to individuals in treatment. We collected a total of 173 surveys between July 11 and August 15, 2016. Participants had to be 18 years of age, speak English, have access to the Internet, and have received infertility treatment within the last 8 years. Due to our extensive outreach efforts to hundreds of thousands of potential participants (through message boards/listservs, blog communities, websites, Facebook, the RESOLVE network, etc.), women and minorities were represented in this sample.

The research team designed a questionnaire through SurveyMonkey and distributed it through email and social media postings. We exported all responses from SurveyMonkey and organized them in an Excel spreadsheet. To further understand the types of support our participants desired, we analyzed the surveys for specific information about greeting cards they might have liked or would like to receive before, during, or after REI treatment. We categorized responses based on preferred materials. We broke feedback into categories for themes, color, messaging, and suggested text and then grouped similar responses and analyzed groupings.

The research team also analyzed the written commentary in the original 173 for types of medical advice offered as support. While we did not ask specific questions about medical advice, our qualitative research on Instagram (IRB #16-07-12, outlined below) suggested that medical advice is often offered as a kind of support. See Table 2 for types of medical advice.

After compiling our findings from this step, we commissioned artist Rowan Reyes of Ursula Wild Design to draft cards based on survey findings. In total, 138 of the original 173 participants indicated an interest in viewing artist-rendered materials and received a Google poll with images to vote on a group of seven cards, which we designed based on initial feedback. Participants were invited to participate in the poll even if they previously stated that they would not be open to receiving these materials. Of the 138 invited, 67 responded and 14 gave us detailed written feedback on the first round of designs. The artist then created a final round of designs based on Google poll feedback.

TABLE 2

ADVICE GIVEN TO INDIVIDUALS UNDERGOING VARIOUS (IN)FERTILITY
TREATMENTS AND SOURCES OF ADVICE

Subject Matter/Message	Medical Practitioner	Partner	Family/ Friend(s)
Relax	0	1	20
Sexual advice	0	1	6
Do not worry, do not stress, try to have fun	0	0	11
Stop trying, don't try or stop trying so hard	0	0	7
Try harder, keep trying	0	0	4
Be patient, persevere, give time	0	0	2
Manage work stress	0	0	2
Lose weight	1	0	0
Eating habits	1	0	1
Consume or do not consume alcohol or drugs	0	0	5
Adoption as cessation of treatment	1	0	1
Use donor eggs or donor sperm	3	0	0
Treatment by specialist	1	1	1
Surgical or procedural	2	0	0
Medication: changes to, discontinuation of, or other	3	0	0

Study 3: "A Rhetorical Analysis of Infertility Messages across Instagram," Approved August 17, 2016, IRB #16-07-12

The purpose of this study was to examine how women use Instagram (IG) to record their IVF journies as well as how they use IG to seek out social support. With the help of research assistant Rachel Ayers, we collected IG posts between October 10 and October 24, 2016. The study population consisted of IG "users" and "followers" who posted comments/info and visual media content on their own or others' IG feeds related to a diagnosis of infertility and/or fertility treatment. The specific demographic of these individuals remains unknown, although individuals sometimes included specific personal information in their feeds, such as demographic location, medical status, insurance information, and doctors' names, reproductive endocrinology and infertility (REI) practice names, and their personal bioinformatics. When individuals share this information, they do so knowingly in the public sphere; the use of hashtags publicizes information for all IG users. We included any IG user who used our chosen hashtags. We did not interact directly with the participants for this study. Finally, to further protect our participants, identifying information was blurred within images.

We gathered data through hashtag use. The research team selected hashtags with the largest number of users connected to REI treatment and IVF, specifically. The first two hashtags are paired with a second hashtag because they are often used interchangeably. We selected the following:

1. #ivfsisters/ #ivfcommunity
2. #IVFfail/ #infertilitysucks
3. #ivfjourney
4. #ivfsuccess

The research team also selected what we termed "outlier hashtags," meaning hashtags that frequently accompany IVF posts but are not always about the IVF journey. These were the following:

1. #ttc
2. #ttcsisters
3. #infertility

Our criteria for selecting posts included that each must have at least two of the total seven hashtags, with at least one main hashtag. Using both initial and outlier hashtags, we collected 199 images and analyzed the first 25 comments (if there were that many) for types of medical advice. After analyzing both pictures and comments, the research team coded for categories of users providing medical advice such as "information on reactions to (in)fertility treatment" and "evidence of pregnancy/pregnancy symptoms." Our final codes included Sharing Medical Advice/Educating, Recommending Doctors/Procedures/Supportive Therapies, and Resisting Technical Expertise through Social/Emotional Support. A spreadsheet was created to track forms of advice and responses to that advice. We have included our conclusions and observations throughout this book.

Quantitative Study across Chapters: Radian6

We identified relevant social media postings using Radian6 (R6), a social media monitor program that draws on content from more than 150 million blogs and 75 to 100 million Twitter users as well as IG (no images), Facebook, and so on. This program, generously provided by Dr. Joseph Mazer and the Social Media Listening Center at Clemson University, enabled us to do searches for nearly every chapter. R6 findings allowed us to examine social media conversations around our topics, which enriched our analysis and provided a quantitative basis for our understanding of social media behavior and claims about the nature of expert advice dissemination.

For each chapter where we used R6, the research team used the program to collect data from a range of social media platforms, including blogs, Facebook, Twitter, and IG. Our focus on social media platforms reflects the increasing popularity of these platforms, which has unquestionably impacted how both individuals and organizations seek and share information. Examining social media platforms provides insight into key lay experts who may be shaping public perception (e.g., popular "mommy bloggers"; Squiers et al., 2011). Blog posts, tweets, and a host of other social media messages are publicly accessible and archived and thus searchable, making compiling representative samples for coding feasible (Squiers et al., 2011).

We took an identical approach to collecting and analyzing data relevant to the topical focus of each chapter. We have included a sample list of search terms and phrases we used in three chapters in Table 3.

Key search term results were evaluated to establish eligibility. For example, posts that specifically mentioned key search terms were included; we excluded duplicates from final tallies. R6 searches produced between hundreds

TABLE 3

A SAMPLE OF INDIVIDUAL AND PAIRED SEARCH TERMS

Chapter	Term
Chapter 1	conception and advice
	Trying to conceive (ttc) and advice
	ttc
	preconception advice
	preconception advice
Chapter 2	ttc and relax
	infertility
	infertility and relax
	"just relax"
Chapter 5	Couney
	NICU
	couney baby
	preemie
	Coney Island and incubator

and thousands of results. To maximize resources, we closely analyzed the top 100 posts with the greatest audience reach, although the research team viewed all results to ensure we were not overlooking potential historiographical touchpoints (e.g., tweets from archives and historical societies). One of the limitations of R6 is that searches extend back a maximum of 90 days. While this assisted us in getting very up-to-date "hits," we could not make any arguments about trends throughout six months, a year, or several years.

Physical and Digital Archival Analysis

We applied for and received IRB approval to view permission-only collections and patient records at the Francis A. Countway Library of Medicine at Harvard and the David M. Rubenstein Rare Book & Manuscript Library at Duke University.[2] All identifying patient information was redacted either by the archives or alternatively by us, during transcription or through blurring images after our visit. As a result, no identifiable patient information exists in this text.

Mindful that websites are always in flux and social media postings (while never absolutely gone) can be edited and deleted, we took screenshots of every web page, comment section or thread, blog post, forum post, and social media posting representing all comments we analyzed (e.g., on FB or IG). We catalogued these images by date and category. Given that not all websites are catalogued with the Wayback Machine (https://archive.org/web/), these digital reference images illustrate the sources that we studied at a particular date and time.

ACKNOWLEDGMENTS

We've heard plenty of "you're doing it wrong" over the last five years (and throughout our lives). But there were many individuals who saw the value in this work, so we extend particular thanks to our "village:"

First to our parents, partners, siblings, and friends for their support and patience and for believing in us before we did.

To our enthusiastic and persistent editors and early readers: Jodi Vandenberg-Daves, Heather Carmack, Kali Basu, and anonymous reviewers. To Jodi for her mentorship and encouragement throughout the project. To Beatrice Burton for her excellent attention to detail. To Rutgers University Press, especially Kimberly Guinta for her vision and support of this project.

For their scholarly generosity: Laura Ellingson, Lynn Harter, Robin Jensen, Tasha Dubriwny, Cris Davis, Ashli Stokes, Erin Willer, Leland Spencer, Patricia Geist-Martin, and medical practitioners Drs. Lauren Johnson and Nancy Teaff. To Richard Leeman for encouraging us to begin and Dan Grano, Ritika Prasad, John David Smith, and Paaige Turner for their expertise, wisdom, and friendship.

To the librarians at the New York Academy of Medicine Library, especially Arlene Shaner, the New York Public Library Manuscript and Archives Division, the Duke University Rubenstein Rare Book Library, and the Francis A. Countway Library of Medicine at Harvard University. To Joe Mazer and the Social Media Listening Center at Clemson University and the Clemson University Library Special Collections and Archives. To Donna Van Der Zee, the Burns Archive, the University of Tennessee, Knoxville (and Isabell Farrell), and the Indiana Historical Society for sharing their images. Special thanks to the University of Tennessee for permission to use the incredible cover image. To Keith Olson of Quality Printing for his assistance with image formatting and editing.

For their institutional support: Jason Edward Black, Kayla Modlin, and the entire UNC Charlotte Communication Studies Department, College of Liberal Arts and Sciences Dean Nancy Guiterrez and Associate Dean Shawn Long, Jürgen Buchenau in the Department of History, and Brian Mosley, Lesley Brown, Joy McAuley, and Peter Szanton. We are grateful for our "home" librarians Donna Gunter, Amanda Binder, and Renee Moorefield. Finally, to the Textbook & Academic Authors Association for grant support for this project.

To our diverse "expert community" for sharing their stories and dialoguing about the depiction of their experiences. This community brought digital conversations to printed text, deepened our thinking, and broadened our perspective. To Rowan Reyes for their support, artistic partnership, and willingness to offer guidance on our language. To those who cared for and loved our children while we wrote, including Julie Appleyard, who also offered her stories and expertise as a registered nurse and doula.

Last but in no way least, to our intrepid student research support, we are so grateful for you: Nathan, Madeleine, Jade, Kendra, Emma, Rachel, Jaclyn, Marissa, Katelyn, Katlyn, Haley, "the Sams," Zach, Bee, and Bre-Ann.

NOTES

INTRODUCTION

1. This IG reference comes from our data collected on how individuals use it for social support during infertility treatment (Institutional Review Board [IRB] #16-07-12).

2. This reference also comes from our data collected on how individuals use IG for social support during infertility treatment, in which we found both particular medical advice and actual medicines exchanged between users undergoing infertility treatment (IRB #16-07-12).

3. When we viewed patient information at different locations, we received IRB approval for access to these data (see the Methodological Appendix for details).

CHAPTER 1 — ON PRECONCEPTION, THE BEGINNING OF THE LIFE CYCLE OF EARLY MOTHERHOOD

1. For the purposes of this chapter, we focused on Shettles instead of Billings because the Shettles Method came up far more often on social media platforms.

2. We are unclear exactly what Dr. Branscombe meant with this directive.

CHAPTER 2 — A STATE OF MIND?

1. The Mayo Clinic defines IVF as a "complex series of procedures used to treat fertility or genetic problems and assist with the conception of a child. During IVF, mature eggs are collected (retrieved) from your ovaries and fertilized by sperm in a lab. Then the fertilized egg (embryo) or eggs are implanted in your uterus. One cycle of IVF takes at least two weeks." Intrauterine insemination (IUI) is a type of AI and a procedure for treating infertility. "Sperm that have been washed and concentrated are placed directly in your uterus around the time your ovary releases one or more eggs to be fertilized" (see Mayo Clinic, 2017a, 2017b). Finally, intracytoplasmic sperm injection (pronounced "icksy") resulted from Dr. Gianpiero Palermro's successful experiments; in 1992, he manually fertilized one egg with one sperm (Barnes, 2014; Johnson, Quinlan, & Marsh, 2018).

2. For more on our qualitative research and survey collection and follow-up, please see the Methodological Appendix.

3. Dr. Melendy (1904) (and others, including Dr. Tyler Smith, whom Melendy cited in her book) recommended that women could not conceive in the middle between the two periods—she also claimed "women are far less likely to conceive midways between the menstrual periods than either before or after them" (p. 337). According to WHO data, this is peak fertility.

4. Carr was the 15th "IVF baby" in the world (Marsh & Ronner, 2010; see also Sullivan, 1981).

5. There are numerous complicating factors in IVF outcomes, which include but are not limited to age, egg quality, autoimmune diseases, smoking, and weight (see SART, 2014).

6. In American medicine, by the 1850s "regular" physicians were also called "allopathic," which often meant white, male practitioners trained in Europe or America or a combination. For more on the structure of American medicine in the nineteenth century and early twentieth, see Bonner (1995), Breslaw (2012), Janik (2014), Morantz-Sanchez (2000), Shyrock (1966), Starr (1982), and Weiner and Hough (2012).

7. Curtis (1924) alleged 12% (p. 123) of couples were sterile, Macomber (1924) claimed 1 in 10 (p. 678), and an editorial in *Journal of Conception* cited 10% (1939, p. 58). Hale (1878) claimed 1 in 8 (12.5%) but added that the "ancient" rate was 1 in 80 (or 0.12%) (p. 48). Bigelow (1883) asserted that between 1 in 6 and 1 in 10 couples were infertile (p. 16). The highest percentages we found were from the early twentieth century, in which Engelmann (1901) maintained an average of 20% and referenced "Sim's law" of 11% being the previously accepted norm (p. 890), but in his statistical analysis he included "relative sterility," or any pregnancy ending in miscarriage (p. 894) and potentially even "artificial sterility" (p. 895), which includes contraceptive use, so the extensive definition here could account for this high of 20%. Gregg (1905) appeared to be referencing Engelmann: "According to our latest observations 20 per cent of American marriages are found to be barren" (p. 60). As Marsh and Ronner (1996, 2010) indicated, available records (including census data) in a large-scale study by Samuel Meaker (1934) titled *Human Sterility* claimed a rate between 10% and 13% (p. 120). However, even Meaker's detailed work was used by some to argue that infertility rates had increased 600-fold (see p. 327, n. 15), despite the fact that Meaker (1934) directly debunked the long-standing myth of increasing fertility rates (p. 9; see also May, 2007). In 1983, Aral and Cates maintained the infertility of a "relatively large number of American couples of reproductive age" and cited 1 in 10 (p. 2327).

8. For more, see Marsh and Ronner's (1996) work on Ernest Henry Starling, Harold Shaw, and Henry H. Harrower (pp. 134–137).

9. Newman (2017) cited a recent study in Australia and noted that the use of oil to "flush" the tubes was a far more effective treatment modality. However, practitioners in the early twentieth century used a variety of substances for flushing; the use of oil in this study is not new, at least in the United States (Marsh & Ronner, 2010, p. 64). Hysterosalpingogram (HSG) also does not offer effective treatment for endocrine or ovulation issues or male-factor issues and has unknown effectiveness on "unexplained" fertility. Again, Newman's inadequately researched claims promulgate the notion that reproductive endocrinology and infertility practitioners are denying patients useful treatments to make money, when in fact any patient undergoing IVF and, in many cases, IUI or even drug therapy has had one or more HSGs and/or may have a condition not impacted by the procedure.

10. Syna (2017), a clinical hypnotherapist, said on the Houston Hypnosis Center website, "In a clinical study, women undergoing in-vitro fertilization who were hypnotized had double the conception rate of the control group who were not hypnotized." However, Syna does not cite a research study or any other reviewable data to support his claims.

11. Mazor (1984) debunked some of the previous assumptions of psychogenic sterility: "Attempts to confirm . . . hypotheses based on psychiatric interviews and psychological tests, were either inconclusive or irreproducible" (p. 24). Mazor offered some of the particular stresses and emotional conflict that arises from infertility and treatment and helpful suggestions for therapists looking to support their infertile patients. Still, the use of the term in 2008 suggests that the idea continues to resurface among traditional medical experts in America.

12. While Louis et al.'s (2011) publication reported on results from a study conducted in the United Kingdom, it was published in *Fertility and Sterility*, an international journal produced by the American Society for Reproductive Medicine (2017).

13. In our research, we interviewed the partner of a person who identified as a trans man. His partner reported that they did not experience discrimination but that heterosexism may have allowed for a more positive experience. The couple sought fertility treatment in a state where hospitals/clinics can deny same-sex couples treatment, but since they presented as male and female, there were no impediments to treatment. Additionally, we interviewed one lesbian couple and one lesbian partner from another couple; the couple detailed the discrimination they faced, while the partner from the second couple had an overwhelmingly positive experience. Again, each situation is unique, and individual experiences vary due to a multiplicity of factors.

14. We acknowledge that not all trans and/or nonbinary people identify using the same term or terms. In this chapter, we try to balance internal consistency with following best practices by using research participants' own names, pronouns, and descriptors for body parts, treatments, and so on. We recognize that some of the language in sources we quote from will, for some, be offensive or at the least nonrepresentative. Again, we want to honor individual identity choices and language, reflect the range of terminology and yet remain consistent, so we rely on quotations more heavily in this passage.

CHAPTER 3 — RED UNDERWEAR, GENES, AND MONSTROSITY

1. For more on the collection and coding methods for our Facebook (FB) materials, please see the Methodological Appendix.

2. We use the term "pregnant individuals," "folk," or "bodies" instead of "women" or "pregnant women" because we acknowledge that not every pregnant person identifies as a woman or female (Hempel, 2016; "My body," 2017; Trans Birth, 2017).

3. For quotations from the Private FB Group (2017) post, pseudonyms are used, based on the first initial of the poster's name, as we noted in the original post that real names would not appear in this book.

CHAPTER 4 — "YOU WOMEN WILL HAVE TO FIGHT FOR IT"

1. In the late nineteenth century and early twentieth, New York experienced a huge influx of immigrants from Southern and Eastern Europe and Russia. The bulk of practicing midwives seemed to be from this new group (Crowell, 1907).

2. For more on the longer history of midwifery and formal obstetrics in urban centers, see Davis-Floyd and Johnson (2006), Dawley (2000), and Starr (1982).

3. As with many names in the late nineteenth and early twentieth centuries, multiple spellings occur across publications. Dr. Kenneth Junor is also listed as Dr. Kenneth Junior, depending on the source.

4. Dr. Krönig says, "The sensitiveness of those who carry on hard mental work is much greater than that of those who earn their living by manual labor" (Tracy & Leupp, 1914, p. 43). Dr. Krönig also said the nervous condition, brought on by this "sensitiveness," belonged to "mothers of a better class" (Ver Beck, 1915, p. 8). Note that in Tracy and Leupp's (1914) article, they give the testimony of a "Scottish noblewoman" and tell the story of an American mother whose baby was presented to her with a ribbon reading, "1st Class," both of which signal the class and social position of patients in the Freiburg clinic (pp. 47–48). For more on notions of class evolution and the nervous conditions of the "highly civilized" in the early twentieth century, see Bederman's (1995) work.

5. One of the ways Twilight Sleep (TS) in Brooklyn differed from TS in Manhattan is that doctors in Brooklyn regularly used narcophen instead of morphine—a change first linked to Dr. Polak in *TBE*: "An exception, in one respect only, to this statement has been encountered in the cases at the Long Island College Hospital. In one or two instances, where morphine has been substituted for narcophen, the babies have shown symptoms of weakness during the first few hours of their lives. As a result, the physicians in charge ordered that narcophen only be used in conjunction with scopolamin, the second drug being used in the treatment" ("'Twilight Sleep' now permanent," 1914, p. 11).

6. See also "Court" (1917), Hamilton (1914, pp. 1, 58), and "Hospital not a nuisance" (1917).

7. Dr. Rongy (1914) noted that many physicians performing TS delivered babies they believed to be "asphyxiated" or not able to breathe, when in fact the newborns were experiencing "oligopnea." Oligopnea is a depression of the "peripheral filaments of the vagus," meaning that "when the child is born it requires a long period to accumulate a sufficient quantity of carbon dioxide to stimulate the respiratory center in the medulla" (p. 634).

8. Some physicians in the United States attempted to use the Siegel Method, a form of TS originating with a Dr. Siegel in Germany. His method sought to find a standardized dosage for the procedure. American doctors who attempted the Siegel Method had little success, because by placing women together in a ward, they found that the women disturbed each other. Many doctors referring to the failures of the TS method were attempting the Siegel Method rather than the Freiburg Method (Leupp & Hendrick, 1915).

9. Ver Beck's (1915) research suggested that American physicians were the most reticent to perform the labor-intensive Freiburg Method.

10. A few obstetricians suggested that a small group of (wealthy) patrons could bring in a full staff for a TS home birth ("Dr. Polak approves," 1914; "'Twilight Sleep' baby," 1914).

11. As Craven (2010) outlined, feminists disagree about available choices in reproductive health. As women of color argued in the 1970s and 1980s, choice extended beyond abortion and contraception; pregnancy and birth had to be informed and supported choices as well (pp. 48–50). There are instances in which white middle-class advocates and women of color worked together to protect traditional midwifery, though this did not represent normative partnerships in the period (pp. 57–58).

12. Ina May Gaskin's description of the Farm Midwifery Center includes the following language: "Birth guided by wisdom and experience for over 40 years . . . women are treated with love and respect, empowering them to fulfill their desire for natural childbirth in a sane and safe home setting" (The Farm, n.d.-a).

CHAPTER 5 — "ONE OF THE MOST CURIOUS CHARITIES IN THE WORLD"

1. Interestingly, while the BBC radio documentary ("Life under," 2016) includes Dr. Jeffrey Baker talking about the consistency of design in Couney's exhibits, including the glass pane set up to separate the incubators, babies, and medical technicians from the viewer, surviving pictures suggest that at the Pan American Exposition in Buffalo in 1901 and the New York World's Fair from 1939 to 1940, there was no pane of glass—instead, visitors stood behind metal poles, similar to those at a zoo or a lookout point ("Baby incubators," 1901; Weglein, Scheir, Peterson, Malsbury, & Schwartz, 2008).

2. For more on the particular challenges premature babies face after birth and into their life and care at home, see "Common Conditions Treated in the NICU" (March of Dimes, 2014).

3. Pediatric medicine emerged in the first half of the twentieth century, so mothers at the turn of the century would not have considered receiving care for premature babies at a hospital. Baker (1996) notes that while this became common first in France, treatment often occurred after parents returned with a languishing baby already days or weeks old.

4. There is ample and excellent research examining the medical narrative of modernity and health conditions, most notably neurasthenia and hysteria. Doctors feared that white individuals, particularly middle- and upper-class women, ailed as a result of their "good breeding" and evolutionary development (Bederman, 1995; Leavitt, 1995; Smith-Rosenberg, 1985; see also Koerber, 2018).

5. In his unpublished dissertation, Dr. Jeffrey Baker (1993) made a similar comment about Dr. Hess, noting that in his incubator ward in Chicago in 1922, Hess oversaw wet nurses "with a paternalism worthy of any of the French obstetricians" (p. 422; see also Baker, 1996). It seems Couney was not unique in his unyielding expectations (see also Hess, 1922, pp. 118–126).

6. Dr. J. Hess and Nurse Lundeen's workplace is referred to with various names, including the Michael Reese Center and the Chicago Lying-in Hospital (see also Baker, 1993; Hess, 1922; Reedy, 2000; "Scolds," 1933; Silverman, 1979).

7. Nearly all of these pieces include information that is easy to dispute. For example, Pascetta (2014) claimed that Couney put his own daughter Hildegarde on display for three months, when newspaper articles from the time make it clear that since Hildegarde was born in the "off-season" her incubator was removed from storage and set up in her parents' bedroom ("Invention saved," 1907; Liebling, 1939).

8. This article also fails to contend with the historic context of the term "white" in the United States and the way this term expanded over time to include previously "nonwhite" ethnic groups (for example, Jewish, Irish, and Italian). This historical trend is, in itself, evidence of white privilege and systemic racism—if the socially constructed concept of "whiteness" provided no material or social benefits, groups would not seek the label. For more on this phenomenon, see Bederman (1996) and Roediger (2007). In the case of Couney, according to A. J. Liebling's (1939) article, Orthodox Jewish and Italian babies

were brought to Coney. Neither of these groups were considered "white" at the turn of the twentieth century or among the professional or lay eugenics promulgators, an ideology that flourished until well after World War II (see Bederman, 1995; Dennett papers, 1874–1945; Kline, 2001). We included Liebling to show ethnic diversity in the exhibits; Prentice (2016a) also noted both class and race diversity in the exhibits. There is still an issue with Brown's (1994) article, which includes the claim that Couney accepted every baby "high or low, rich or poor, black or white . . . this institution for the preservation of infant life makes no distinction," but fails to provide the source of this quotation; there are no notes or references. However, in Brown's (1994) article, a picture appears to show three premature triplets of color sharing an incubator, which helps to substantiate his claim (p. 30). Still, given the lack of scholarly rigor, we cite Brown with caution and reservation.

CHAPTER 6 — NOT JUST BABY BLUES

1. Throughout the text we use the term "mother" when we are quoting from historical documents, articles, or interviewees (e.g., as a form of self-identification). We realize not all postpartum bodies identify as mothers; where possible, we remove gender-specific language. For example, in online posts, unless an individual self-identifies, we do not assume the person is cis female.

2. The fundus is the bottom part or base of an organ (The Free, 2017). In 1913, *The Modern Hospital* advised physicians to keep patients' genitals clean with "1/2 per cent lysol . . . after birth of child patient should be assisted to turn on back from side with her knees closed and the nurse's hands on the fundus uteri. Fundus should be held, not manipulated, however, for 30 minutes. Then and not until then, accoucher should deliver placenta. Fundus should be held for another thirty minutes before putting abdominal binder on" (Hornsby & Schmidt, 1913, p. 394). It is likely the anonymous women, family members, husbands, and/or neighbors mentioned holding the fundus in these patient records were involved in these immediate postpartum practices.

3. Historian Regenia Morantz-Sanchez (2000) also examined Boston and New England maternity cases, though she examined the inpatient cases in both systems. Her book was originally published in 1985; we reviewed the revised 2000 version.

4. As per our IRB agreement with Francis A. Countway library in this collection (Boston Lying-In, 1832–1981) as well as the New England collection (New England Hospital, 1885–1900), we were not permitted to photograph any materials or record any patient names, addresses, or other identifying information. As such, we could not include page numbers or any other specific information in in-text citations in this chapter. For more on these collections, see our Selected Bibliography and Master Reference List. For more on our archival research, see the Methodological Index

5. By the early twentieth century, hospitals such as Boston Lying-In were, in fact, using aseptic measures, even with outpatients, so deaths from puerperal fever were already improving from the mid-nineteenth century, though doctors in private practice sometimes resisted these changes and had for years, and maternal mortality rates did not show a marked increase until after the 1930s (Breslaw, 2012; Morantz-Sanchez, 2000; Morbidity, 1999). In the outpatient records we studied there is an extensive entry by a resident outlining his training in sanitary and aseptic setup for delivery and postbirth procedure (Boston Lying-In, 1832–1981).

6. This study did not give a background on prematernal health conditions, which may also impact outcomes (see Global, 2016).

7. For more on our R6 research, please see the full description in the Methodological Appendix.

8. Aurora679's (2017) BabyCenter forum post prompted all the responses in a comment chain. In the text above we provide other commenters' platform/account names, but we cite the original post, which includes the comments, rather than citing each individual comment.

CHAPTER 7 — MEMENTO MORI IN THE VICTORIAN ERA AND ON SOCIAL MEDIA

1. All quotations in this chapter reflect the punctuation, spelling, and grammar of the original.

2. For more on the various literature claiming and exploring parental emotive distance, see Pollock's (1983) research on parent-child relations, specifically the first section of the book, "Past Children: A Review of the Literature on the History of Childhood" (pp. 1–31).

3. Well aware of the impact of racial stereotypes, prejudice, and what would come to be called structural racism, W. E. B. Du Bois dedicated space in his publication *The Crisis* to the issue of parenting and instilling notions of black worth, value, and beauty into the "colored child." Beginning in the mid-1920s, *The Crisis* also published pictures of black babies, infants, children, and young adults to display the beauty, resilience, and power of the black or "colored" body. These pictures, in which dimpled babies smile from cozy blankets, are stark opposites to memento mori, yet they too seek to capture the purity and angelic nature of childhood in the late nineteenth and early twentieth centuries (see Du Bois, 1926; Kelly, 1922, pp. 251–255; for more images, see the November 1922 issue of *The Crisis*, specifically pp. 247–250, 265, 267).

4. One commenter said, "You would think it would be common sense, but no. Common sense fled academia long ago. They teach that people didn't love their little ones like we do now. I wish I was making this up, but no. It's commonly believed," and most commenters agreed in this thread, with one outlier who said, "I have read hundreds of 19th-century journals and letters. People did love their children as much as modern people loved theirs; however, they were used to children dying" (The Thanatos Archive, 2017).

5. In Romer and International Photography Center's (2005) collection, images 1457, 1461, 1462, 1560, 1564, and 1565, all titled "Unidentified Child," illuminated the need for parental assistance in keeping toddlers still long enough to capture them in the daguerreotype process (pp. 422–423, 432). Other images, such as 1511, 1559, and 1556, also titled "Unidentified Child," exhibit babies and young children unassisted (Romer & International Center of Photography, 2005, images 428, 432). As Iepson (2013) noted, unassisted prints exhibited the idealized children of the time, capable of mastering their desire to move long enough to get a usable image. For more on grief and the death of children in Victorian America, see Jalland (1996).

6. In 2017, Johnson, Quinlan, and research assistant Zachary Fandl created a codebook for memento mori images of children (perceived as) age five and under; Fandl coded six books for images.

7. Some cultural traditions, such as several indigenous American tribes, the Church of Jesus Christ of Latter-day Saints, Old Order Amish, Orthodox Jewish, and Muslims, forbid postmortem images (Blood & Cacciatore, 2014b; Chichester, 2005; Clements et al., 2003; Lundquist, Nilston, & Dykes. 2004).

8. The article titled "A Brief History of Memorial Photography" (Burns & Burns, 2015) links modern-day memento mori to Victorian practices. However, this article is available only to members with a paid subscription to the magazine, which makes it inaccessible to the wider public unless they know it exists and seek access to it. There is certainly nothing wrong with paying for articles and keeping magazines afloat; we are simply pointing to the specificity of the publication and how this piece (and the publication) likely does not have a wide readership.

9. James Van Der Zee's name appears with multiple capitalizations, including Vanderzee and VanDerZee, across available sources. We chose the capitalization style used on the cover of his book *The Harlem Book of the Dead* and approved by his widow, Donna Van Der Zee.

CHAPTER 8 — "BETTER BABIES"

1. Throughout this chapter, we use the term "better babies contest," unless a particular event used a proper noun (e.g., WPFF Better Baby Contest). Some contests called their events "better baby contests," but structure and emphasis of all these events remained largely the same throughout the nation.

2. Although the term "millennial parents" is not defined by the author, we are referring to millennials as researchers typically do: using the early 1980s as starting birth years and the mid-1990s to early 2000s as ending birth years (Pew Research Center, 2010).

3. This quotation came from an undated document in Mrs. Frank de Garmo's papers at the University of Tennessee, Knoxville. Given the years she worked on these contests, we would estimate the date to be between 1908 and 1918.

METHODOLOGICAL APPENDIX

1. Please see chapter 1, which discusses infertility—both the content and our footnotes deal with the heteronormativity and ableism in these constructions and terminologies.

2. IRBs remained internal to these libraries. As such, we were given documented permission but not specific IRB numbers.

MASTER REFERENCE LIST

This list includes sources we cited in multiple chapters in the book. Sources cited once are included in the Selected Bibliography. For more on our reference organization, please see the introduction.

Apple, R. D. (1995). Constructing mothers: Scientific motherhood in the nineteenth and twentieth centuries. *Social History of Medicine, 8,* 161–178. doi:10.1093/shm/8.2.161

Ayala, S., & Freeman, L. (2016). The placental microbiome: A new site for policing women's bodies. *International Journal of Feminist Approaches to Bioethics, 9,* 121–148. doi:10.3138/ijfab.9.1.121

Baker, J. P. (2000). Historical perspective: The incubator and the medical discovery of the premature infant. *Journal of Perinatology, 20*(5), 321–328.

Barnes, L. W. (2014). *Conceiving masculinity: Male infertility, medicine and identity.* Philadelphia, PA: Temple University Press.

Bartholomew, M. K., Schoppe-Sullivan, S. J., Glassman, M., Kamp Dush, C. M., & Sullivan, J. M. (2012). New parents' Facebook use at the transition to parenthood. *Family Relations, 61*(3), 455–469.

Bederman, G. (1995). *Manliness and civilization: A cultural history of gender and race in the United States, 1880–1917.* Chicago: University of Chicago Press.

Bonner, T. N. (1995). *Becoming a physician: Medical education in Britain, Germany and the United States, 1750–1945.* New York: Oxford University Press.

Boston Lying-In Hospital Records (1832–1981). MC 87; Vols. 52, 58, 109. Boston Medical Library in the Francis A. Countway Library of Medicine, Boston, MA.

Bredl, K., Hünniger, J., & Jensen, J. L. (Eds.). (2014). *Methods for analyzing social media.* London, UK: Routledge.

Breslaw, E. (2012). *Lotions, potions, pills, and magic: Health care in early America.* New York: New York University Press.

Briggs, P., Burford, B., de Angeli, A., & Lynch, P. (2002). Trust in online advice. *Social Science Computer Review, 20,* 321–332. doi:10.1177/089443930202000309

Calkin, M. M. (2015). *Making pretty: Examining contemporary identity construction through Instagram* (Unpublished doctoral dissertation). San Francisco State University, San Francisco, CA.

Callahan, A. (2012, June 8). Why care about breastfeeding research? Retrieved from https://scienceofmom.com/2015/10/22/should-your-baby-sleep-in-your-room-for -how-long-balancing-sleep-safety-and-sanity/

Callahan, A. (2013, October 2). The magic and the mystery of skin-to-skin. Retrieved from https://scienceofmom.com/?s=skin+to+skin

Callahan, A. (2015). *Science of mom: A research-based guide to your baby's first year*. Baltimore, MD: Johns Hopkins University Press.

Caton, D. (1999). *What a blessing she had chloroform: The medical and social response to the pain of childbirth from 1800 to the present*. New Haven, CT: Yale University Press.

Centers for Disease Control and Prevention. (2014). Trends in out-of-hospital births in the United States, 1990–2012. Retrieved from https://www.cdc.gov/nchs/products /databriefs/db144.htm

Chandra, A., Copen, C. E., & Stephen, E. H. (2014). Infertility service use in the United States: Data from the national survey of family growth, 1982–2010. *National Health Statistics Reports, 73*, 1–21. Retrieved from http://www.cdc.gov/nchs/data/nhsr/nhsr073 .pdf

Craven, C. (2010). *Pushing for midwives: Reproductive rights in a consumer era*. Philadelphia, PA: Temple University Press.

Crenshaw, K. (1991). Mapping the margins: Intersectionality, identity politics and violence against women of color. *Stanford Law Review, 43*, 1241–1299. doi:10.2307/1229039

Curry, L. (1999). *Modern mothers in the heartland: Gender, health, and progress in Illinois, 1900–1930*. Columbus: Ohio State University Press.

Dennett, M. W. (1874–1945). Mary Ware Dennett Papers, 1874–1945. Personal papers, Schlesinger Library, Radcliffe Institute, Cambridge, MA.

Derkatch, C. (2016). *Bounding biomedicine: Evidence and rhetoric in the new science of alternative medicine*. Chicago: University of Chicago Press.

Dubriwny, T. N. (2012). *The vulnerable empowered woman: Feminism, postfeminism, and women's health*. New Brunswick, NJ: Rutgers University Press.

Dubriwny, T., & Ramaduri, V. (2013). Framing birth: Postfeminism in the delivery room. *Women's Studies in Communication, 36*, 243–266. doi:10.1080/07491409.2013.830168

Eastin, M. S. (2001). Credibility assessments of online health information: The effects of source expertise and knowledge of content. *Journal of Computer Mediated Communication, 6*(4). doi:10.1111/j.1083–6101.2001.tb00126.x

Edison Research. (2013). Moms and media 2013. Retrieved from http://www.edison research.com/wp-content/uploads/2013/05/Moms-and-Media-2013-by-Edison -Research.pdf

Ehrenreich, B., & English, D. (1978). *For her own good: 150 years of the experts' advice to women*. New York: Anchor Books.

Ehrenreich, B., & English, D. (2005). *For her own good: Two centuries of the experts' advice to women* (2nd ed.). New York: Random House.

Ellis, C. (2004). *The ethnographic I: A methodological novel about autoethnography*. Walnut Creek, CA: AltaMira Press.

Epstein, R. H. (2010). *Get me out: A history of childbirth from the garden of Eden to the sperm bank*. New York: Norton.

Feiler, B. (2017, November 4). App time for nap time: The parennials are here. *New York Times*. Retrieved from https://www.nytimes.com/2017/11/04/style/millennial-parents-par ennials.html?smid=fb-nytimes&smtyp=cur

Foss, K. A. (2010). Perpetuating "scientific motherhood": Infant feeding discourse in *Parents* magazine, 1930–2007. *Women & Health, 50*, 297–311. doi:10.1080/03630242.2010.4 80905

Foucault, M. (1995). *Discipline and punish: The birth of the prison* (A. Sheridan, Trans.). New York: Random House.

Fram, S. M. (2013). The constant comparative analysis method outside of grounded theory. *Qualitative Report, 18*, 1–25.

Gaskin, I. M. (2002). *Spiritual midwifery*. Summertown, TN: Book Pub Co. (Original work published 1975)

Grant, J. (2012). *Raising baby by the book: The education of American mothers*. New Haven, CT: Yale University Press.

Guttmacher, A. F. (1962). *Pregnancy and birth: A book for expectant parents*. New York: Viking Press.

Hempel, J. (2016, September 12). My brother's pregnancy and the making of a new American family. *Time*. Retrieved from http://time.com/4475634/trans-man-pregnancy -evan/

Hoberman, J. M. (2012). *Black and blue: The origins and consequences of medical racism*. Berkeley: University of California Press.

Hoffert, S. D. (1989). *Private matters: American attitudes toward childbearing and infant nurture in the urban north, 1800–1860*. Urbana: University of Illinois Press.

Hulbert, A. (2004). *Raising America: Experts, parents, and a century of advice about children*. New York: Vintage Books.

Janik, E. (2014). *Marketplace of the marvelous: The strange origins of modern medicine*. Boston, MA: Beacon.

Jensen, R. E. (2016). *Infertility: Tracing the history of a transformative term*. University Park: Pennsylvania State University Press.

Johnson, B., & Quinlan, M. M. (2015). Technical vs. public spheres of knowledge: A feminist analysis of women's rhetoric in the Twilight Sleep debates of 1914–1916. *Health Communication, 30*, 1076–1088. doi:10.1080/10410236.2014.921269

Johnson, B., & Quinlan, M. M. (2017). High-society framing: *The Brooklyn Eagle* and the popularity of Twilight Sleep in Brooklyn. *Health Communication, 32*, 60–71. doi:10.10 80/10410236.2015.1099505

Johnson, B., Quinlan, M. M., & Marsh, J. S (2018). Telenursing and nurse-patient communication within Fertility, Inc. *Journal of Holistic Nursing, 36*, 38–53. doi:10.1177 /0898010116685468

Johnson, S. A. (2014). "Maternal devices," social media and the self-management of pregnancy, mothering and child health. *Societies, 4*(2), 330–350. doi:10.3390/ soc4020330

Kata, A. (2010). A postmodern Pandora's box: Anti-vaccination misinformation on the Internet. *Vaccine, 28*(7), 1709–1716.

Kellogg, J. H. (1891). *Ladies' guide in health and disease: Girlhood, maidenhood, wifehood, motherhood*. Battle Creek, MI: Good Health Publishing.

Kerber, L., Kesslar-Harris, A., & Sklar, K. K. (Eds.). (1995). *U.S. history as women's history: New feminist essays*. Chapel Hill: University of North Carolina Press.

Khouri, J. S., McCheyne, M. J., & Morrison, C. S. (2018). #Cleft: The use of social media amongst parents of infants with clefts. *Cleft Palate-Craniofacial Journal, 55*, 974–976.

Kline, W. (2001). *Building a better race: Gender, sexuality, and eugenics from the turn of the century to the baby boom*. Berkeley: University of California Press.

Koerber, A. L. (2018). *From hysteria to hormones: A rhetorical history*. University Park: Pennsylvania State University Press.

Kukla, R. (2005). Pregnant bodies as public spaces. In C. Wiedmer & S. Hardy (Eds.), *Motherhood and space: Configurations of the maternal through politics, home, and the body* (pp. 283–305). New York: Palgrave Macmillan.

Leavitt, J. W. (1986). *Brought to bed: Childbearing in America 1750–1950*. New York: Oxford University Press.

Leavitt, J. W. (Ed.). (1999). *Women and health in America: Historical readings*. Madison: University of Wisconsin Press.

Leavitt, J. W., & Numbers, R. L. (Eds.). (1997). *Sickness and health in America: Readings in the history of medicine and public health*. Madison: University of Wisconsin Press.

Lincoln, Y. S., & Guba, E. G. (1985). *Naturalistic inquiry*. Beverly Hills, CA: Sage.

Madge, C., & O'Connor, H. (2006). Parenting gone wired: Empowerment of new mothers on the Internet? *Social & Cultural Geography, 7*(2), 199–220.

Marsh, M., & Ronner, W. (1996). *The empty cradle: Infertility in America from colonial times to present*. Baltimore, MD: Johns Hopkins University Press.

Marsh, M., & Ronner, W. (2010). *The fertility doctor: John Rock and the reproductive revolution*. Baltimore, MD: Johns Hopkins University.

McMillen, S. G. (1990). *Motherhood in the old south: Pregnancy, childbirth, and infant rearing*. Baton Rouge: Louisiana State University Press.

Melendy, M. R. (1904). *Vivilore: The pathway to mental and physical perfection; the twentieth century book for every woman*. Chicago. Retrieved from https://archive.org/details/vivilorepathwaytoomeleuoft

Morantz-Sanchez, R. (2000). *Sympathy and science: Women physicians in American medicine*. Chapel Hill: University of North Carolina Press.

Morbidity and Mortality Weekly Report. (1999, October 1). 1900–1999: Healthier mothers and babies. *Achievements in Public Health, 48*(38), 849–858. Retrieved from https://www.cdc.gov/mmwr/preview/mmwrhtml/mm4838a2.htm

Morse, J. M. (1995). The significance of saturation. *Qualitative Health Research, 5*, 147–149. doi:10.1177/104973239500500201

"My body is awesome": Trans man expecting first child. (2017, June 8). Retrieved from http://fox5sandiego.com/2017/06/08/my-body-is-awesome-trans-man-expecting-first-child/

New England Hospital for Women and Children Maternity Records (1885–1900). B MS b19.3; Vols. 13 & 37. Boston Medical Library in the Francis A. Countway Library of Medicine, Boston, MA.

Ovia Fertility Tracker & Ovulation Calculator App. (2017). Retrieved from http://www.oviahealth.com/

Pew Research Center. (2016). Social media update. Retrieved from http://www.pewinternet.org/2016/11/11/social-media-update-2016/pi_2016-11-11_social-media-update_0-03/

Reedy, E. A. (2000). *Ripe too early: The expansion of hospital based premature infant care in the United States, 1922–1950* (Unpublished doctoral dissertation). University of Pennsylvania, Philadelphia.

Reedy, E. A. (2007). *American babies: Their life and times in the 20th century.* Westport, CT: Praeger.

Reyes, R. (2017). Personal communication.

Ridgway, J. L., & Clayton, R. B. (2016). Instagram unfiltered: Exploring association of body image satisfaction, Instagram #Selfie posting, and negative romantic relationship outcomes. *Cyberpsychology, Behavior, and Social Networking, 19,* 2–7. doi:10.1089/cyber.2015.0433

Sandelowski, M. (1984). *Pain, pleasure, and American childbirth: From the Twilight Sleep to the Read Method, 1914–1960* (13th ed.). Westport, CT: Greenwood.

Sandelowski, M. (1993). *With child in mind: Studies of the personal encounter with infertility.* Philadelphia: University of Pennsylvania Press.

Sandelowski, M. (2000). *Devices & desires: Gender, technology and American nursing.* Chapel Hill: University of North Carolina Press.

Scolds mothers of babies born prematurely: Can't tell them anything, Says Dr. Couney, incubator expert. (1933, December 17). *Brooklyn Daily Eagle,* p. 12.

Seigel, M. (2014). *Rhetoric of pregnancy.* Chicago: University of Chicago Press.

Shryock, R. H. (1966). Women in American medicine. In R. H. Shryock (Ed.), *Medicine in America: Historical essays* (pp. 182–185). Baltimore, MD: Johns Hopkins University Press.

Sillence, E., Briggs, P., Harris, P., & Fishwick, L. (2006). Going online for health advice: Changes in usage and trust practices over the last five years. *Interacting with Computers, 19,* 397–406. doi:10.1016/j.intcom.2006.10.002

Smith-Rosenberg, C. (1985). *Disorderly conduct: Visions of gender in Victorian America.* New York: Knopf.

Squiers, L. B., Holden, D. J., Dolina, S. E., Kim, A. E., Bann, C. M., & Renaud, J. M. (2011). The public's response to the US Preventive Services Task Force's 2009 recommendations on mammography screening. *American Journal of Preventive Medicine, 40,* 497–504.

Starr, P. (1982). *The social transformation of American medicine: The rise of a sovereign profession and the making of a vast industry.* New York: Basic Books.

Stern, A. M., & Markel, H. (2002). *Formative years: Children's health in America, 1880–2000.* Ann Arbor: University of Michigan Press.

Strauss, A., & Corbin, J. (1998). *Basics of qualitative research: Techniques and procedures for developing grounded theory* (2nd ed.). Thousand Oaks, CA: Sage.

Sublette, J. W. (Ed.). (1993). *The letters of Anna Calhoun Clemson* (Unpublished doctoral dissertation). Florida State University, Tallahassee.

Thon, F. M., & Jucks, R. (2017). Believing in expertise: How authors' credentials and language use influence the credibility of online health information. *Health Communication, 32,* 828–836. doi:10.1080/10410236.2016.1172296

Tomes, N. (2002). Epidemic entertainments: Disease and popular culture in early-twentieth-century America. *American Literary History, 14,* 625–652. doi:10.1093/alh/14.4.625

Tracy, M., & Boyd, M. (1914, October). More about painless childbirth. *McClure's Magazine,* pp. 56–69.

Tracy, M., & Boyd, M. (1915). *Painless childbirth: A general survey of all painless methods, with special stress on "twilight sleep" and its extension to America.* New York: Frederick A. Stokes Company.

Trans Birth. (2017). Retrieved from http://www.transbirth.com/

Twilight Sleep Association. (1914). *Aim: To promote all safe and efficacious means of securing painless childbirth* [Pamphlet]. New York: Frederick A. Stokes Company. Jarvis-Robinson Family Papers (Box 29, Folder Twilight Sleep). Yale Collection of Western Americana, Beinecke Rare Book and Manuscript Library.

Ulrich, L. R. (1990). *A midwife's tale: The life of Martha Ballard, based on her diary, 1785–1812.* New York: Knopf.

Vandenberg-Daves, J. (2014). *Modern motherhood: An American history.* New Brunswick, NJ: Rutgers University Press.

Washington, H. A. (2006). *Medical apartheid: The dark history of medical experimentation on black Americans from colonial times to the present.* New York: Doubleday.

Weedon, C. (1996). *Feminist practice and poststructuralist theory* (2nd ed.). Malden, MA: Wiley-Blackwell.

Weiner, M. F., & Hough, M. (2012). *Sex, sickness, and slavery: Illness in the antebellum South.* Urbana: University of Illinois Press.

Wolf, J. H. (2001). *Don't kill your baby: Public health and the decline of breastfeeding in the nineteenth and twentieth centuries.* Columbus: Ohio State University Press.

Wolf, J. H. (2009). *Deliver me from pain: Anesthesia and birth in America.* Baltimore, MD: Johns Hopkins University Press.

Zelizer, V. A. R. (1994). *Pricing the priceless child: The changing social value of children.* Princeton, NJ: Princeton University Press.

SELECTED BIBLIOGRAPHY

The list below is organized by document type and contains all the sources we used for this book which were not included in our Master Reference List. While this selected bibliography does include all our sources, we are calling it a "selected" bibliography because it does not reflect Master Reference List sources or utilize full citations, just titles. This format allows us to illustrate the extensive number of secondary, tertiary, archival, social media, digital, and digitized sources we accessed during our work. For more on our digital record, please see the Methodological Appendix. Full citations by chapter are located on our website: www.johnsonquinlanresearch.com.

ARCHIVAL RESOURCES

Articles

Regulations governing the practice of midwifery in the City of New York

Conference Papers

The care of premature infants: Historical perspective

Digital Archives

The Burns Archive
North American Women's Letters and Diaries
The Thanatos Archive

Educational Pamphlets

Those denied a child: A guide for husbands and wives seeking parenthood

Institutional Records

Maternal mortality in New York City: A study of all perpetual deaths, 1930–1932
New York World's Fair 1939–1940 Records, New York Public Library

Personal Papers

Mrs. Frank [Mary] de Garmo Papers
Thomas Green Clemson Family Papers

Professional Papers

Louise Hortense Branscomb Papers
Robert Latou Dickinson Papers

UNPUBLISHED DISSERTATIONS/THESES

Disciplining mommy: Rhetorics of reproduction in contemporary maternity culture
The machine in the nursery: The premature infant incubator and the origins of neonatal medicine in France and the United States, 1880–1922
New mothers and social media: The effects of social media consumption and production on social support and parental stress
Postmodern relationships: Death and the child in the antebellum American visual culture
Shifting expectations: Medicine, nature and disability in pregnancy texts
"You women will have to fight for it": Early twentieth-century feminism and Twilight Sleep
"What to inspect when you're expecting": Critically examining constructions of women in *What to Expect When You're Expecting*

ACADEMIC MONOGRAPHS

Addresses and papers of Theodore Roosevelt
At the breast: Ideologies of breastfeeding and motherhood in the contemporary United States
Baby meets world: Suck, smile, touch, toddle: A journey through infancy
Barren in the promised land: Childless Americans and the pursuit of happiness
Better baby contests: The scientific quest for perfect childhood health in the early twentieth century
Bikini-ready moms: Celebrity profiles, motherhood and the body
Birthing a slave: Motherhood and medicine in the antebellum South
The birth of the clinic: An archaeology of medical perception
Blessed events: Religion and home birth in America
Bodies: Exploring fluid boundaries
Body/politics: Women and the discourse of science
Centuries of childhood: A social history of family life
Changing images of the family
Childbirth: Changing ideas and practices in Britain and America 1600 to the present
Children in the house: The material culture of early childhood, 1600–1900
Communicating in the clinic: Negotiating frontstage and backstage teamwork
The construction of social reality
Conversations of science, culture, and time
The criminalization of a woman's body

Death, memory and material culture

Death in the Victorian family

Doing harm: The truth about how bad medicine and lazy science leave women dismissed, misdiagnosed, and sick.

The Eagle and Brooklyn, 1841–1955

Engaging crystallization in qualitative research: An introduction

Expecting better: Why the conventional pregnancy wisdom is wrong—and what you really need to know

Families of handicapped persons: Research, programs and policy issues

The focal encyclopedia of photography: Digital imaging, theory and application, history and science

Forgotten children: Parent-child relations from 1500 to 1900

The Golden Age of the newspaper

Good old Coney Island: A sentimental journey into the past: The most rambunctious, scandalous, rapscallion, splendiferous, pugnacious, spectacular, illustrious, prodigious, frolicsome island on earth

The great influenza: The story of the deadliest pandemic in history

Great myths of child development

Guide to a healthy pregnancy

The Harlem book of the dead

A history of American childhood

The hour of our death: The classic history of western attitudes towards death over the last one thousand years

How pop culture shapes the stages of a woman's life: From toddlers-in-tiaras to cougars-on-the-prowl

How to choose the sex of your baby: Fully revised and updated

Infertility: Medical, emotional, and social considerations

The infertility of women, the nervous system in sterility: Some of the requirements of treatment

An international study of maternal care and maternal mortality

Key concepts in developmental psychology

Killing the black body: Race, reproduction, and the meaning of liberty

Lying-in: A history of childbirth in America

The machine in the nursery: Incubator technology and the origins of newborn intensive care

Mainstreaming midwives: The politics of change

Mediated moms: Contemporary challenges to the motherhood myth

Medical talk and medical work: The liturgy of the clinic

Medical visions: Producing the patient through film, television, and imaging technologies

Medicine as culture: Illness, disease and the body in western societies (2nd ed.)

Midwifery

Miracle at Coney Island: How a sideshow doctor saved thousands of babies and transformed American medicine

The mommy myth: The idealization of motherhood and how it has undermined women

A most important picture: A very tender manual for taking pictures of stillborn babies and infants who die

The motherhood business: Consumption, communication and privilege

Mothers who deliver: Feminist interventions in public and interpersonal discourse

Necessary but not sufficient: The respective roles of single and multiple influences on individual development

New medical technologies and society: Reordering life

Objects of the dead: Mourning and memory in everyday life

Of woman born: Motherhood as institution and experience

On female body experience: "Throwing like a girl" and other essays

On photography

Our bodies, our crimes: The policing of women's reproduction in America

Passed on: African American mourning stories, a memorial

Perfect motherhood: Science and childrearing in America

Photography and death

The political geographies of pregnancy

The politics of reality: Essays in feminist theory

Poverty in policy in American history

Pregnancy and power: A short history of reproductive politics and America

Raising a baby the government way: Mothers' letters to the Children's Bureau, 1915–1932

Raising baby by the book: The education of American mothers

A rebel came home: The diary and letters of Floride Clemson, 1863–1866

Rhetorics of motherhood

The sacred remains: American attitudes toward death, 1799–1883

Save the babies: American public health reform and the prevention of infant mortality

The secret: Daily teachings

Secure the shadow: Death and photography in America

Silent travelers: Germs, genes, and "the immigrant menace"

Sleeping beauty: Memorial photography in America

Sleeping beauty II: Grief, bereavement and the family in memorial photography, American & European traditions

Sleeping beauty III: Memorial photography, the children

The social construction of reality: A treatise in the sociology of knowledge

The system of professions: An essay on the division of expert labor

Taking charge of your fertility: The definitive guide to natural birth control, pregnancy achievement, and reproductive health

To be young was very heaven: Women in New York before the First World War (1st ed.)

To serve the living

A true likeness: The black South of Richard Samuel Roberts, 1920–1936

Twenty-five years of sex research: History of the National Research Council Committee for Research in Problems of Sex

Unraveling the double-bind

Volatile bodies: Toward a corporeal feminism

Voyages in childhood

The wages of whiteness: Race and the making of the American working class

White feminists and contemporary maternity: Purging matrophobia

Who cares? Women, care, and culture

Women as mothers

The world split open: How the modern women's movement changed America

The wrong prescription for women: How medicine and media create a "need" for treatments, drugs, and surgery

Young America: the daguerreotypes of Southworth & Hawes

EDITED VOLUMES

Biomedicalization: Technoscience, health and illness in the US

A century of eugenics in America: From the Indiana experiment to the human genome era

Childbirth and authoritative knowledge: Cross cultural perspectives

Conceiving the future: Pronatalism, reproduction, and the family in the United States

Documents of life and the undead: The 'undead,' online postmortem photographs and critical humanist ethics

Double stitch: Black women write about mothers and daughters

The embryology of behavior: The beginning of the human mind

Encyclopedia of North Carolina

Marginalized reproductions: Ethnicity, infertility and reproductive technologies

Methods for analyzing social media

Power/knowledge: Selected interviews and other writings, 1972–1977

Slave narratives, A folk history of slavery in the United States from interviews with former slaves

Standing in the intersection: Feminist voices, feminist practices in Communication Studies

Throwing like a girl and other essays in feminist philosophy

MEDICAL REFERENCE VOLUMES:

Diagnostic and statistical manual of mental disorders (DSM-I)

Proceedings of the SIGCHI conference on Human factors in computing systems

Williams obstetrics (24th ed.)

What a young wife ought to know (Vol. 3)

POPULAR/BESTSELLING (THE TWENTY-FIRST CENTURY)

Belly laughs: The naked truth about pregnancy and childbirth (10th ed.)

The happiest baby on the block: The new way to calm crying and help your newborn baby sleep longer

Ina May's guide to childbirth

The mommy plan: Restoring your post-pregnancy body, naturally using women's traditional wisdom

The pregnancy countdown book: Nine months of practical tips, useful advice, and uncensored truths

HISTORICAL MONOGRAPHS/MEDICAL REFERENCE VOLUMES (THE NINETEENTH, EARLY TWENTIETH CENTURIES)

Amnesia and analgesia in parturition

Baby incubators: A clinical study of the premature infant, with especial reference to incubator institutions conducted for show purposes

Clinical notes on uterine surgery: With special reference to the management of sterile condition

Diseases of women, especially those causing sterility

Expectant motherhood: Its supervision and hygiene

The guidance of mental growth in infant and child

History of the college of physicians and surgeons in the city of New York

Human sterility: Causation, diagnosis, and treatment. A practical manual of clinical procedure

Infancy and human growth

Infant and child in the culture of today: The guidance of development in home and nursery school

The modern hospital: Its inspiration: Its architecture: Its equipment: Its operation

The National Standard Dispensatory: Containing the natural history, chemistry, pharmacy, actions, and uses of medicines: Including those recognized in the pharmacopoeias of the United States, Great Britain, and Germany, with numerous references to other pharmacopoeias: In accordance with the Eighth Decennial Revision of the United States Pharmacopoeia, as amended to 1907

Nostrums and quackery, Vol. 2

The nursling: The feeding and hygiene of premature and full-term infants

Plain home talk about the human system—The habits of men and women the causes and prevention of disease—Our sexual relations and social natures: Embracing medical common sense applied to causes, prevention, and cure of chronic diseases

Premature and congenitally diseased infants

Prenatal care

Private sex advice to women: For young wives and those who expect to be married

The question of rest for women during menstruation

Scopolamine-morphine anesthesia

The souls of black folk

Theories of developmental concepts and applications

The truth about Twilight Sleep

FILMS/DOCUMENTARIES

American Experience

ACADEMIC JOURNALS

Advances in Sex Research

African Journal of Reproductive Health

American Heritage

American Journal of Maternal/Child Nursing

American Journal of Obstetrics and Diseases of Women and Children

American Journal of Obstetrics and Gynecology

American Journal of Public Health

Archives of Pediatrics & Adolescent Medicine

Association of Women's Health, Obstetric and Neonatal Nurses

Atlantic Journal of Medicine

Atlantis: Critical Studies in Gender, Culture & Social Justice

Berkeley Journal of Sociology

BioMed Central Psychology

The British Journal of the History of Science

British Journal of Medical Psychology

British Medical Journal

The Bulletin of the History of Medicine
Clinical Nursing Research
Cognitive Science
Communication Monographs
Communication Quarterly
Complementary Therapies in Clinical Practice
Cultural Studies Review
Cyberpsychology, Behavior, and Social Networking
Cyberpsychology: Journal of Psychosocial Research on Cyberspace
Death Studies
Departures in Critical Qualitative Research
Digital Literature Review
Discourse, Context, & Media
The Doula
Feminist Media Studies
Fertility and Sterility
Gynecological Endocrinology
Hastings Center Report
Health Affairs
History of Photography
Hospital Physician
Human Reproduction
Illness, Crisis, and Loss
Journal of Allergy and Clinical Immunology
Journal of American Folklore
Journal of American Medical Association
Journal of Andrology
Journal of Assisted Reproduction and Genetics
Journal of Business and Technical Communication
Journal of Contraception
Journal of Education and Health Promotion
Journal of Emergency Nursing
Journal of Genetic Psychology
Journal of Language and Social Psychology
Journal of Law and Religion
Journal of Loss and Trauma
Journal of Material Culture
Journal of Medical Internet Research
Journal of Midwifery & Women's Health
Journal of Nursing
Journal of Nutrition
Journal of Obstetric, Gynecologic, & Neonatal Nursing
Journal of Perinatal Education
Journal of Perinatal and Neonatal Nursing
Journal of Personality and Social Psychology
Journal of Psychosocial Nursing and Mental Health Services
Journal of Social History

Journal of Special Education
Journal of Sport and Social Issues
Journal of the American Medical Association
Journal of Visual Communication in Medicine
Journal of Women's Health
Journal of Women's History
Lancet
Law and History Review
Maternal and Child Health Journal
MCN: The American Journal of Maternal Child Nursing
Medical Care
Medical Anthropology Quarterly
Molecular Reproduction and Development
Nature
NeoReviews
Nepal Medical College Journal
New England Journal of Medicine
New Literary History
Nursing Inquiry
Obstetricia et Gynecologica Scandinavica
Past & Present
Patient Education and Counseling
Patterns of Prejudice
Pediatrics
Pharmacy and Therapeutics
Proceedings of the American Philosophical Society
Proceedings of the National Academy of Science
Public Library of Science One
Quarterly Journal of Speech
Revue Française d'Allergologie
Rhetoric Review
Science News
Seminars in Fetal and Neonatal Medicine
Seminars in Perinatology
Signs
Signs and Society
Social Media + Society
Social Science & Medicine
Sociology
Sociology of Health and Illness
Survey
Texas Review of Entertainment and Sports Law
Text and Performance Quarterly
Victorian Literature and Culture
Visual Communication Quarterly
Visual Studies
Women's Studies

Women & Criminal Justice
Women & Language
Women, Gender, and Families of Color

HISTORICAL JOURNALS (NINETEENTH, EARLY TWENTIETH CENTURIES)

Charities and the Commons
Journal of Human Lactation
Lancet—Clinic
Medical Record
Milwaukee Medical Journal
Obstetric Gazette
Philadelphia Medical Times
Philosophical Transactions (1683–1775)
Psychoanalytic Quarterly
Psychosomatic Medicine
Surgery, Gynecology, and Obstetrics

MAGAZINES

Cosmopolitan
Indiana Magazine of History
Newsweek

HISTORICAL MAGAZINES (REFERENCED FROM THE NINETEENTH, EARLY TWENTIETH CENTURIES)

Crisis
Ladies' Home Journal
Modern Mechanics and Inventions
National Magazine (Boston)
New Yorker Magazine
Pacific Rural Press
Scientific American
Women's Home Companion

NEWSPAPERS

Denver Post
Irish Independent
New York Herald
Salt Lake Tribune
St. Joseph News-Press

HISTORICAL NEWSPAPERS (REFERENCED FROM THE NINETEENTH, EARLY TWENTIETH CENTURIES)

Brooklyn Eagle
Charlotte Daily Observer
New York Herald
New York Times

PERSONAL COMMUNICATION (THE TWENTY-FIRST CENTURY)

Amy, 2014
Anonymous, May 2017
Anonymous, February 2017
B. Allen, April 2017
C. Hayes, June 2017
C. Masi, April 2017
D. Myrick, June 2017
E. A. Burns, March 2017
E. Miller Quinlan, April 2017
E. Willer, March 2017
G. Harris, February 2017
Hilary, December 2017
Jaime, November 2017
Kandace, November 2017
Karen, November 2017
L. Johnson, July 2017
Lorelai, November 2017
Meredith, November 2017
M. Medina, August 2017
M. Michalik, March 2017
N. Teaff, October 2014
Sandra, December 2017

SOCIAL MEDIA PLATFORMS

Facebook.com
　　Malinda Nichols Daniel, October 2016
　　WeAreWoman.us, September. 2017
　　Various private groups
LinkedIn.com
　　A Heart to Hold
Twitter.com
　　Twitter accounts:
　　@BabyWeConnect
　　@ICEA_org
　　@nilmdtsHQ
　　@StongMamaClub
　　@ToMakeAMommy
Vimeo.com
　　GloZell Green
Youtube.com
　　"The Craziest Thing I Tried to Get Pregnant," 2017 [video]

WEBSITES

Business/Commerce

BabyCenter
BirthFit™
Chennia Acupuncture
The Farm Midwifery Center
I Love Fashion + Retail
Inner Peace Acupuncture
Genetics and IVF Institute
Houston Hypnosis
La Belle Dame
Omnicore Agency
Rhythms Acupuncture and Chinese Medicine Center for Women's Health
Skinner, Inc. Auctioneers

Commerce Customer Reviews/Comments

Amazon Author Pages, Frans X. Plooji
Amazon Customer, Amazon Customer Review: What to expect when you're expecting
Beatrice, Amazon Customer Review: Mayo Clinic guide to a healthy pregnancy
Cathy G., Amazon Customer Review: Mayo Clinic guide to a healthy pregnancy
Erica, Amazon Customer Review: The pregnancy countdown book
Jesse C., Amazon Customer Review: The happiest baby on the block
Lisa W., Amazon Customer Review: The pregnancy countdown book
Mommy Division, Amazon Customer Review: Ina May's guide to childbirth
Rob, Amazon Customer Review: What to expect when you're expecting

eBusiness Publications/eCourses

Before the Bump
eMarketer
Fertility
From Maiden to Mother
Last Chance for Beautiful Babies
Mind Body Mana
Naturally Knocked Up
Organic Conceptions
Unlock Your Fertility
The Yes, You Can Get Pregnant eCourse

SMARTPHONE APPLICATIONS (APPS)

Kindara, Inc.
National Center on Birth Defects and Developmental Disabilities, Milestone Tracker
    Mobile App
What to Expect When You're Expecting
The Wonder Weeks

INSTITUTIONAL WEBSITES

Governmental, International

National Center for Complementary and Integrative Health (NCCIH)
National Center for Health Statistics, FastStats, Infertility
National Center for Health Statistics, Infant Health Data
National Center for Health Statistics, Vital Statistics, Report 4
National Center on Birth Defects and Developmental Disabilities, Child Development Facts
World Health Organization (WHO) recommendations on postnatal care of the mother and newborn
World Health Organization, Reproductive Health
U.S. Department of Health and Human Services

Governmental, Historical (the nineteenth and early twentieth centuries)

Library of Congress

Nonprofit Organizations

American Society for Reproductive Medicine
The ART of Infertility
Baby-Friendly USA
Boston Children's Hospital
Cleveland Clinic
Coney Island History
Cystic Fibrosis Foundation
Gesell Institute of Child Development
Graham's Foundation
Healing Hearts: Baby Loss Comfort
A Heart to Hold
Integrative Fertility Symposium
March of Dimes
Mayo Clinic
The Mindful Fertility Project
Now I Lay Me Down to Sleep
Reproductive Facts (American Society for Reproductive Medicine)
RESOLVE: The National Infertility Association
Scraps of the Heart Project
Society for Assisted Reproductive Technology
Washington Parish Free Fair
World Professional Association for Transgender Health

ONLINE MEDIA

News Sites

ABC News
Blaze
British Broadcasting Company (BBC)
Business Insider
Bustle

Buzzfeed
Cable News Network (CNN)
Clued In (of Medium)
Daily Mail
Deadline
Digital Trends
Evonomics
Gizmodo
Health Impact News
Huffington Post
Medical News Today
Medscape
Mobi Health News
National Public Radio (NPR)
National Right to Life News Network
OKCFox; Fox Corporation Affiliate
ProPublica
Quora
Quartz
Slate
TechCrunch
10News, WTSP (CBS Corporation Affiliate)
Verge
WDBJ7; CBS Corporation Affiliate
WMC Actions News 5; The National Broadcasting Company Affiliate
WSOC-TV Charlotte

Online Newspapers

Davis Enterprise
Los Angeles Times
NY Daily News
Star Tribune
Washington Post

Online Magazines

Atlantic
Forbes
Invention and Technology Magazine
Mental Floss
Mothering
New Orleans Magazine
Now I Lay Me Down To Sleep
Parents
People Magazine
Smithsonian Magazine
Still Standing Magazine
USA Today

Us Magazine
U.S. News
Vela Magazine
Vital
Wired

Online Television

TLCgo (of The Learning Channel [TLC])

BLOGS

Public/Organizational Blogs

Belly Bloom Birth Services
BabyCenter Community Forum
The Mighty
NOLA Blog (of New Orleans Times-Picayune)
Science of Us (of New York Magazine online)
SheKnows Media Community
What to Expect Community Forum
Women's Health Today
Women's Mental Health Matters (of Psychology Today online)

Individual/Personal

theBohoWife
CarlyMarie: Project Heal
Cori's Cozy Corner
Fertility Friend
Scary Mommy
Ways to Help Get Pregnant

INDEX

ABOUT THE AUTHORS

BETHANY L. JOHNSON (MPhil, MA) is an instructor in history and an associate member to the graduate faculty and research affiliate faculty in the Department of Communication Studies at the University of North Carolina at Charlotte. She studies how science, medicine, and health discourses are framed and reproduced by institutions and individuals from the nineteenth century to the present. She has published in interdisciplinary journals such as *Health Communication*, *Women & Language*, *Departures in Critical Qualitative Research*, and *Women's Reproductive Health.*

MARGARET M. QUINLAN (PhD) is an associate professor in the Department of Communication Studies and core faculty in the interdisciplinary Health Psychology Ph.D. Program at the University of North Carolina at Charlotte. She explores how communication creates, resists, and transforms knowledges about bodies. She critiques power structures in order to empower individuals who are marginalized inside and outside of healthcare systems. She authored approximately 40 journal articles and 17 book chapters and co-produced documentaries in a regional Emmy Award–winning series.